Pneumopedics *and* Craniofacial Epigenetics

Biomimetic Oral Appliance Therapy *for* Pediatric *and* Adult Sleep Disordered Breathing

Pneumopedics *and* Craniofacial Epigenetics

Biomimetic Oral Appliance Therapy *for* Pediatric *and* Adult Sleep Disordered Breathing

Dr G Dave Singh DMD PhD DDSc

World Scientific

NEW JERSEY • LONDON • SINGAPORE • BEIJING • SHANGHAI • HONG KONG • TAIPEI • CHENNAI • TOKYO

Published by

World Scientific Publishing Co. Pte. Ltd.

5 Toh Tuck Link, Singapore 596224

USA office: 27 Warren Street, Suite 401-402, Hackensack, NJ 07601

UK office: 57 Shelton Street, Covent Garden, London WC2H 9HE

Library of Congress Cataloging-in-Publication Data
Names: Singh, G. Dave, author.
Title: Pneumopedics and craniofacial epigenetics : biomimetic oral appliance therapy for pediatric and adult sleep disordered breathing / G Dave Singh.
Other titles: Epigenetic orthodontics in adults
Description: New Jersey : World Scientific, [2021] | Preceded by: Epigenetic orthodontics in adults / G. Dave Singh, James A. Krumholtz. Chatsworth, Calif. : SMILE Foundation, 2009. | Includes bibliographical references and index.
Identifiers: LCCN 2020042486 | ISBN 9789811225345 (hardcover) | ISBN 9789811225352 (ebook for institutions) | ISBN 9789811225369 (ebook for individuals)
Subjects: MESH: Sleep Apnea, Obstructive--genetics | Sleep Apnea, Obstructive--therapy | Airway Remodeling | Maxillofacial Development--genetics | Craniofacial Abnormalities--therapy | Biomimetic Materials--therapeutic use
Classification: LCC RC737.5 | NLM WF 143 | DDC 616.2/09--dc23
LC record available at https://lccn.loc.gov/2020042486

British Library Cataloguing-in-Publication Data
A catalogue record for this book is available from the British Library.

For any available supplementary material, please visit
https://www.worldscientific.com/worldscibooks/10.1142/11967#t=suppl

Printed in Singapore

Biography

Professor G. Dave Singh is a US citizen who was born, educated, and trained in England, UK. He holds three doctorates, including Doctor of Dental Medicine (University of Newcastle, UK — validated at the University of Puerto Rico, USA); a PhD in craniofacial development (University of Bristol, UK), and a third Doctorate in Orthodontics (University of Dundee, UK). Dr Singh was awarded a grant by the British Society for Developmental Biology (University of Oxford, UK) and later he was appointed to the Board of Examiners, Royal College of Surgeons of England, London. He was also Visiting Professor at: the University of Saskatchewan, Canada; the University of Airlangga, Indonesia; the University of Health Sciences, Antigua; University Sains Malaysia, Kelantan; and Adjunct Professor, Portland State University, USA. On the basis of being an "outstanding professor" supported by Harvard University, the University of Michigan, and the University of Hawaii, he was invited to relocate to the Center for Craniofacial Disorders, USA where he led a NIH-funded program of clinical craniofacial research. Currently, he is a Board Member of the American Sleep and Breathing Association, Member of the World Sleep Society, Academic Fellow of the World Federation of Orthodontists, and Fellow of the International Association for Orthodontics, where he was awarded prizes in 2005, 2013, and 2014. He has published over 200 articles in the peer-reviewed medical, dental, and orthodontic literature, has published 7 books/chapters, and has coined terms such as pneumopedics, craniofacial epigenetics, and craniofacial sleep medicine, which focuses on a curative approach to obstructive sleep apnea in both children and adults. He has lectured and presented his work at numerous medical, dental, and orthodontic conferences in North America, Asia, Europe, Australia, and Africa. Dr Singh was the Founder and Chief Executive Officer of BioModeling Solutions, Inc., where he obtained 8 US patents, 2 Canadian patents, and 2 international patents. He also obtained FDA registrations and clearances for his patented family of biomimetic oral appliances known as the Daytime-Nighttime Appliance (DNA appliance®) system. Currently, he is Founder and Chief Medical Officer, Vivos Therapeutics, Inc. Dr Singh was the 2019 recipient of the US Invisible Disabilities Association award for "providing the possibility of healthy lives for millions living with illness, pain and disability". In 2020, Dr Singh was given a lifetime achievement award as one of the world's top 100 doctors in orthodontics for his work on sleep apnea "exemplifying leadership, excellence, and entrepreneurship in service to humanity and the advancement of global health".

Contents

Foreword

I've been privileged to know early on that I wanted to devote my entire career toward the study of sleep and its disorders when I was a freshman at Stanford University and enrolled in a class taught by one of the pioneers of sleep medicine and research, Dr William C. Dement. Dr Dement and his colleagues initiated the organized, scientific study of sleep in 1952 with the discovery of rapid eye movement (REM) sleep. Since that time, there has been an explosion of new discoveries and findings in the fields of sleep medicine and sleep research.

Given this accumulated knowledge, one might mistakenly believe that at the present time there would be a paucity of new lines of investigation in these areas. This premise would be incorrect, as evidenced by this book, *Pneumopedics and Craniofacial Epigenetics*, by Dr G. Dave Singh. This new book, which is the second edition of *Epigenetic Orthodontics in Adults*, published over a decade ago, greatly amplifies and expands the work of the prior edition and introduces new concepts, such as pneumopedics and biomimetics, as well as new diagnostic and therapeutic approaches for patients with dental, orthodontic, and sleep problems.

My personal interest in this book stems from my medical observations and clinical research in the limitations of current treatment of sleep-related breathing disorders, especially obstructive sleep apnea. I first met Dr Singh in the fall of 2018, when we discussed his work on upper airway remodeling as a treatment for obstructive sleep apnea. This treatment is an attractive one, especially when contrasted with other therapeutic approaches, particularly positive airway pressure, which obligates patients to a lifelong commitment of wearing a device nightly to maintain its success in improving patient outcomes.

Pneumopedics and Craniofacial Epigenetics is a remarkable book, and could not have been written without training and experience in dental medicine, orthodontics, and craniofacial development; Dr Singh holds doctorates in all three of these fields. He takes the reader on a journey of exploration, starting with a foundation in the genetics, epigenetics, and development of the craniofacial complex, and then new craniofacial diagnostic and therapeutic approaches, which tap his years of experience using his pneumopedics and craniofacial epigenetics (PACE) protocol. Despite the complexity of the subject matter and the fact that the book is first and foremost a scholarly text with references that takes a deep dive into each topic, the terms, concepts, diseases, and treatments are explained in a manner that is easy to understand.

The successful growth of sleep medicine, dental medicine, and medicine itself relies on the continuous exploration and acquisition of knowledge, and medical practitioners, especially trainees, collectively need to learn about cutting-edge diagnostic and therapeutic approaches that can revolutionize the practice of medicine and improve the quality of life for countless numbers of patients.

Clete A. Kushida MD PhD
Division Chief and Medical Director, Stanford Sleep Medicine
Neurologist and Professor, Department of Psychiatry and Behavioral Sciences
Stanford University Medical Center
Director, Stanford Center for Human Sleep Research
Stanford University
California, USA

Preface

Since the first edition of this book was published over a decade ago, several significant changes have occurred both in terms of our scientific understanding and clinical experience of epigenetics. The previous version of this book was based on the novel idea of 'epigenetic orthodontics in adults', but new advances have allowed us to move past that concept on several fronts. Primarily, orthodontics is currently viewed as a specialty of dentistry that is mostly concerned with dentoalveolar correction of the teeth. Put simply, most people regard orthodontics as 'straightening the teeth' in children/young adults. However, this procedure cannot be done in isolation since the teeth are, ostensibly, attached to the underlying bone. Therefore, bone remodeling is a pre-requisite for orthodontic tooth movement. Bone remodeling may be achieved either non-surgically or surgically, which is referred to as orthopedics. Interestingly, bone remodeling in the craniofacial region is accompanied by an additional phenomenon, namely pneumatization, which is the mechanism of paranasal sinus formation, whereby bone tissue is replaced by morphologic (functional) spaces filled with air. Moreover, these sinuses form part of the upper airway, and this realization led me to postulate the novel concept of Pneumopedics®, which I defined as non-surgical, upper airway remodeling. Note that remodeling refers to the development of specific but potentially irreversible structural changes in tissue. Therefore, one of the major objectives of this book is to introduce the principles of pneumopedics, and to appreciate the principles of non-surgical, upper airway remodeling. In turn, the pneumopedic developmental mechanism includes both epigenetic orthopedics for bone formation and bone remodeling, as well as epigenetic orthodontics, which can be viewed as cosmetic treatment with systemic health benefits. In other words, while upper airway changes are induced, clinically identifiable changes occur in the hard tissues, dental tissues, and soft tissues of the craniofacial complex in both adults and children.

These clinical, craniofacial corrections are achieved through 'biomimetic oral appliance therapy', which introduces further ideas. Notably, biomimetics or biomimicry is a science that studies natural models and then uses these designs and processes to solve human problems. There are numerous examples of biomimetics in general, and biomimetic dentistry in particular; for example, dental materials that mimic the behavior of natural tooth tissues, such as enamel and dentin. More specifically, the natural (biomimetic) model of the human body plan is based on bilateral symmetry on the outside with directional asymmetry on the inside, such as an asymmetric heart. Symmetry is dependent on a midline and humans can be considered to have three midlines; soft tissue, hard tissue and dental midline. Since humans exclusively consist of soft tissue when embryonic pattern formation occurs at about 3–4 weeks in utero, the soft tissue midline can be considered as the true midline for humans. Post-natally, the random departure from biologic symmetry is referred to as fluctuating asymmetry, which can mimic directional asymmetry if the extent of deviation is clinically noticeable. In addition, the human body plan also has a specific number of organelles, for example: 46 XY chromosomes; ten fingers, and 32 permanent teeth. Variations from the normal number of chromosomes, digits, or teeth produce recognizable genetic/clinical anomalies; for example, trisomy 21 (Down syndrome), syndactyly, and oligodontia/hypodontia. Significantly, tooth enamel is derived from surface ectoderm so, technically, teeth are on the outside of the body and thus subject to bilateral symmetry. In addition, the teeth are not normally found outside the oral cavity of the craniofacial region. This localization of dental tissues is due to a process called 'temporo-spatial patterning', involving site-specific gene expression at or during certain time periods of life, especially during embryonic and fetal stages. These patterns of gene expression lead to developmental mechanisms that result in natural growth and development. It is worth noting that the genes that a person inherits and is born with are kept for the life of that individual. Therefore, it is, at least hypothetically, possible that these genes could be modulated at later time points for continued growth and development, perhaps as part of the ageing process. Moreover, renewed gene expression might permit someone to achieve their 'genetic potential'. I defined genetic potential as the capacity of reaching the optimal outcome in the prevailing conditions, subject to a viable population(s) of stem cells. This idea would depend on an epigenetic response, whereby genes are influenced by external factors, such as dietary components, to provide a slightly different outcome, identifiable as phenotypic variation. Specifically, I defined craniofacial epigenetics as using a person's natural genes to correct and straighten the jaws, teeth, soft tissues, and functional spaces, painlessly, using biomimetic appliances.

Historically, hundreds if not thousands of appliances or devices have been used by the dental profession for a wide variety of applications. In the specialty of orthodontics, devices are still classified as being either removable, fixed, or functional appliances. This is an empiric classification of convenience, which simply notes that devices can or cannot be removed from the mouth by the patient, while there is still no general consensus of what constitutes a 'functional' appliance. Nevertheless, the overall necessity here is to understand how these appliances might work to produce their results. This requirement led me to introduce the word 'biomimetic' to describe a specific family of devices that rely on epigenetic phenomena to achieve their results. In other words, these appliances are intended to mimic nature, and replicate craniofacial growth and development that is encoded at the level of the human genome. Consequently, bearing in mind the concept of temporo-spatial patterning, these devices are not designed to be worn for 24 hours per day, but instead follow the circadian rhythm of human physiology, including hormones that influence growth, sleep, and other physiologic functions in both children and adults.

Applying these concepts over the past decade or so, numerous adult and pediatric patients have been treated using the pneumopedics and craniofacial epigenetics (PACE) protocol, sometimes as a potential cure for selected cases of sleep disordered breathing, including obstructive sleep apnea in a multi-disciplinary setting. The scene is now set to establish a full-time residency program in a University-Hospital with a view to creating a new specialty of craniofacial sleep medicine/Pneumopedics with Board examinations conducted by professional academies for dentists that successfully complete their training programs. It is my hope that this textbook will be on the recommended reading list and its contents will form part of the core curriculum.

Acknowledgements

Bryan Ferre Front cover design; Dr Bikram S. Thind; the late Dr William Harris; the late Dr Gabriela Lipka; Dr Chris Chapman: Figure 5, Figure 13, and Figure 79; Dr Dennis Alleman: Figure 6; Dr Tammarie Heit: Figure 7, Figure 21, Figure 64, Figure 70, and Figure 102; Dr Sue Wendling: Figure 8, Figure 9, Figure 11, and Figure 29a; Dr Sam Cress: Figure 12 and Figure 13; Dr Scott Lozanoff: Figure 15; Dr Jon Caulfield: Figure 16; Dr Hwasub Hwang: Figure 17 and Figure 50; Dr Charin Hwang: Figure 17 and Figure 50; Dr Carmen Cadilla: Table 1; Dr HeeNam Kim: Table 2 and Figure 38; Dr Kwangyeon Kim: Figure 19; Dr Payam Ataii: Figure 23; Dr Edna Santos: Figure 29b; Dr Mike Safranek: Figure 29c; Dr Neal Murphy: Figure 36 and Figure 37; Dr Mike Williams: Figure 36 and Figure 37; Dr TerryLynn Tennant: Figure 41b; Dr Myles Preble: Figure 41a and Figure 42; Dr Bradley Sievert: Figure 43; Dr Bill Payne: Figure 44; Dr Alex Pavlenko: Figure 45a; Dr Lihua Zhang: Figure 45b, Figure 47b, and Figure 69; Dr Dennis Klemp: Figure 48 and Figure 105; Dr Sang Min Lee: Figure 49, Figure 52, Figure 63, and Figure 65; Dr Felix Liao: Figure 53; Dr David Arnold: Figure 57; Dr Shamshudin Kherani: Figure 59a; Dr Han: Figure 59b; Dr Martha Cortes: Figure 62; Dr Prabu Raman Figure 77; Dr John Utama Figure 97 and Figure 106; Dr John Utama: Figure 97 and Figure 106; Dr Ravindra Chandrasekhar: Figure 101; Dr Claire Stagg; Dr Richard Teel; Dr Scott Neish; and Dr Steven Lin.

Glossary

3D axial springs: Patented components of biomimetic devices with a compressible 3D spring design fabricated from a super-elastic nickel-free alloy; have the capability of exerting cyclic, intermittent signals, which can enhance bone development and tooth alignment.

Adipogenesis: The biologic process of fat deposition/fat cell formation through mesenchymal stem cell differentiation.

Allometry: Size-related shape change, e.g. those that occur during normal growth and development. In other methods of assessment, e.g. cephalometric analysis, it is not possible to dissociate size changes from shape changes, which can obscure interpretation of perceived results.

Angiogenesis: The biologic process for the formation of new blood vessels.

Anisotropy: Directionality or polarity during size change, which contributes to shape changes.

Anterior nasal spine (ANS): A cephalometric landmark defined as the anterior-most point of the two maxillary bones at the intermaxillary suture.

Apnea: A period of time during sleep when a patient stops breathing for at least 10 seconds, which is used to diagnose obstructive sleep apnea (OSA).

Apnea-hypopnea index (AHI): The combined number of apnea-hypopnea events per hour, which is used to define the severity of OSA.

Apoptosis/programmed cell death: A biologic process used to produce programmed cell death. For example, separation of the digits during in utero limb development.

Attention deficit hyperactivity disorder (ADHD): A chronic primarily pediatric condition showing a range of behavioral disorders, including poor concentration, hyperactivity, and impulsivity.

Basion: A cephalometric landmark defined as the midpoint of the anterior margin of the foramen magnum, which is often used to calculate the length of the cranial base.

Biomimetics/biomimicry: A science that studies natural models and then uses these designs and processes to solve human problems. An interdisciplinary field in which scientific principles from engineering, chemistry, and biology, etc. are applied to the development of materials, systems, or machines that mimic biological processes

Biomimetic oral appliances: A family of devices that rely on epigenetic phenomena to mimic nature, and putatively replicate craniofacial growth and development that is encoded at the level of the human genome.

Biomimetic orthodontics/epigenetic orthodontics: A way of aligning the teeth by trying to copy the way the teeth and upper airway grow and develop naturally. Cosmetic orthodontic treatment with systemic health benefits.

Body mass index (BMI): Defined as the weight/body mass in kilograms divided by the height in meters squared (kg/m^2).

Complexity: A mathematical/statistical theory that examines uncertainty and non-linearity, emphasizing interactions and feedback loops that constantly change systems, e.g. the human genome.

Structural complexity: The craniofacial context of dental tissues (teeth); hard tissues (jaw bones); soft tissues (tongue/lips) and functional spaces (upper airway, etc.), contributing to clinical craniofacial heterogeneity.

Compensation: Correction of a biologic defect or deficiency by an increased response/function of another component or unimpaired parts of the same system. A process in which a tendency for a change in a given direction is counterbalanced by another change so that the original defect of structure/function is less evident.

Developmental compensation: Correction of a biologic defect or deficiency by a response during physiologic growth and development, which often occurs to permit compromised function; for example, crowding/malocclusion.

Postural compensation: Correction of a biologic defect or deficiency by a structural response of another component or unimpaired parts of the same system, which often occurs to permit compromised function; for example, forward head posture.

Carabelli's tubercle: The evolution of a sixth cusp on the first permanent maxillary molar, described in certain modern human sub-populations.

Cervical subluxation: Chiropractic term meaning that the cervical vertebrae are not well-aligned, and can impinge on spinal nerves of the intervertebral disks, facet joints, etc., to cause referred pain in the head, neck, shoulders, arms, etc.

Chondrocranium: A series of cartilages that largely constitute cranial base developmental.

Clasp: Orthodontic components used for retention to attach an appliance to the teeth such as: Adams clasps, ball clasps, Crozat clasps, delta clasps, and C clasps that engage the mesial and distal undercuts of the teeth for device retention.

Craniocaudal gradient: The developmental pattern of changing spatial proportions over time, especially during early growth and development. For example, the first branchial arch appears and gives rise to various structures prior to the second branchial arch. The gradual increase in size of the neurocranium/brain relative to the rest of the body during early human growth and development and childhood.

Craniosynostoses/craniosynostosis: A group of conditions in which the craniofacial sutures are unable to grow normally because of the inheritance of mutated genes that render the cell membrane receptors non-functional. Condition in which the sutures are synostosed/fused and unable to produce bone.

Decompensation: A correction of the functional spaces enclosed by dysmorphic structures, achieved surgically or non-surgically (through appropriate spatial signaling), to allow the structures to remain or grow/remodel into new/enhanced spatial matrices. Corrective surgical and/or other non-surgical clinical procedures used to enhance function and/or esthetics.

Deformational plagiocephaly/positional plagiocephaly: Cranial asymmetry associated with changes in child-rearing practices. For example, when a baby spends too much time lying on his/her back.

Dehiscence/fenestrations: Bone loss/perforations of the cortical plates of the jaw bones due to excessive pressure/force being exerted on the roots of the teeth. For example, during rapid palatal expansion using fixed orthodontics.

Differentiation/cytodifferentiation: A developmental mechanism by which (stem) cells change from being non-specific to cells that are functionally or morphologically distinguishable. For example, mesenchymal stem cells that form osteoblasts.

Distal stop: Orthodontic wire applied to the distal surface of a tooth to prevent tooth movement.

Mesial stop: Orthodontic wire applied to the mesial surface of a tooth to prevent tooth movement.

Occlusal stop: Orthodontic wire applied to the occlusal surface of a tooth to prevent eruptive tooth movements. Occlusal stops or rests usually pass over the distal marginal ridge of the last standing molar or sometimes lie in the disto-palatal groove of the first permanent molar. In these cases, the job of the occlusal stops is to prevent the mandible from occluding in its habitual position, precipitating a change in the spatial matrix.

Distraction osteogenesis: A surgical procedure initially used to elongate long bones of the legs, involving the phases of osteotomy, latency (initiation of wound healing), distraction (of the callus), and consolidation (ossification), which is now used in the correction of craniofacial syndromes, etc.

Dryopithecus pattern: The five-cusped tooth morphology of lower molar teeth of modern humans.

Endothelial dysfunction: A reduced availability of nitric oxide that results in a myriad of disorders. Commonly, the endothelial vessel walls become stiffer, while vasorelaxation is diminished, which is often associated with hypertension.

Enuresis: Involuntary urination, especially by children at night.

Primary nocturnal enuresis: A developmental or neurologic abnormality of the urogenital tract associated with involuntary urination.

Secondary nocturnal enuresis: Involuntary urination in which the etiologic factors are external to a normally developed urogenital tract.

Nocturnal polyuria: An increased amount of urine production, necessitating frequent urination at night.

Natriuresis diuresis: A physiologic process involving atrial natriuretic hormone (ANP), a cardiac hormone that can precipitate bed-wetting in children.

Epigenetics: The study of phenotypic changes that occur via mechanisms other than DNA sequence alteration. External factors above and beyond the genome that can affect growth and development.

Craniofacial epigenetics: Using a person's natural genes to correct and enhance the jaws, teeth, soft tissues, and functional spaces, painlessly, using biomimetic appliances. Treatment aimed at the overall health of the craniofacial region, by providing treatment protocols that address the condition's underlying signs of symptoms.

Epigenetic orthopedics: Physiologic bone formation and bone remodeling achieved non-surgically.

Epigenome: The chemical groups surrounding the DNA and its associated proteins, histones, and chromatin. The local environment of the genome, which is like a covering or layer that consists of specific structures. A complex system of switches that regulates how genes are controlled.

Excessive daytime sleepiness (EDS): An inability to maintain wakefulness or alertness during daytime, leading to feeling tired all the time. An essential symptom of narcolepsy.

Expansion: A developmental process during which hyaluronan (hyaluronic acid/hyaluronate), a hydrophilic macromolecule binds water and, as a result, the extracellular spaces undergo expansion and the tissue gets larger. For example, neonatal brain growth.

Palatal expansion/rapid palatal/maxillary expansion: An orthodontic technique used to widen the dentoalveolar arch in the transverse axis.

Facial perception: A person's understanding and interpretation of human facial features, in relation to neural information processing, which provides a basis for human social exchange. For example: She looks pretty but he looks mean.

Facial recognition: The human capability of identifying or verifying another person from seeing only their face (or an image of their face), which is largely unaffected by reasonable changes in lighting, viewing angle, and distance. Biometric (not biomimetic) software that mathematically maps human facial features and stores the data as a 3D model. The software uses deep learning algorithms to compare a new digital 3D image to the stored model to verify a person's identity.

Finite element analysis: An engineering technique applied to medicine by describing structures through discretization of the domain as a set of nodes/points, allowing computerized predictions on how a system might react/behave to real-world physical effects, including surgery, growth, and development, etc.

Form/morphology: The integration of size and shape information.

Function: The normal workings of a particular organ system. For example, the masticatory apparatus during swallowing; the respiratory tract during breathing; the neurologic system while sleeping, etc.

Functional appliance/myofunctional appliance: An historic misnomer. Removable devices used in pediatric cases to reposition the mandible similar to mandibular advancement appliances used for adult obstructive sleep apnea.

Functional space: In mathematics, a metric space whose elements are defined by specific functions. Clinically, a metric space whose elements are defined by physiologic function. For example, a synapse of the nervous system, Posselt's envelope of mandibular movement, the nasal airway, the periodontal space, the upper and lower temporo-mandibular joint (TMJ) spaces, etc.

Genetic potential: The capacity of a biologic system to reach an optimal outcome in the prevailing conditions, subject to a viable population(s) of stem cells.

Glabella: A cephalometric landmark defined as the most prominent point of the frontal bone in the mid-sagittal plane.

Soft tissue glabella: A cephalometric landmark defined as the most prominent point on the skin of the frontal bone (forehead) in the mid-sagittal plane.

Glycocalyx: A cell membrane component that consists of carbohydrate moieties of membrane glycolipids/glycoproteins. These molecules contribute to cell–cell recognition, cell communication, and cellular adhesion.

Gonion: A cephalometric landmark defined by bisecting the angle formed by the tangents to the posterior border and lower border of the mandible.

Gonial angle: Formed by three landmarks on the mandibular profile (condylion-gonion-pogonion), which gives an indication of the morphology/phenotype of the mandible.

Growth/development: The net outcome of genetic inheritance and environmental modulation, resulting from cell migration, proliferation, differentiation, and biosynthesis of extracellular matrix in specific, temporo-spatial directions and magnitudes, producing identifiable morphologies. A quantitative increase in size and/or mass and/or complexity.

Homology: The condition that describes how certain regions of the mammalian genome are highly conserved throughout evolution.

Headgear effect: A relative restriction/restraint/retraction of anterior growth within the midface, by exerting a growth-inhibitory effect on the maxilla, producing supposed improvements in facial balance following treatment with various functional/myofunctional appliances.

Hyperplasia: Cell proliferation through mitotic cell division, resulting in an increased number of cells.

Hypertrophy: An increase in individual cell size so that the overall tissues, e.g. muscles, get bigger.

Hypopnea: A reduction in airflow (say 30–50%) during sleep accompanied by oxygen desaturation (say 3–4%) of the blood and often associated with arousal, which is used to diagnose the severity of OSA.

Induced maxillary morphogenesis: A clinical technique to restore midfacial bone volume to accommodate 16 maxillary teeth *inter alia*.

Infradentale: A cephalometric landmark defined as the antero-superior point of the mandibular central incisor alveolus in the mid-sagittal plane.

Intercanthal angle: Formed by the intersection of two lines that pass through the lateral and medial canthi (corners of the eyes on both sides). A positive (V-shaped) intercanthal angle suggests that there is sufficient midfacial volume since the floor of the orbit is the roof of the maxilla.

Isotropy: Uniform size change in all directions.

Kinetic chain: An engineering concept used to describe the interrelated groups of body segments, connecting joints, and muscles working together to perform movements. A series of overlapping segments that create a system which allows movement of one joint to affect the movement of another. It is used in sports medicine, musculoskeletal and neuro-rehabilitation, as well as prosthetics and orthotics.

Klinorhynchy: Craniofacial evolutionary adaptations for speech secondary to cranial base flexion, resulting in a prognathic facial profile so that the jaws do not impinge on the upper airway.

Labiomental angle: Angle formed between the orthodontic landmarks inferior prolabiale, soft tissue point B, and soft pogonion, which indicates the extent of mandibular retrognathia.

Leptin: A hormone that is crucial to appetite and weight control, which is predominantly synthesized by adipocytes (fat cells) and enterocytes in the small intestine. It helps regulate energy balance by inhibiting hunger and diminishes fat storage in adipocytes.

Lordosis: The normal convex curvature of the cervical and lumbar regions of the spine.

Mallampati score: In anesthesia, the Mallampati score/classification is used to predict the ease of intubation. It is also used to classify tongue/soft palate posture as a simple test/predictor of obstructive sleep apnea; the higher the score, the increased likelihood of OSA, although is not highly predictive.

Malocclusion: A solution for a complex, adaptive system to remain in equilibrium or homeostasis.

Microbiome: Combined population of microorganisms in a particular environment or region of the body, e.g. the oral microbiome. Cumulative population of microorganisms that reside on or within human tissues/systems/biofluids, such as the gastro-intestinal tract.

Nasion: Cephalometric landmark defined as the most anterior point of the frontonasal suture.

Soft tissue nasion: Landmark corresponding to nasion on the skin at the bridge of the nose.

Neural crest cells: A sub-population of cells that originates at the developing neural tube and leaves the central nervous system to populate the developing craniofacial regions. These cells give rise to the connective tissues of the head and neck region as well as other tissues, e.g. cardiac cells, melanocytes, and autonomic (nerve) ganglia.

Obstructive sleep apnea (OSA): Medical condition characterized by pauses in breathing during sleep due to upper airway collapse, which can be associated with a myriad of serious health issues.

Occlusion/bite: The end point of the body with respect to the plantar surfaces of the feet, and within these two boundaries all functional spaces for physiologic processes must be accommodated.

Neuromuscular bite registration: The use of transcutaneous electrical nerve stimulation (TENS) to relax the muscles of mastication in order to achieve the physiologic rest position of the mandible.

Phonetic bite registration/sibilant phoneme registration: A protocol to therapeutically reposition the mandible using the 's' sound to determine the minimum speaking distance.

Ontogeny: The complete life period of an individual, including ageing.

Opisthion: A cephalometric landmark defined as the midpoint of the posterior margin of the foramen magnum.

Oral myofunctional therapy/oral myology: A program of specific exercises supervised by an oral myofunctional therapist that targets the tongue, facial muscles, and oropharynx to reinforce the proper resting posture of the tongue, lips, and jaws with the goal of facilitating proper breathing.

Orthodontics: A specialty of dentistry primarily concerned with dentoalveolar correction of the teeth.

Orthodontic extrusion: The utilization of light orthodontic forces to enhance the eruption of teeth, during which the entire attachment apparatus relocates coronally with the crown of the tooth.

Orthodontic intrusion: The utilization of light orthodontic forces so that the crown and entire attachment apparatus of the tooth relocates apically, with no change in the clinical crown height.

Oxygen desaturation index (ODI): The number of times per hour of sleep that the blood's oxygen level drops by a certain degree (say 80%) from baseline. The ODI is typically measured as a percentage of the time of decreased oxygenation of the blood while asleep.

Parasomnia: A group of sleep disorders defined as undesirable physical events or experiences that occur during the initiation of sleep, during sleep, or during arousal from sleep.

Pattern formation: A critical process and developmental mechanism during the early embryonic development that gives rise to the body plan, including polarity (e.g. right-side/left-side) and the midline, etc.

Pcrit: The critical pressure at which the upper airway collapses. Airway obstruction may be induced when nasal pressure is decreased below Pcrit.

Periodontal ligament: An historical misnomer since it is not a true ligament but somewhat analogous to a modified craniofacial suture. A soft fibrous connective tissue located between the cementum of the tooth root and the alveolar bone of the tooth socket to help support teeth.

Pharyngeal stent: An extension extending from the posterior border of a biomimetic oral appliance to prevent upper airway collapse by the tongue, soft palate/uvula, or lateral pharyngeal walls.

Pogonion: A cephalometric landmark defined as the most anterior point of the chin button.

Prolabiale: A cephalometric landmark defined as the most anterior point of the lower lip.

Prognathic/prognathism: A phylogenetic condition in which the maxilla and mandible are preferentially located anterior to the anterior cranial base subsequent to klinorhynchy to avoid upper airway obstruction.

Pharyngoplasty: A group of surgical procedure using superior or inferior pharyngeal flaps or uvulopharyngopalatoplasty (UPPP) to compensate for various velopharyngeal dysfunctions.

Pneumatization: The physiologic mechanism of paranasal sinus formation, whereby bone tissue is replaced by epithelial-lined cavities/functional spaces filled with air.

Pneumopedics: Non-surgical upper airway remodeling, without using drugs, injections, or pain.

Point A/subspinale: A cephalometric landmark defined as the deepest point of the concavity below the anterior nasal spine and above prosthion.

Soft subspinale/Soft tissue point A: A cephalometric landmark defined as the deepest point of the concavity below the anterior nasal spine and above prosthion on the profile of the upper lip.

Point B/supramentale: A cephalometric landmark defined as the deepest point of the concavity below infradentale and above the chin.

Soft infradentale/Soft tissue point B: A cephalometric landmark defined as the deepest point of the concavity of the lower lip and above the chin.

Posterior nasal spine (PNS): A cephalometric landmark defined as the posterior-most point of the two palatine bones at the intermaxillary suture.

Procrustes superimposition: A mathematical method of superimposition deploying a rotation, translation, and scaling procedure that is re-iterated till the fit of two or more objects cannot be improved.

Prolabiale: A cephalometric landmark defined as the most anterior point of the upper lip.

Pronasale: A cephalometric landmark defined as the most anterior point on the tip of the nose.

Prosthion: A cephalometric landmark defined as the antero-inferior point of the maxillary central incisor alveolus in the mid-sagittal plane.

Rapid maxillary/palatal expansion (RME/RPE): An orthodontic procedure which fractures the two halves of the maxilla in the midline, precipitating a midline diastema between the maxillary central incisors. A dento-alveolar technique which splits the midpalatal suture in the transverse plane while attempting to widen the hard palate medio-laterally in pediatric cases.

Respiratory disturbance index (RDI): Combined number of apneas, hypopneas, and RERAs per hour of sleep. RDI includes respiratory effort-related arousals (RERAs) and may help confirm the typical symptoms of pediatric OSA.

Respiratory effort related arousal (RERA): A sleep disorder characterized by upper airway flow reduction that does not meet the criteria of apnea or hypopnea but is associated with arousal from sleep.

Retrognathia: Developmental compensation of the mandible, often resulting in a posteriorly positioned mandible, an increased overjet, and Class II malocclusion. Note that maxillary protrusion is often not associated with mandibular retrognathia.

Relapse: A physiologic response to a violation of equilibrium or balance so that a biologic system regresses to homeostasis.

Remodeling: The development of specific but potentially irreversible structural changes in tissues.

Screw-fin mechanism: A patented component of some biomimetic oral appliances that permits mandibular advancement. The vertical flange of the screw-fin mechanism found on the lower component of the device engages an acrylic slot of the upper component, permitting mandibular repositioning.

Sella: A cephalometric landmark defined as the center of the sella turcica in the mid-sagittal plane.

Shape: The properties of an object that remain invariant when size information is removed.

Signal transduction: A cascade of events that, starting with a growth factor (ligand) that undergoes binding at its specific cell membrane receptor, leads to particular functional or morphologic changes, usually through a cascade of secondary intra-cellular messengers.

Mechano-transduction: A physical signal, such as mechanical loading pathways, which induce specific functional or morphologic changes through a cascade of secondary intra-cellular messengers.

Size: Displacement of two-dimensional or three-dimensional space that can be quantified through measurement.

Sleep bruxism: A movement disorder associated with sleep arousals and characterized by a rise in sympathetic-cardiac activity, rhythmic masticatory muscle activity (RMMA), and tooth grinding.

Sleep disordered breathing/Sleep-related breathing disorders: Spectrum of disorders ranging from primary snoring, upper airway resistance syndrome, to mild-moderate-severe obstructive sleep apnea, including pediatric obstructive sleep apnea. Upper airway dysfunction during sleep characterized by snoring and/or increased respiratory effort secondary to increased upper airway resistance and/or upper airway collapsibility associated with obstructive sleep apnea.

Sleep hygiene: Habits and practices that are conducive to sleeping well on a regular basis.

Somniloquy: A rare sleep disorder defined as talking (dialogues, monologues, gibberish, or mumbling) while asleep without being aware of it. Somniloquy differs from catathrenia, which is a rare condition characterized by monotonous, irregular groans that occur during prolonged expiration while asleep (sleep-related groaning).

Spatial matrix: An arena, site, system, or region in which development events unfold as gene-environmental interactions proceed, e.g. the developmental dynamics of the orofacial complex.

Spinal moment arm: The perpendicular distance from a pivot to a point undergoing torque.

Stridor: Abnormal, high-pitched sounds produced by turbulent airflow through a partially obstructed airway at the level of the supraglottis.

Sudden infant death syndrome (SIDS)/crib death: Unexplained death of an otherwise healthy baby, typically less than one year old, usually during sleep.

Suture: A joint between two bones formed by intramembranous ossification. Sutures harbor populations of mesenchymal stem cells that are depleted subject to heterochronicity (genetically controlled differences in the timing or duration) so that some craniofacial sutures synostose later than others.

Periodontal suture: The periodontium appears to represent a modified suture and within the sutural boundaries (100–400μm) resides a population(s) of periodontal stem cells.

Talon: Phylogenetic feature which produces a four-cusped maxillary molar tooth morphology.

Torus mandibularis: Bony exostoses on the medial aspect of the mandible usually in the premolar region. Typically, bilateral, but unilateral torus mandibularis has recently been described.

Torus palatinus: Bony exostoses in the midline of the maxilla, usually anterior to the transverse palatal suture.

Trigone: Phylogenetic feature, which produces a three-cusped component of a maxillary molar tooth.

Temporo-spatial patterning: Site-specific gene expression at or during certain time periods of life, especially during embryonic and fetal stages.

Thyromental angle: Lateral profile photographic feature formed by: soft pogonion; the deepest point of the concavity below the chin and above the neck; and the laryngeal prominence (the most anterior point of the thyroid cartilage).

Tooth support: Physiologic tooth movement, which can be observed as an adaptation to intermittent axial forces (loading and unloading) without any orthodontic tooth movement.

Upper airway: The combined regions of the nasopharynx, oropharynx, and hypopharynx, excluding the laryngopharynx, and contiguous with the trachea and the lower airway further distally.

Upper airway resistance syndrome (UARS): A sleep disorder characterized by the narrowing of the airway and oxygen desaturation of the blood associated with disruptions/arousals during sleep.

Vertical drift: A known feature of ageing sometimes referred to as being ‘long in the tooth’. This expression alludes to a horse’s gums receding with age and making the teeth appear longer. Clinically, vertical drift is associated with a reduced functional space for the mandible due to encroachment by the maxilla, resulting in an increased frequency of crowding of the lower anterior teeth with age.

Wireframe DNA appliance: Biomimetic oral appliance in which the palatal acrylic and screw system is replaced with a double omega loop design. The device has anterior and posterior omega loops, which permit widening of the palate without using a screw system.

Chapter 1

Introduction

Summary: This chapter introduces the novel principles of craniofacial epigenetics, Pneumopedics®, and biomimetic oral appliance therapy. It outlines factors within the craniofacial region that can be affected by the epigenetic approach. It looks at the new concept of pneumopedics, which is defined as non-surgical upper airway remodeling since the goal of pneumopedics is to enhance the upper airway without using surgery, drugs, injections, or pain. This goal is a quest of biomimetic appliances, which are based on the science of biomimicry. Specifically, it is suggested that biomimetic oral appliance therapy may be utilized for the treatment of sleep disordered breathing in both children and adults.

The objectives of this book are threefold: first, to introduce the principles of craniofacial epigenetics; second to appreciate the principles of Pneumopedics, and the third is to gain knowledge of biomimetic oral appliances. Although the human genome has been sequenced, there are, in fact, factors above and beyond the genome that can affect growth and development, which is referred to as Epigenetics in this book, and we are going to realize how the craniofacial region can be affected by the epigenetic approach. The second idea is to look at the concept of Pneumopedics in a little more detail. Historically, we've held the view of orthodontics as a method to straighten teeth; and the idea of orthopedics, which is to surgically remodel bone; and now we have the concept of Pneumopedics, which is to non-surgically remodel the upper airway. Therefore, the goal of this novel technique is to enhance the upper airway without using surgery, drugs, injections, or pain. The question then arises, how are we going to do that? Consider orthodontic appliances that we've used in the past have been classified as either removable, fixed, or functional appliances. This classification does not indicate how the appliances actually work. Removable appliance simply means that patients can take the devices in and out of the mouth, unlike fixed appliances that cannot be removed by the patient. On the other hand, there is still debate in the literature on how functional appliances work exactly. In contrast, we are going to look at biomimetic oral appliances, based on the science of biomimicry or biomimetics. Biomimetics, in this context, is a way of copying or replicating the way the body grows and develops naturally. Specifically, we use biomimetic oral appliances for the treatment of sleep disordered breathing (SDB), so the overall objective of this book is to apply these novel concepts to the clinical management of patients diagnosed with obstructive sleep apnea (OSA) in a multi-disciplinary setting. This protocol includes other professionals working in a team that may include a medical physician, such as a sleep specialist. It may also include other therapists, such as an oral myofunctional therapist; and a chiropractor, perhaps with additional training, such as an atlas-orthogonist and, maybe, a nutritionist or naturopath, etc. as needed. The central part of this team is a dentist/orthodontist with special training in craniofacial sleep medicine, with the aim of achieving maximum medical benefit for a particular patient.

To best understand the idea of epigenetics in a bit more detail, we can ask the question, what is epigenetics? In the literature, epigenetics is defined as the study of phenotypic changes that occur via mechanisms other than DNA sequence alteration; in other words, it's a way to change or vary the phenotypic outcome without changing the underlying genome and its sequence of base pairs. This is a relatively new idea and it's important to understand how this phenotypic variation can be achieved. During epigenetic modification, it is thought that biochemical changes are mediated via covalent attachments of chemical groups surrounding the DNA and associated proteins, histones, and chromatin. In other words, there is a local environment surrounding the DNA, which is like a covering or layer that consists of specific structures, such as proteins, histones, etc., referred to as the epigenome. The idea is that these biochemical groups behave like epigenetic tags. These tags are mechanisms that are available to permit interactions with the external environment, and this gene-environmental interaction induces epigenetic modification, resulting in phenotypic variation. Thus, epigenetic modification includes different types of biochemical changes, such as ADP-ribosylation, acetylation, methylation, phosphorylation, sumoylation, and ubiquitination, etc. All of these effects are complex biochemical reactions, and there are numerous studies that specifically describe these kinds of molecular genetic interactions. For example, let's consider methylation. The current medical advice to women of childbearing age includes folate supplementation of the diet prior to and during pregnancy. Folate and folic acid act as methyl (CH_3) donors, producing methylation of the local genes. Methylene-tetrahydrofolate reductase (MTHFR) is the enzyme necessary for this methylation. This enzyme converts folate and folic acid into an active form that the body can use. Note that the MTHFR gene produces this enzyme, but a genetic mutation can inhibit its function. In non-affected individuals, it has been found that over a period of time methylation via this mechanism significantly decreases the risk of neural tube defects, such as spinal bifida, cleft palate, etc. This is the first and most well-researched example of epigenetic modification, but historically we have been doing this type of modification for a long time, by simply adding nutrients and various other factors to the diet — although we didn't know or understand the underlying corrective mechanisms. More recently, the mechanisms of epigenetic modification have become more fully understood, and we can now apply these mechanisms to the craniofacial region, which is known as craniofacial epigenetics. But first, we need a working definition of what we mean by craniofacial epigenetics. I defined craniofacial epigenetics as deploying a person's natural genes to correct and straighten the jaws, the teeth, the soft tissues, and functional spaces, painlessly using biomimetic oral appliances. The emphasis here is on the person's natural genes as we are not employing any form of transgenics or genetic modification; we're not introducing any new genes from a different species into the native genome. Instead, we are targeting the genes that are naturally inherited, the genes that a child is born with, the genes that are kept for a lifetime. However, we're going to signal those genes indirectly by working with their local environment, with the epigenome. In the same way that the human genome was sequenced in 2003, molecular geneticists have now started to sequence the epigenome. It's a complex system of switches that regulates how genes are controlled, i.e. upregulated or switched on, modulated, down-regulated, or switched off.

In the craniofacial region there are several complex structures, such as the bones of the jaws, the dental tissues of the teeth, the craniofacial soft tissues, such as the tongue and lips, etc. and, significantly, there are functional spaces, such as the sinuses and upper airway. In fact, you can regard the whole of the human body as a system of functional spaces, and by regulating those spaces we can modify functions or how those systems behave. For example, if you have an artery that undergoes vasoconstriction, you can increase blood pressure, and you may need to do that if you're exercising, for example. Similarly, nerve transmission requires the presence of a synaptic space because an absence of a mere 9nm of space means that neurotransmitters can't reach the post-synaptic region. Another key aspect of craniofacial epigenetics is that this modification of the structures is done painlessly. For example, when children are growing and developing, typically they don't complain of pain. In other words, they are in a physiological state, and we would like to do our clinical corrections in that state also. On the other hand, if you are inducing pain by using surgery or orthodontic brackets, you are inducing inflammation, and inflammation is not healthy for the body. It now understood that conventional orthodontic brackets and wires utilize the inflammatory process to move teeth. Alternatively, if at all possible, we'd like treatment to be a pain-free procedure, and that is the mode of biomimetic oral appliances. Thus, biomimetic appliances try to replicate the way the body normally grows and develops. Biomimetics is a science that studies natural models, and then uses these processes to solve human problems. So what is the natural model for the human body that we are trying to replicate? The human body is characterized by being bilaterally symmetrical on the outside and asymmetric on the inside. We also know that the human body plan consists of site-specific patterns; for example, two eyes, ten fingers, 32 teeth, etc. The biomimetic approach is simply trying to replicate this natural body plan as far as possible, unlike previous approaches that have reduced bodily components, for example appendectomy, the extraction of wisdom or premolar teeth, etc. Bearing in mind the body's design, what processes are available to solve clinical issues such as malocclusion, temporo-mandibular joint (TMJ) problems, snoring, and obstructive sleep apnea (OSA)? The processes we want to utilize are developmental processes, and these developmental processes are encoded by genes. We keep these genes for life and if there were a way that we could communicate with the genes, through the epigenome perhaps, then we may have a potential mechanism of being able to address specific clinical problems. In this way, we can think about biomimetic orthodontics and Pneumopedics as a way of straightening the teeth by trying to copy the way the upper airway and teeth grow and develop naturally. The full dental complement in a modern human consists of 32 teeth symmetrically aligned in occlusion, which will produce a broad and attractive smile; essentially, if the teeth are well aligned and symmetric, we are providing cosmetic treatment with a view to overall, systemic health. Therefore, those teeth are going to be accommodated in well-developed jaw bones, and behind those jaws we find the upper airway. Now, if the jaws are well-developed, then the upper airway will likely be well-developed, with concomitant oxygenation of the blood during daytime wakefulness and also during sleep.

Thus, we expect to get tangible health benefits to a greater or lesser extent over the length of the person's life. Therefore, biomimetic orthodontics can be regarded as cosmetic treatment with health benefits.

Another question that arises is, what makes craniofacial epigenetics different from traditional dentoalveolar orthodontics? One major difference is that craniofacial epigenetics is aimed at the overall health of the craniofacial region, and it does so by providing appropriate treatment protocols that address the underlying signs of symptoms of malocclusions, temporo-mandibular dysfunction (TMD), OSA, atlas subluxation, etc. As a whole, the craniofacial region encompasses the brain, the upper airway, the temporo-mandibular joints, the tongue, as well as the jaws and teeth. Pertinently, these structures neither exist in isolation nor do they function in seclusion. In other words, if you have jaw pain, you are unable to chew, swallow, and speak properly because of the pain. Similarly, the overall health of the craniofacial region includes brain health. For example, over a long period of time, chronic, neurologic diseases, such as dementia, cognitive impairment, Parkinson's disease, and even concussions, can take their toll on the quality and quantity of a person's life. Conditions that may affect cognitive function need to be addressed early, so it's important to be able to optimize those functions during childhood, and the way that is accomplished is by taking a craniofacial approach. Let's say we want to use the teeth and jaws to protect brain function of a person who's playing team sports. It's essential to prevent that athlete from getting a minor traumatic brain injury or concussion, and one way to do that is by aligning the jaws and teeth to a more optimal position. This positional alignment can be obtained through development, but may also be achieved in the short term by using, for example, an oral orthotic or sports mouthguard (Singh *et al.*, 2009). We're looking at the underlying etiology of a condition with a view to prevention; not symptomatic relief. Accordingly, if a patient attends a clinic and their main concern is that the teeth are not straight, and it's found that they have a malocclusion on examination, then there's an underlying cause of why those teeth are crowded. Our aim is to find the reason(s) for that before we unravel the teeth, because medically we want to know what made those teeth move into an irregular position with respect to the rest of the body in the first place. Similarly, if a patient attends a clinic and complains of TMJ pain, we want to know what is causing that pain, why is the joint in that position, and what do we need to do to correct the current symptoms, as well as long term management. Another craniofacial example would be a patient diagnosed with obstructive sleep apnea. Why does this patient have OSA? What is the site(s) of obstruction and the severity of the condition? By looking at the overall health of the craniofacial region, we look for the underlying etiology of the issue, to formulate an appropriate treatment protocol that addresses the signs and symptoms of a particular condition.

I'm often asked how did these concepts actually arise and where did these ideas come from? The story is that I was invited to relocate to the Center for Craniofacial Disorders, USA from the UK. In this Center we were looking after babies and children with specific craniofacial abnormalities, such as cleft lip, cleft palate, and other rare and complex craniofacial conditions. We developed novel 3D modeling software and analysis for use with non-invasive 3D imaging hardware (Singh *et al.*, 2005). Using these sophisticated modeling techniques, we were able to take a group of babies and by imaging their facial structures we were able to produce the average 3D model of a typical baby's face. Next, we repeated this procedure for babies born with cleft lip and palate. Importantly, we were able to take those babies and non-surgically correct the nasal deformity, using a nasal stent in a procedure called nasoalveolar molding (NAM). After the NAM procedure had been finished, we took the 3D model of those babies where the nose, lip, and palate had been corrected and compared the models. We found that when we superimposed the post-treatment 3D model of the children with cleft lip/palate and the control group, the two models were virtually indistinguishable (Singh *et al.*, 2007). Furthermore, principal components analysis showed that the two groups overlapped in statistical shape-space; in other words, these were not two groups of 'objects' but simply an array of one set of 3D objects. Therefore, by using a non-surgical method, we were able to make babies who were born with cleft palate have a similar facial morphology as regular babies. But then we needed to understand how the epigenetic change in facial phenotype was achieved in this study. Part of the answer lies in a developmental mechanism known as temporo-spatial patterning (Chaplain *et al.*, 1999). Put simply, the body has a genetic blueprint so various components/systems are going to fit into a certain spatial pattern, according to the body plan. In cleft lip and palate, a genetic mutation means that the structures are found in a slightly different position due to changes in gene expression during a very early part of pre-natal development. What we were able to do non-surgically was put the structures close to where we thought they needed to be based on *a priori* bilateral symmetry, for example. In other words, we used a nasal stent to open up the deformed nares/nasal cartilage to allow the baby to breathe through the nose. Next, we gently molded the palatal segments together using an oral plate, so the baby could breathe through the nose and feed through the mouth simultaneously, just as in breast-feeding, following the biomimetic principles outlined above. When approximately 1mm of space was left between the major and minor palatal segments, our team's plastic surgeon would surgically close the palate and then allow the baby to grow. Similarly, when there was about 1mm of space left between the two sides of the cleft lip, we would ask our team's plastic surgeon to close the lip surgically without any post-operative tension. By following this procedure, we found that the children tended to heal slightly more symmetrically, and our 3D assessments showed that after a period of time there was virtually no difference between the infants treated in that manner and those babies who are born in the normal condition. Therefore, we believe that the process of temporo-spatial patterning is helping to correct the craniofacial region in those specific children, using an epigenetic mechanism for correction.

The reverse of the above findings is also true in that there can also be detrimental epigenetic changes in the craniofacial region, such as nasal obstruction following allergic rhino-sinusitis. In one study (Parsons *et al.*, 2015), a genetic mutation of the cranial base was induced in mice. As expected, there was a change in morphology of the cranial base but this was accompanied by an epigenetic change in facial shape even though the facial genes of these mice were not targeted. This finding is somewhat similar to some clinical syndromes. In Down syndrome or trisomy 21, temporo-spatial patterning is disrupted presumably because of the extra copy of chromosome 21 and its attendant genes. The epigenetic effect of this mutation is the characteristic facies that are recognizable in children born with Down syndrome. It appears as though the cranial base dysmorphology correlates with facial changes such that these children appear to have macroglossia, which predisposes them to an increased risk of SDB (Ng *et al.*, 2006). Current thought is that if the midfacial deficiency could be addressed, then the associated OSA may also be corrected. Another more common example of an epigenetic craniofacial change is adenoid facies or long face syndrome. Typically, this condition develops secondary to nasal obstruction and is associated with mouth-breathing due to adenoidal and tonsillar hypertrophy. The spatial change in the position of the mandible leads to an epigenetic effect such that the midface grows downward predominantly, since the tongue is lying in the floor of the mouth and not molding the hard palate. The clinical features of long face syndrome include a 'gummy smile' or vertical maxillary excess, anterior open bite, and often a marked antegonial notch, producing a steep mandibular plane angle, although not all of these features might be seen in a specific case because of complexity. In other words, although there is a finite number of clinical features associated with adenoid facies, it's difficult to predict which ones will be present in a particular case. On the other hand, if features such as gummy smiles are epigenetic in their nature, then it ought to be possible to reverse or reduce these effects without using surgery. In fact, there are some studies that support this contention.

The chief concern in the case illustrated in Figure 1 is twofold; first the patient was concerned by the cosmetic appearance of the gummy smile,

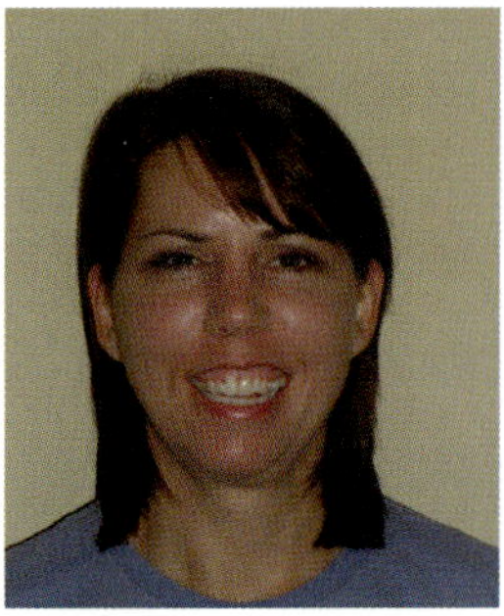

Figure 1a: Pre-treatment appearance.

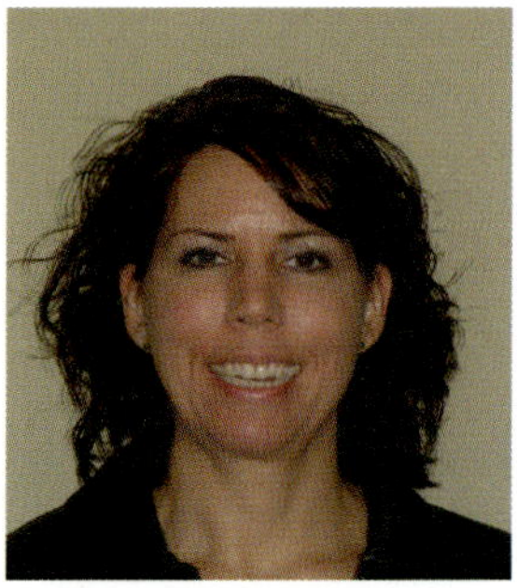

Figure 1b: Mid-treatment changes.

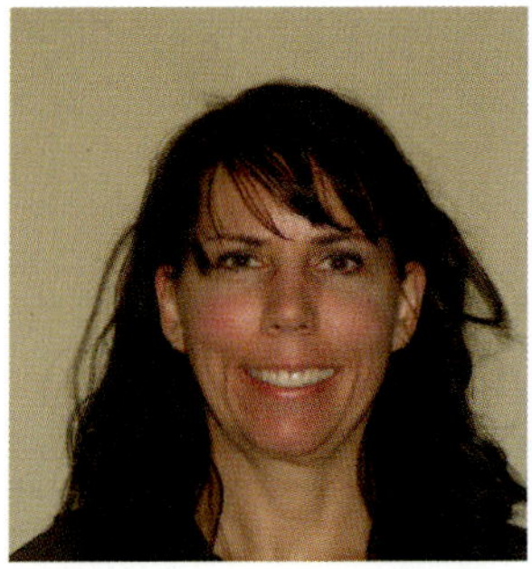

Figure 1c: Post-treatment appearance.

and second there was a functional issue in terms of the anterior open bite (Fig. 1a). Previous consultations with various professionals had indicated that the main treatment option available for this adult was to have surgery, but this particular patient wasn't keen on taking a surgical approach. Instead, biomimetic treatment was initiated (Harris and Singh, 2013).

Fig. 1b shows the effects on the facial appearance midway through treatment. Notably, an increase in nasal symmetry is discernible and the gummy smile has been reduced. The nasal change is essential for correction since the mode of breathing has changed from mouth-breathing to nasal breathing since the nasal obstruction has been addressed. At the end of treatment (Fig. 1c), the gummy smile has been resolved and the anterior open bite has been dramatically improved. Overall, the finished case, which took about 14 months, appears to have addressed the underlying cause of the condition. Pre-treatment (Fig. 1a), the left naris was obstructed, and the patient probably opened her mouth to breathe, becoming a habitual mouth breather. The chronic open-mouth posture allowed the maxilla to drift vertically downward into that spatial matrix and produced the gummy smile (vertical maxillary excess). In addition, the tongue was lying in the floor of the mouth since the palate was too narrow, and following the path of least resistance thrust forward, thereby perpetuating the gummy smile. Therefore, the underlying reason why this patient presented with a gummy smile and anterior open bite probably relates to the left-sided nasal obstruction and the inability to breathe through the nose. Midway through treatment the nares appear to be fairly symmetric (Fig. 1b) and these correlations of form and function support the notion of craniofacial homeostasis. In other words, functional space has been recaptured, and if the patient is able to breathe through the nose, she is less likely to keep the lips apart. In order to maintain this new functional outcome, however, it's important for the patient to undergo myofunctional therapy to train the tongue to stay in the palate since upper arch development now provides that space. Thus, by the end of treatment there is improved symmetry, a broader smile and the mandible has been brought into position for final occlusion, using some limited fixed appliance therapy. Therefore, even though the option of seeing a patient when they are very young is sometimes missed, there may still be non-surgical solutions available at a later age.

Preferentially, we would see babies the day after they were born in the Center for Craniofacial Disorders. Postnatally, on day one, our medical colleagues would examine the baby to make sure there were no other syndromic abnormalities, specifically cardiac defects for example. If the baby was diagnosed with isolated cleft lip and/or cleft palate, we would see that case almost immediately and start the impression-taking stage of the procedure. Unfortunately, that doesn't always happen, and by the time we see some children they are already teenagers with a history of surgical correction for cleft lip and/or cleft palate in some, if not, all cases. In these types of cases a midfacial deficiency is not uncommon, and the lower jaw appears to be prominent while the midface is set further back. Therefore, in young subjects that were born with cleft lip and palate, which was surgically repaired, the midface often needs to be brought forward in order to improve the facial profile. Nowadays, a relatively established procedure called distraction osteogenesis is deployed. This technique basically has four stages. Phase one is osteotomy, for example, Le Fort II, where the entire midface is dislocated or disimpacted, to allow the midface/maxilla to be repositioned surgically. Stage two is latency, where the bone fracture is allowed to heal to a certain extent with concomitant stem cell differentiation. Stage three is distraction, where a mechanical screw system is used to distract or stretch the callus and allow tissue remodeling. Phase four is consolidation, allowing the bone to heal in the new spatial matrix and the newly formed bone regenerate to be remodeled, along with histogenesis. This type of procedure has been done both on the mandible, on the midface, and in combination in the craniofacial region at specific sites for anomalies of the human face and jaws. It's an interesting technique that was discovered or pioneered by a Russian orthopedic surgeon (Ilizarov *et al.*, 1982). Originally, we studied the outcomes of these procedures using MRI scans since 3D cone-beam CT scans were not widely available at that time. Pre-treatment, the facial profile typically looked concave due to a deficiency of the maxilla and/or the midface (Fig. 2a), so if we were to plot the position of subspinale (point A: the most concave point of the maxilla) in 3D space it would be relatively retruded compared to the rest of the facial profile. Post-treatment, we often noticed the position of this point changed dramatically, being placed

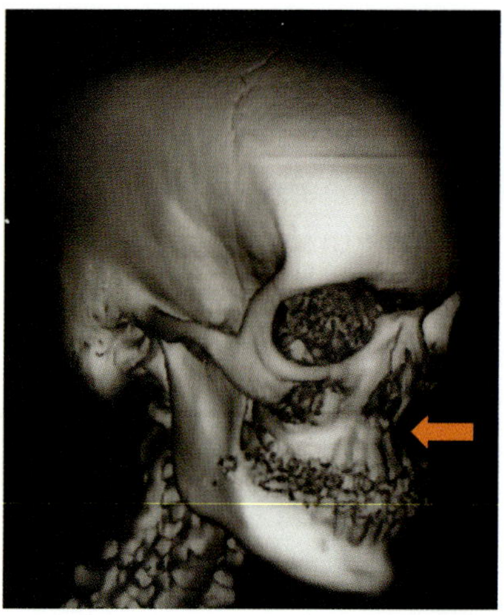

Figure 2a: Pre-treatment MRI scan showing position of subspinale (orange arrow).

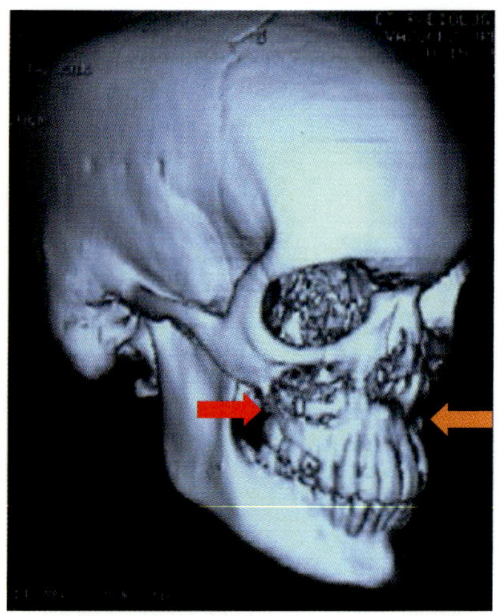

Figure 2b: Post-treatment MRI scan showing osteotomy site (red arrow). Note change at subspinale.

further forward, as if supported by bone growth (Fig. 2b). Therefore, we looked for features that might suggest that the whole bony deficiency had been addressed and/or corrected.

An important feature I observed was the site of the initial osteotomy; the surgery had been done further distally (pterygopalatine disjunction) to disarticulate the maxilla (Fig. 2b). Typically, the surgical sites healed normally, so we have to ask the question: how did the anterior aspect of the maxilla change (subspinale: point A; Fig. 2a) when it was not directly surgically manipulated? The most probable answer that arises is that the anterior region of the maxilla had undergone remodeling, so the entire body of the maxilla found itself in a different spatial relationship to the mandible compared to the pre-operative conditions. That a change in spatial relations allows remodeling of the maxilla to occur was predicted by the spatial matrix hypothesis (Singh, 2004; 2007; 2009), giving these patients a more normal look post-treatment. But, according to the spatial matrix hypothesis, other (functional) improvements should follow. One of the things that we observed looking at the teenagers is that they would come back for the review/follow-up appointment with a smile, and they appeared be happier/healthier people. This made me wonder what was going on at a deeper level. In terms of the facial changes, they obviously looked better but we surmised they probably had improved self-esteem and more confidence. I wanted to know if there were any other morphologic features that might correlate the clinical observations to the structural changes that we had achieved using distraction osteogenesis. I took the mid-sagittal slice from the MRI scans from a sample of patients, and then using the software that we had developed, I computed the average 3D midfacial slice from that group of patients, pre-treatment and post-treatment. Then using Procrustes superimposition (Singh *et al.*, 1997), which is a mathematical method that we had utilized previously, I superimposed those two slices, and then applied an engineering technique (pseudo-colored finite element analysis; Singh *et al.*, 2004) to localize and quantify any changes that might have occurred post-treatment.

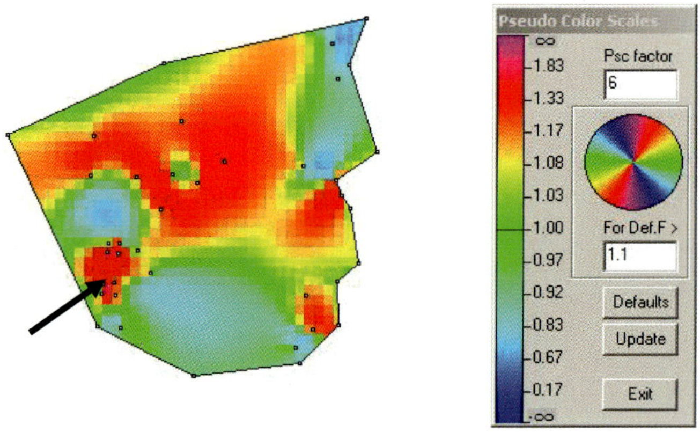

Figure 3: Note the increase in upper airway size (black arrow).

As expected, we found an improved facial profile; there was an increase in midfacial size, and the mandible had moved into a better position (Fig. 3). Specifically, in the midfacial region there was an increase in midfacial bone volume. We expected that finding because we disarticulated the maxilla and allowed the bone to heal, but then the most interesting finding for me was that behind the jaws I found another red region, indicating an increase in volume. That red region was superimposed on the upper airway (Fig. 3 arrow). I realized that when the jaws are surgically manipulated to make the maxilla larger and move it forward, the upper airway expands to fill the new space, similar to pneumatization of the paranasal air sinuses during normal growth and development. That was the first time I had the idea in terms of what we now call Pneumopedics. The question then arose, how can we provide this procedure on a non-surgical basis to verify the epigenetic premise of the correction? In addition, another question was: Would we be able to provide this hypothetical, non-surgical procedure to adult patients as well as in children?

The most significant aspect of the preliminary study on teenagers was that they all had some genetic mutation affecting midfacial growth and development, including craniosynostoses, such as Apert syndrome. Although these craniofacial anomalies are rare, and most people have normally functioning genes in the midfacial region, a very large portion of the population exhibits midfacial hypoplasia, which is often symptomatically addressed by the extraction of healthy wisdom teeth and/or premolar teeth in an orthodontic attempt to relieve dental crowding. However, the mechanism of midfacial development may be largely dependent on sutural homeostasis, including the eruption of teeth. It was once believed that the craniofacial sutures synostose (fuse) during early adulthood, but some studies using more modern techniques have cast doubt on this assertion (Kokich, 1986; Williams *et al.*, 2011). It is understood that the craniofacial sutures provide a method of midfacial morphogenesis compliant with functional forces. In other words, during functional activities, such as breast-feeding, mastication, swallowing, speaking, etc., the sutures are gently stretched, sometimes beyond 400μm, which is thought to represent a biologic boundary of mammalian sutural homeostasis (Kambara, 1977). In response, stretch-sensitive genes are activated in the stem cells residing in and around the craniofacial sutures (even in adults; Kaltschmidt *et al.*, 2012), causing these cells to differentiate into osteoblasts (Zhao *et al.*, 2015). These osteoblasts, in turn, lay down new (woven) bone, increasing the midfacial bone volume, which is interpreted as facial growth. Remodeling then ensues in accord with temporo-spatial patterning so that the appropriate bone shape is produced following the genetic blueprint of the individual, at least empirically. But, midfacial growth and development is accompanied by a special feature not seen elsewhere in the body. As the maxilla grows, the teeth erupt and vacate the body of the bone. Instead of bony in-filling, epithelial-lined cavities or maxillary sinuses are formed, a developmental process called pneumatization. The ostia of these sinuses recapitulate their phylogeny and during ontogeny they grow away from their points of origin and sites of drainage. Therefore, the maxillary air sinus may not drain well, or its ostium may become obstructed in various conditions, such as rhinosinusitis (Hwang *et al.*, 2019). In contrast, mammalian teeth have a unique developmental ability, i.e. eruption throughout the life of an individual, sometimes called continuous eruption in rodents or passive eruption in humans. Interestingly, an historical misnomer has been beguiling the dental profession for centuries. Once the term 'periodontal ligament' entered professional parlance, it wreaked havoc on our understanding of the developmental dynamics of tooth eruption. **Put simply, the 'periodontal ligament' does not have the development, structure, or function of a ligament**. Studies have shown that ligaments have a bimodal fiber diameter distribution, indicating old (large) and new (small) fibers within an extracellular matrix. On the other hand, the fibers within the periodontium show a normal distribution and have a small fiber diameter (approx. 40µm), indicating constant turnover so that fibers do not have time to mature into large diameter fibers. Moreover, the periodontium is surrounded by intramembranous bone, and one definition of a suture is a joint between two bones formed by intramembranous ossification. Thus, the periodontium appears to represent a modified suture and within that sutural boundary (100-400µm) resides a population(s) of periodontal stem cells (Rai *et al.*, 2013). The mean width of the periodontal space is approx. 250µm (0.25mm), which is the width typically found on a small, periapical radiograph. If this sutural width is decreased, bone resorption ensues to maintain the functional space, but if the space is increased by the suture being stretched, bone deposition is activated to maintain homeostasis. This homeostatic mechanism would also explain the phenomenon of orthodontic relapse. So how does this information relate to the teenagers' change in behavior mentioned above? Put simply, an oral device capable of stretching the craniofacial sutures ought to be able to initiate bone formation *de novo*. This new bone would increase the midfacial bone volume in normal patients who don't have any genetic mutations associated with craniosynostoses. Concurrently, there would be an increase in nasal airway volume, since the roof of the mouth is the floor of the nose. This epigenetic change would allow the maxillary teeth to be repositioned and, consequently, following the cranio-caudal gradient, the mandible would follow the maxilla and most likely move antero-inferiorly, thus alleviating any upper airway obstruction. Simultaneously, the upper airway would show changes in size and shape, following the process of pneumatization alluded to above. With consequent airway remodeling, the pneumopedic process would be completed with subsequent elimination of the signs and symptoms of obstructive sleep apnea and other conditions of sleep disordered breathing. Our preliminary studies appear to support this epigenetic mechanism, as predicted by the spatial matrix hypothesis.

In fact, Figure 4 illustrates some of the principles noted above in one of the very first patients that was treated using a biomimetic appliance. This patient was a teenager with no known genetic anomalies. The chief concern was that she had a deep overbite (Fig. 4a). After wearing the biomimetic appliance for several weeks, an improvement in the degree of vertical overlap was noted (Fig. 4b), and the extent of mouth opening also improved (Fig. 4c and Fig. 4d), which indicated that the position of the intra articular disk of the TMJ was probably repositioned during this procedure, allowing increased and improved mouth opening. Presumably, the shape-change of the upper arch permitted a subsequent spatial change of the lower arch, but the teeth still remained fairly well aligned. The study models of the upper arch (Fig. 4e and Fig. 4f) suggested that the upper arch was remodeled, and we suspect that the bone underwent remodeling, which permitted the mandible to move downward and forward. This translation, in turn, improved the facial profile (Fig. 4g and Fig. 4h), and we suspect that since the mandible moved forward the upper airway may have been improved. This case study was one of our first experiences of using a DNA appliance in a teenager (Singh and Lipka, 2009).

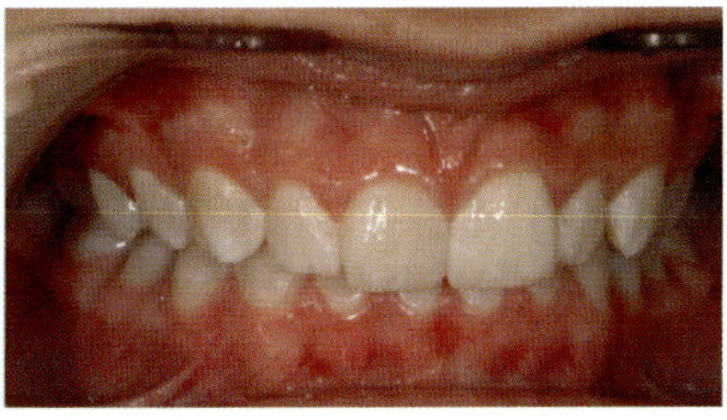

Figure 4a: Pre-treatment occlusion with deep bite.

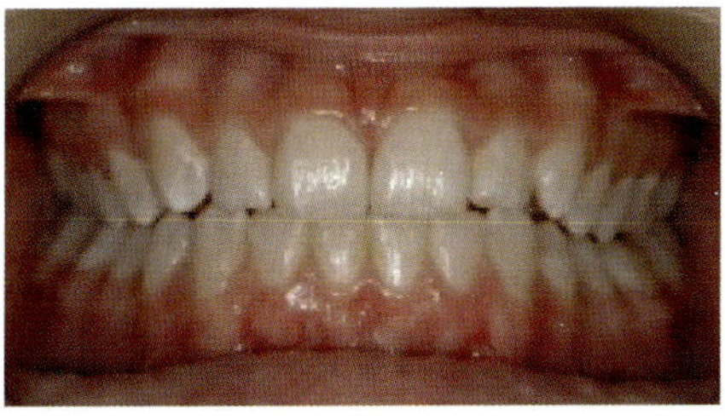

Figure 4b: Mid-treatment occlusion with improved overbite.

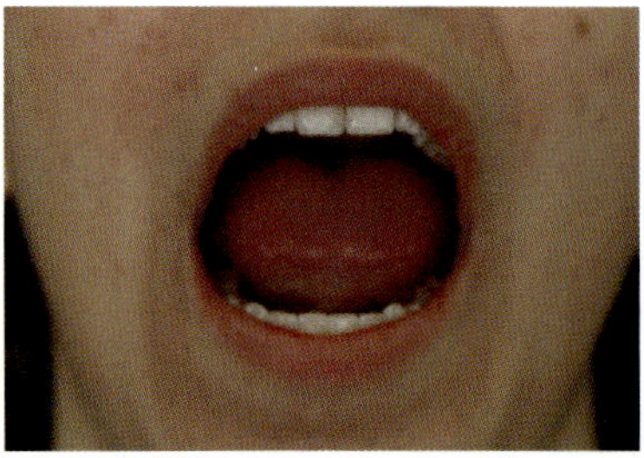

Figure 4c: Pre-treatment maximum mouth opening.

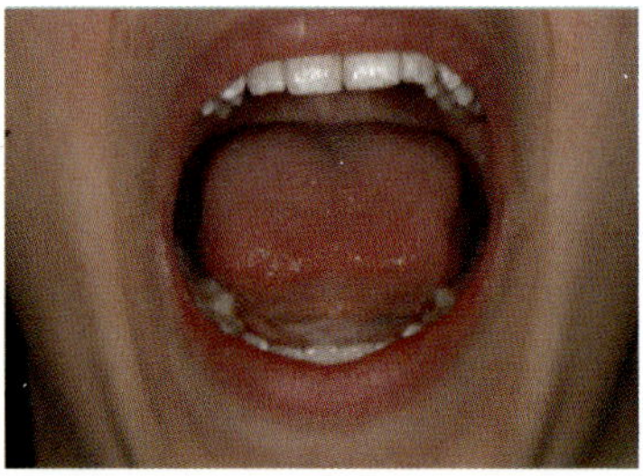

Figure 4d: Mid-treatment maximum mouth opening.

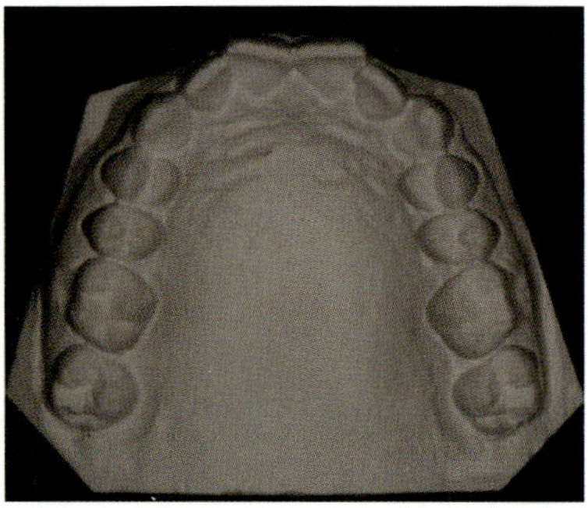

Figure 4e: Pre-treatment upper study model.

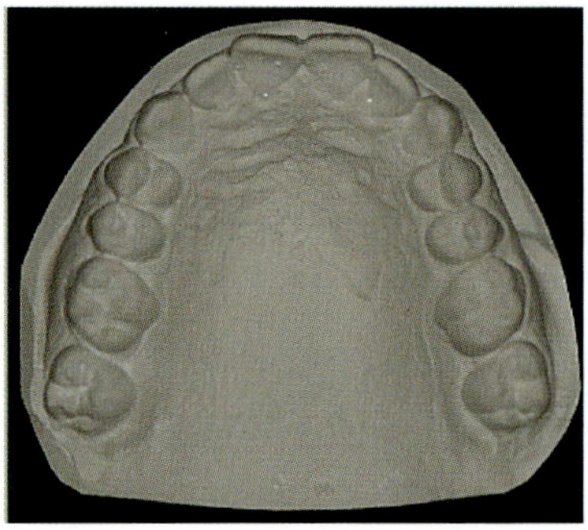

Figure 4f: Mid-treatment upper study model.

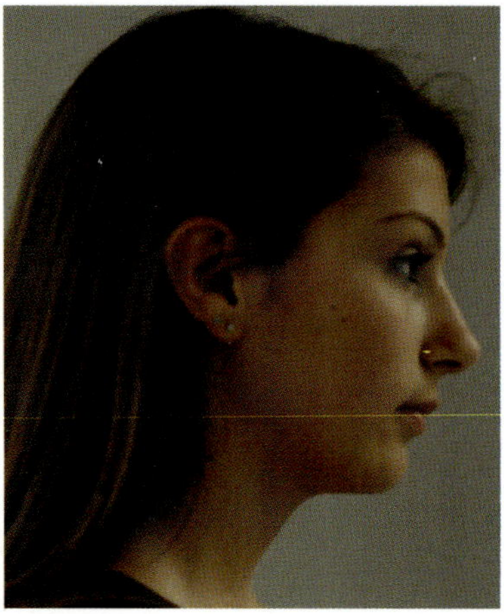

Figure 4g: Pre-treatment lateral facial profile.

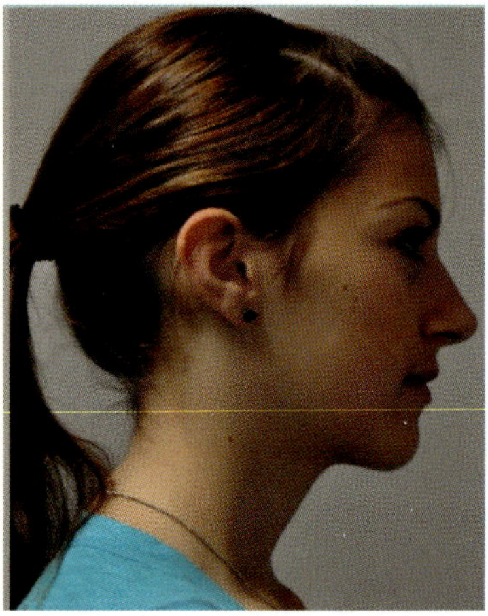

Figure 4h: Post-treatment lateral facial profile.

However, even though individual cases are illustrative, there needs to be a scientific basis to help us explain how these changes might occur on a molecular, cellular, or tissue level, and we need to be able to test and make predictions about the proposed mechanism(s). Taking these ideas together, I developed the spatial matrix hypothesis, first published at the University of Michigan, Craniofacial Growth Series (Singh, 2004), and then in an abbreviated form in the *British Dental Journal* (Singh, 2007). It was also re-published in the first version of this book (Singh and Krumholtz, 2009). The central idea is to contemplate how craniofacial components can grow and develop, in an attempt to achieve a resolving synthesis between the Darwinian genomic thesis and the epigenetic antithesis. According to Moss' old functional matrix hypothesis, during growth the spatial and functional relationships of the craniofacial elements are maintained through remodeling at the bony surfaces. In other words, when the maxilla and mandible are growing, their relationship is being modified through the remodeling process, and that growth depends on the spatial relations of the maxilla and the mandible. Thus, the positions of the jaws and their functional alignment during swallowing, speaking, mastication, breathing, sleeping, etc. is being monitored through proprioceptive capabilities. In fact, during tooth eruption, the bony surfaces of the maxilla and mandible are also modified to produce the periodontium (periodontal 'ligament') to house and attach the teeth. But this bony remodeling is also required to permit functions such as swallowing, speech, mastication, etc. while the teeth are erupting as a child grows. Simultaneously, therefore, the jaws undergo environmentally induced epigenetic changes. These environmental influences include things like bottle feeding, pacifier use, digit-sucking, etc. In other words, even though the jaws follow a genetic blueprint in terms of the growth and development, genes are being expressed slightly differently, producing an increased overjet, for instance, in response to the newly introduced environmental factor; for example, thumb-sucking at a particular age. This activity produces a change in the early morphologic relationship with the jaws developing into a Class II malocclusion, by increasing the overjet. This malocclusion now represents a 'new solution' or phenotypic variation that differs from the temporo-spatial body plan encoded by genes. This new solution also represents a departure from the genetically encoded developmental body plan, which includes 32 teeth symmetrically arranged in a Class I occlusion for all modern humans. Certain patterns of gene expression would allow that condition to be achieved in the absence of detrimental influences from the environment. But, in this example of a Class II case, the environment has induced phenotypic changes through a process called developmental compensation. Developmental compensation occurs to permit compromised function. In other words, characteristic functions of the mandible and maxilla can be achieved but not to the optimal extent. For example, the mouth can be opened but not to the full range; biting is possible but the teeth are crowded; mastication is achievable but pain and a diagnosis of temporo-mandibular joint dysfunction is present; daytime mouth-breathing is accompanied by snoring or obstructive sleep apnea at nighttime, etc. All of these clinical features represent developmental compensation. The body had to compensate for the fact that these structures were in a slightly different position compared to what was expected based on temporo-spatial patterning or the ideal body plan. Conversely, in conditions such as cleft lip and palate, structural asymmetry is often evident. A correction of the functional spaces enclosed by these dysmorphic structures is required, preferably non-surgically, to then allow the structures to grow or remodel into those new spatial matrices. This corrective procedure can be summarized as (clinical) decompensation. Decompensation is required through treatment with appropriate spatial signaling to re-establish the genomic foundation for optimal form and function. For example, if the mandible is retrognathic, it needs to be re-positioned anteriorly into a new spatial relationship with a maxilla that will allow that correction. It is now thought that changing the spatial relations of the mandible permits genes to be re-expressed, which in turn try to replicate the pattern formation for the best form and function. A study by Fuentes *et al.* (2003) provides further details of this working hypothesis in terms of molecular genetics, explaining how we might achieve clinical correction in these types of cases.

Historically, skeletal decompensation has been largely achieved surgically. For example, in a severe case of Class III malocclusion or severe anterior open bite, orthognathic surgery is often suggested. However, prior to the skeletal components being corrected by the surgeon, orthodontic decompensation is often first performed by the orthodontist. For example, Katiyar *et al.* (2010) reported orthognathic treatment of an adult patient with skeletal Class III malocclusion. The malocclusion was first decompensated using orthodontics and the jaw relationship was then normalized surgically using a bilateral sagittal split osteotomy. However, Kim *et al.* (2017) consider that facial asymmetries often involve 3D dentoalveolar compensations that relate to skeletal discrepancies. Thus, it is not always possible to achieve the pre-surgical orthodontic goals, but dentoalveolar decompensations are needed to help correct the underlying skeletal discrepancy. Therefore, we need to understand what we're trying to achieve through conventional fixed orthodontics, which is based on the idea of 'straightening the teeth' and having nice looking smile esthetics. Traditional orthodontic brackets and wires can induce pain and inflammation during the treatment process (Roberts and Hartfield, 2004). Actually, the clinical practice of orthodontics is based on one word — the condition called malocclusion, which we now believe is an example of craniofacial developmental compensation. A malocclusion is a diagnosis. If a patient visits a dental office, is examined by a dentist or an orthodontist and the teeth are found to be not well-aligned, then they are maloccluded, and there may be a specific class of malocclusion. To understand this concept better we need to re-examine the definition of malocclusion.

Reviewing various orthodontic textbooks, we realize that there is no real consensus on the definition of malocclusion. Each textbook appears to have its own definition and some of these are more complete and some less so. It is important to formulate a definition that is encompassing, in a broader aspect. In the *British Dental Journal* (Singh, 2007), I defined **malocclusion as a solution for a complex, adaptive system to remain in**

equilibrium or homeostasis. In this regard, the craniofacial region exhibits complexity. There are at least two types of complexity; first, there is structural complexity and second, there is also mathematical complexity. Structural complexity in the craniofacial context includes dental tissues (teeth); hard tissues (e.g. the jaw bones, etc.); soft tissues, such as the tongue, the lips, etc.; and, in addition, there are functional spaces such as the upper airway, the TMJ joint spaces, the periodontal 'ligament' spaces, etc. So craniofacial structures have a fair degree of complexity. On the other hand, statistical or mathematical complexity can be illustrated by using dice. If dice are thrown, a combination is achieved, say, 7. But if the same dice are thrown again, the chances are a different combination might be obtained, say 11; thus, despite a finite number of outcomes, it's impossible to predict which combination (number) will be obtained. Thinking about the human genome, there are numerous potentially different outcomes from combinations of the same sets of genes. Put simply, a patient may inherit genes from one parent predisposing to a large jaw (Class III tendency) and perhaps genes predisposing to small teeth (hypodontia) from the other parent. Although the phenotypic outcome may be difficult to predict, clinically, spacing or crowding irregularities of the teeth may be precipitated based on the idea of complexity. In view of that perspective, a clinician has to understand what approach might best allow correction of that condition. The second part of the new definition of malocclusion suggests that this system is not static, it is adaptive and undergoing constant remodeling. Because of this adaptive capability, bone can be remodeled, and subsequently the teeth can be repositioned in a new 3D spatial matrix. Ideally, the dental arches would become more symmetric and an enhanced level of equilibrium or homeostasis might be attained. In that respect, the craniofacial system is no different from other systems in the body, for example blood pressure, body temperature, etc., in that it is also subject to homeostasis.

On the other side of the coin, however, we need a definition for occlusion. Consulting various orthodontic textbooks on the topic, we find a large number of descriptions for the word occlusion but there appears to be no consensus for a definition at this point. Here, I define **occlusion (or the 'bite') as being the end point of the body with respect to the plantar surfaces of the feet, and within these two boundaries all functional spaces for physiologic processes must be accommodated**. Therefore, the occlusion can be regarded as the relationship of surface enamel, which can come into precise contact. Note that since the enamel is derived from surface ectoderm, in terms of developmental biology it is technically on the outside of the body. During embryologic development, each human being starts life as a flat embryonic disk. This disk undergoes curvature (reversal), so that the rostral-most ectoderm forms the bucco-pharyngeal membrane that undergoes apoptosis to form the primitive oral cavity (stomatodeum). From this ectodermal lining, epithelia differentiate into the oral mucosa of the hard palate and the enamel of the teeth, *inter alia*. Enamel, thus, represents one end point of the body. The other end point of the body is the plantar surfaces of the feet, where the feet actually touch the ground. Between those two boundaries, there needs to be sufficient (functional) space for all physiologic processes. For example, specific functional spaces are needed for nerve transmission. These take the form of synapses, whereby the endplates are separated by 9nm of space, which permits neurotransmitters to traverse the gap to the post-synaptic membrane. Without this minute space, which is genetically encoded, nerve transmission would be impossible. Functional space is also needed for blood flow. For example, if the blood supply needs to be improved to an organ or system, an increase in blood pressure is required. Through an elaborate system of vasoconstriction and vasodilatation, blood pressure can be precisely regulated by changing the caliber of the lumen (functional space) of certain blood vessels. Thus, the entire functional space of an organism is captured by two finite boundaries. Now, we can't change the fact that both feet touch the ground since that boundary is set by gravity. We can, however, change the occlusion. A small change even to a slight extent may be able to provide the body with an increased or decreased amount of functional space, and that change could have repercussions throughout the entire systemic structure of the human body. These were the observations of Fonder (1984) and many subsequent scientists that experimented on small mammals (D'Attilio *et al.*, 2005). It was found that placing a small, unilateral bite block in the animal's mouth causing occlusal interference, led to disastrous results further distally in the animal's spinal alignment. There is one case study where a patient who had 'occlusal equilibration' by dentist became almost completely handicapped (Kent, 2006). While these extreme outcomes are thankfully very rare, the significance of the occlusion to systemic health should not be overlooked since idiopathic scoliosis is thought to be associated with occlusal disharmony (Ben-Bassat *et al.*, 2006), which can be induced by a device with a unilateral bite block.

Deficient craniofacial (functional) space will not permit the accommodation of all the teeth, which leads us to revisit the idea of epigenetic orthodontics. It is broadly agreed that 'form follows function'. For example, a cheetah is streamlined to run at fast speeds. Taking the same equation and turning it the other way around, if form follows function then **deformity follows dysfunction**. Dysfunction in this context is detected through abnormal behavior; for example, abnormal (mouth) breathing, abnormal (reverse) swallowing, abnormal sleep (apnea), etc. Conversely, clinically, it is easier to identify the deformity (for example, the teeth are crowded) but it's less easy to identify a dysfunction that precipitated the deformity; for example, unusual, changed, or different behavior while breathing, swallowing, eating, etc. Note that these behavioral changes are components of the environmental factors that precipitate a deformity, in that together they may lead to the formation of a malocclusion. In terms of treatment, should we simply correct the deformity or should we also address the dysfunction? Ideally, of course we should do both, but classically when a patient goes to a dental or orthodontic office, we are primarily concerned with straightening the teeth and reducing the degree of deformity. If we're going to simply 'straighten the teeth', then we need to know with respect to what axis? The answer, of course, is with respect to the antero-posterior, medio-lateral, and supero-inferior body axes, which are genetically determined during axis formation and patterning during the earliest weeks of embryonic life. If we try to straighten the teeth in isolation, we can decrease the degree of deformity but that might not result in a stable outcome in the long term because the teeth might not be well aligned with respect to the rest of the body. Hence the need for orthodontic retainers for life. In fact, the post-cranial parts of the body may not be well-aligned either. Therefore, we need the musculo-skeletal system to be well aligned, and that brings the dental profession into collaboration with different professionals, such as chiropractors, osteopaths, etc. Furthermore, if a child goes to a dental/orthodontic office, we have some further choices: we can do the treatment correction during active growth; or we can do the treatment after growth has been 'completed'. Classically, a young child will go to the orthodontic office and the treatment will be done during the growth phase to correct the cause of the deformity. Sometimes, however, the orthodontist or dentist might say let's wait until the growth has been completed, and then correct the effects of the deformity once the child 'stops growing'. In fact, if we look more carefully, we find that humans never stop growing, even as adults. When an embryo becomes a fetus, and the fetus becomes a baby, and the baby comes a child, the rate of growth decreases, and it continues to decrease throughout life. Note that the rate of decrease itself decreases during puberty, which looks like a growth spurt. But the bottom line is that humans never stop growing, even as adults — we just grow older. In fact, the ageing process varies throughout various systems of the body. During the ageing process, there is vertical drift of the midface and the jaw bones can get smaller via mechanisms similar to systemic osteoporosis. It is also thought that the ageing process is related to telomeres, which are found at the ends of chromosomes. Telomere length itself is vulnerable to inflammation, which is thought to be a consequence of insufficient or poor-quality sleep (Cribbet *et al.*, 2014). In any case, if we accept the epigenetic antithesis, then throughout the life of the individual the genetic potential can be harnessed for clinical corrections. In this context, **I define genetic potential as the capacity to achieve an optimal outcome in the prevailing conditions subject to a viable population(s) of**

stem cells. The optimal outcome is what we are trying to achieve in each particular case, and that is the aim of biomimetic corrections.

Compensation

We discussed decompensation above, but in order to understand how a patient might present clinically, we need to consider also the concepts of homeostasis and compensation. In Figure 5 both images of the body are in a state of homeostasis or (structural) balance, but the one on the right (Fig. 5b) is 'working harder' to maintain homeostasis. This extra work is referred to as compensation. The body on the left side (Fig. 5a) is symmetric and well-aligned in the midline and, therefore, a huge amount of energy is not being used to maintain that position of harmony, balance, and equilibrium. In contrast, the body on the right side (Fig. 5b) is highly asymmetric and, consequently, a lot more energy is being expended to actually hold that position without falling over. This an example of structural or postural compensation, but the human body undergoes different types of compensation. The prior example illustrates postural compensation, but another example is developmental compensation. During development, structures may drift away from the midline and become asymmetric; for example, the spine, jaws, and teeth. This positional or spatial change is less

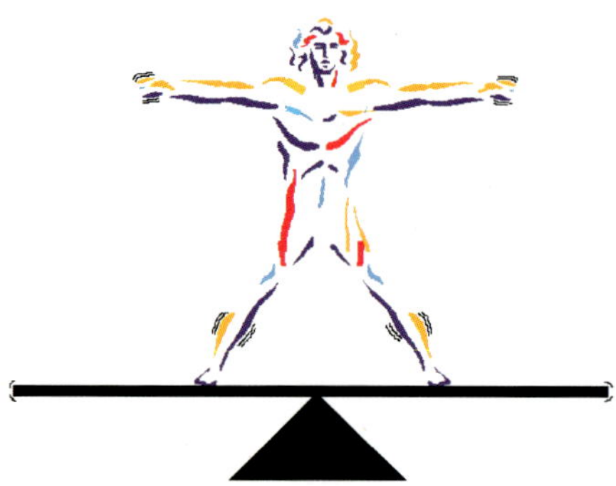

Figure 5a: Postural balance/homeostasis without compensation.
Courtesy: Dr Chris Chapman

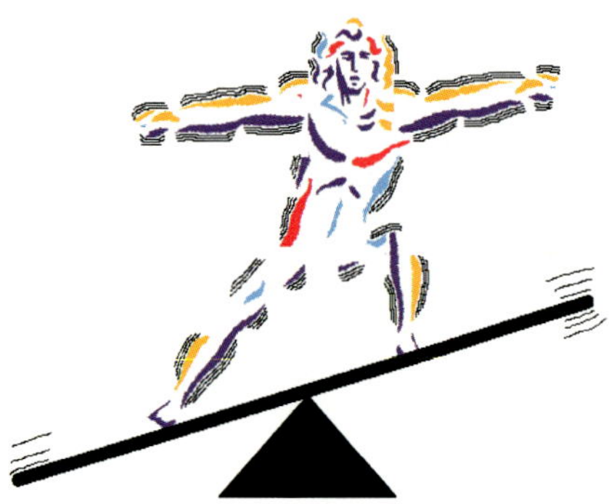

Figure 5b: Postural balance/homeostasis with compensation.

efficient; it requires more energy to remain in homeostasis or metabolic balance. Thus, the human body can undergo developmental compensation, producing a less efficient outcome, which requires more energy to sustain it and remain in homeostasis or balance. Since the body has a cranio-caudal gradient of development, a patient may therefore present at a dental office in a combined state of descending developmental compensation and/or ascending postural compensation. These two gradients most likely meet where the head joins the post-cranial skeleton, at the atlas vertebra (C1), which is the first bone below the mandible.

Now, let's extend this metaphor to the occlusion. Earlier, it was noted that the occlusion represents one of the endpoints of the body with respect to the plantar surfaces of the feet. In this example (Fig. 5), the body is balanced by standing over a pivot point. As a physical metaphor, the pivot point represents the occlusion. If the pivot or point of balance is changed slightly there will be a large change in the overall body posture to remain balanced on the beam. Extending the idea of the pivot, if a small change is made in the occlusion and the way in which the teeth meet, we could expect systemic changes throughout the rest of the body. As mentioned previously, in one case, minor occlusal equilibration led to catastrophic systemic consequences (Kent, 2006). In fact, in my definition, a malocclusion is a solution for a complex, adaptive system to remain in equilibrium or homeostasis. As indicated earlier, developmental compensation proceeds in a cranio-caudal gradient, while postural compensation proceeds in the opposite direction from the ground up, with the two gradients likely intersecting at the level of C1. In either case, decompensation is required. Going from general to specific, it seems rational to first align/decompensate the body (perhaps through chiropractic or some other physical therapy), next align/decompensate the jaws (through epigenetic orthopedics), and finally align/decompensate the teeth (through epigenetic orthodontics). Following this sequence may help to maintain the patency of the upper airway. Note that decompensation is widely practiced in cases of orthognathic surgery. In these severe cases, conventional orthodontic brackets and wires are first used to decompensate the teeth. Next, the surgical intervention uses the occlusion to help the surgeon place the jaws in the best perceived position, often for esthetic purposes. While this procedure usually produces good cosmetic outcomes, there is a risk that the upper airway can be compromised (Chang *et al.*, 2017; He *et al.*, 2019). Alternatively, it seems reasonable to first undertake non-surgical (epigenetic) orthopedics, and then realign the teeth using an (epigenetic) orthodontic approach, in an effort to maintain the integrity of the upper airway.

The antithesis of homeostasis is another concept to think about; the idea of relapse or lack of stability. Relapse is one of the chief concerns of both patients and their caregivers in terms of orthodontic treatment. If we have a clear understanding of what relapse is then we may know how to prevent it from occurring. Relapse occurs if there is a violation of homeostasis. In other words, following clinical orthodontic correction, the teeth appear to be regularly aligned but they may not necessarily be in a state of homeostasis with respect to the rest of the body. In these cases, the craniofacial system regresses to a level of homeostasis that can be more readily maintained (malocclusion), which appears as relapse clinically. As an analogy, let's consider someone holding a 10kg weight vertically with one arm over their head. This posture can be maintained for a short while, but then fatigue ensues, and the weight can no longer be maintained in that position. As a result, the whole system eventually regresses to a level of homeostasis. This analogy appears as relapse to the orthodontic observer, which is why fixed or removable retainers are prescribed for life in most cases. Consider further if the weight was maintained in that vertical position for several minutes each day for several years. In this case, remodeling of the arm bones, including increased bone density and/or mass would likely occur, as well as increased muscle mass and tone. These musculo-skeletal changes represent an epigenetic response, and the same principle could be applied to structures of the craniofacial region.

Returning now to the orthodontic example, when the teeth were first moved, brackets and wires were utilized to apply forces to move them into a corrected position. At de-bonding, the brackets and wires are removed and some of those teeth later drift back into less favorable positions. Now the interesting thing is that when the teeth were first moved into alignment, orthodontic brackets and wires were utilized, but where were forces applied to move these teeth into a relapsed position? Moreover, can't those 'invisible' forces be used to move the teeth into the corrected position without brackets and wires? This notion is currently partially encapsulated by the practice of oral myofunctional therapy. It's important to explain that type of tooth movement compared to the orthodontic tooth movement achieved with braces. Consider the idea that developmental mechanisms that permit relapse in the absence of homeostasis also permit orthodontic corrections. In other words, the periodontium has the capability of constant turnover, which enables the teeth to remain in occlusion through 'passive eruption' when the enamel is worn down through long-term use. In addition, because of craniofacial developmental compensation, the teeth develop and erupt in an irregular position or malocclusion. However, temporo-spatial patterning suggests we can use inherited developmental mechanisms to correct them into a new position of increased homeostasis. And these are the same developmental mechanisms that will permit relapse in the absence of homeostasis. In other words, in some cases after orthodontic alignment, the teeth are in a position that is untenable and can't be maintained; thus, developmental mechanisms move the teeth back into their original positions during relapse in order to produce a more stable outcome or homeostasis. Therefore, the same developmental mechanisms in reverse could be used to correct and improve the position of the teeth because the genetic potential of the system resides there throughout life. As mentioned previously, genetic potential is achieving the optimal outcome in the prevailing conditions, subject to a viable population of stem cells. It is now thought that the periodontium is populated with mesenchymal stem cells that can undergo differentiation into osteoblasts that can regenerate new bone (Rai *et al.*, 2013), which can then be remodeled through appropriate signaling.

In addition, certain patients have an increased predisposition or requirement for orthodontic treatment. The form of the jaws and the teeth are largely inherited through genes. If the father or the mother had a large mandible, it's possible that the children will inherit a similar type of jaw morphology because they inherited the genes for that condition from the parents. But in addition, we know that the genes are affected epigenetically by environmental factors such as function, diet, etc. As a second analogy, consider someone who has decreased muscle tissue or muscle tone. If that person starts a gym program and they start working out or start weightlifting, over a period of time they're going to change the form of their muscles. They're going to increase muscle volume (through hypertrophy) and muscle tone (Chambers *et al.*, 2020) and they're going to increase bone mass (Woo *et al.*, 1981) as well as bone density (Ayalon *et al.*, 1987). These tissue changes are achieved through environmental factors that interact with genes that are responsible for regenerating muscle and bone tissue. The same idea applies, to a greater or lesser extent, to the craniofacial region on an epigenetic basis; it's a gene-environmental interaction to a large extent. Clinically, even though a jaw may appear to have a small phenotype, we can modify that outcome by providing appropriate spatial and functional signals, which will allow the jaw to redevelop and achieve a new level of enhanced homeostasis, although the tongue and other muscles will need to be re-trained to maintain that new spatial matrix. Thus, the main aim is to enhance craniofacial homeostasis by harnessing developmental mechanisms, which are encoded by genes. In other words, the jaws can undergo remodeling throughout life, which is most often seen as part of the ageing process. Classically, the upper jaw undergoes 'vertical drift' with age. This remodeling throughout life changes the spatial matrix and encroaches on the functional space of the mandible. Subsequently, the lower incisor teeth appear to become more crowded as the remodeling process goes on throughout the life of the individual. In fact, lower incisor crowding is a feature often seen in relapsed orthodontic cases. To prevent this type of relapse, many orthodontists utilize fixed, bonded retainers on the lingual aspect of the lower anterior teeth or removable retainers. An alternative approach would be to prevent or decrease the degree of vertical drift of the maxilla. In order to achieve this, a retainer is required for the upper arch, and that is provided by nature at the outset: **the tongue**. Through oral myofunctional therapy, the tongue can be trained to sit in the palate, instead of in the floor of the mouth. At rest, homeostasis is achieved with the tongue sitting in the roof of the mouth with the lips gently together, while breathing through the nose with the teeth lightly in occlusion. This optimal form and function may require foundational correction. For example, if the tongue is restricted, it may not be able to contact the palate, and if the palate is too narrow, it may not be able to accommodate the tongue. Therefore, an epigenetic approach may need to be adopted for craniofacial correction.

Sutural homeostasis

The main aim of pneumopedics and craniofacial epigenetics is to enhance craniofacial homeostasis, and in order to achieve this there is a need to harness developmental mechanisms. Those developmental mechanisms are encoded by the genes of the human genome. These are the genes that we inherit, that we are born with, and keep for life. Specifically, two examples of developmental mechanisms encoded by these genes are: sutural homeostasis and pneumatization. The first mechanism suggests that sutures in the craniofacial region are subject to some form of control or monitoring, known as sutural homeostasis (Borke *et al.*, 2003). As with any other biologic system, the craniofacial suture system requires a state of balance or equilibrium. As mentioned previously, if any system is not in a condition of balance, it is less energy efficient and prone to relapse. But the bigger question arises: Why do humans even possess craniofacial sutures? Sutures are not found elsewhere in the body. Thus, their presence in the craniofacial regions suggests some additional, local requirements or functionality. The craniofacial region of *Homo sapiens* is characterized by a large and fragile brain. In terms of phylogeny, the human brain evolved rapidly over a relatively exceedingly small evolutionary time scale. Human accelerated regions (HARs) are five segments of the human genome that show homology, i.e. are conserved throughout evolution; but they show an unexpected degree of variation and are markedly different in *Homo sapiens* (Pollard *et al.*, 2006). For example, HAR1 shows the largest degree of difference when human and chimpanzee genomes are compared. Importantly, HARs comprise genes known to produce proteins important in neural development. For example, HAR1F is thought to be active in human brain development since it is expressed specifically in neurons of the developing human neocortex (Pollard *et al.*, 2006). Although the concept of 'ontogeny recapitulates phylogeny' has not passed the test of time, it can be postulated that a relatively rapid developmental mechanism is required to protect the rapidly expanding neonatal brain. Initially, endochondral ossification was the original developmental mechanism for bone formation. In this process, bone is developed from precursor cartilage templates. These templates are referred to as 'primary cartilages' since they have a long evolutionary history. There are numerous named primary cartilages, which constitute the cranial base, the axial skeleton, and the long bones, etc. While endochondral ossification requires the conversion of a cartilage precursor into bone, intramembranous ossification bypasses this requirement with the formation of bone from stem cells within the membranes directly. These intramembranous bones are predominantly found in the craniofacial region, including the frontal bone, the parietals, the maxilla, etc. and are separated from each other by sutures.

Consider now two plates of bone covering the brain and developed by intramembranous ossification. As the brain expands, the two plates of bone are pushed apart. This tension is detected by stretch-sensitive genes, which permit the differentiation of sutural stem cells into osteoblasts that, in turn, lay down osteoid, which is mineralized into new bone (Zhao *et al.*, 2015). But there has to be some control mechanism that determines the amount of new, intramembranous bone to be deposited. In this case, temporo-spatial patterning is deployed. The definition of a suture is joint formed between two bones that undergo intramembranous ossification. Here the concept of sutural homeostasis is invoked. It is thought that the typical sutural width varies between 100μm and 400μm with an average width of about 250μm (or 0.25mm). In other words, when the separation of the two bony plates by brain expansion exceeds say, 400μm, bony deposition ensues at the sutural edges. Conversely, when the separation of the two bony plates is less than say, 100μm, bone resorption ensues to maintain sutural homeostasis. Thus, the function of the sutures is simply to lay down new bone in response to spatial changes, and although cranial sutures may be stretched by expansion of brain tissue, the circum-maxillary sutures may be stretched by tongue function or the eruption of the teeth. Note that the average width of the periodontal 'ligament' is approx. 0.25mm (or 250μm), suggesting that it may, in fact, represent a stem cell containing (modified) periodontal suture (Rai *et al.*, 2013). Nevertheless, the overall premise is to use the craniofacial sutures to enhance bone formation, which can be remodeled to attain a better state of balance or homeostasis during growth and development, including ageing.

Pneumatization

The second craniofacial, developmental mechanism to consider is pneumatization, which actually occurs concurrently whilst the sutures are laying down new (woven) bone. Note that the craniofacial region is unique because the cranial and midfacial regions are characterized by sinuses, epithelial-lined cavities within specific intramembranous bones filled with air. These sinuses are formed by pneumatization, so when the new bone is remodeled, the sutures will remain in a state of balance or sutural homeostasis. The concept is to use these sutures to enhance cranial and midfacial bone formation, so that pneumatization will follow. Thus, as the bones in the skull get larger, they won't get heavier because bone volume is being replaced by air. In that respect, the paranasal sinuses might represent the proximal-most part of the upper airway. Therefore, it can be surmised that redeveloping the midfacial structures indirectly targets the upper airway. There are, however, other thoughts to explain the existence of paranasal sinuses in the human skull. These ideas include resonance for vocalization and a 'crumple zone' at the front of the skull to protect the fragile brain, sitting on the cranial base behind the (prognathic) human jaws, against trauma. In any case, in the event that the skull bones were not pneumatized, it's estimated that the typical weight of the human skull (12lbs; 5.4kg) could increase to 32-42lbs (14.5-19kg). This increased loading of the anterior segments of the spine and intervertebral disks could compress the thoracic cavity and cause the spine to deviate from the optimal sagittal posture and undergo pathological remodeling. Indeed, this type of postural compensation often occurs in patients who adopt a forward head posture to maintain an open upper airway. As noted previously, compensated states in the body are less energy efficient than decompensated states, and sophisticated mechanisms are activated, conserving energy, leading to more permanent adaptations, which are observed as postural compensation as well as endogenous adaptation. In this case, these mechanisms provoke remodeling in the axial and appendicular skeleton according to the neural escalator model (Burwell *et al.*, 2008), which is essentially an epigenetic response. Thus, the aim of redevelopment of the midfacial structures is, in fact, to indirectly target the upper airway and avoid detrimental sequelae of both developmental and structural compensation.

The above sequence of events leads to the next idea, which is biomimetic correction. Biomimetics is a science that uses natural models to address clinical problems. In our application, we're trying to copy the way the jaws grow and develop so the 32 teeth have more space to be better aligned. In addition, the tongue would have more functional space, enhancing the level of craniofacial homeostasis by optimizing the upper airway. In other words, we're trying to copy the way the body naturally grows and develops, without trying to expand transversely at the expense of other structures in the midfacial region. Thus, we are aiming for a biomimetic correction with the hard tissues, soft tissues, dental tissues, and functional spaces of the craniofacial region in a state of dynamic balance. Moreover, in addition to the structural changes, there may also be a functional or physiologic correction. For example: changing a mouth breather to a nasal breather during the day, breathing better during sleep, improved swallowing patterns, and sufficient speaking space, etc. Despite these claims, functional correction may or may not occur clinically. While some patients respond quickly and respond well to appliance therapy, there are others that react more slowly, and it takes them longer to achieve clinical results. This spectrum of response is best explained by the term complexity. Complexity is a component of the chaos theory, which suggests that while there are a finite number of outcomes, it's difficult to predict what the actual outcome will be. As an analogy, consider 10 children chosen at random and asked to run 100m. Typically, one child finishes first, others finish later but everyone gets there in the end, all things being equal. Clinically, the results are no different; some patients respond really well and produce a pleasing result, but some cases are more challenging, and it takes more time and effort to obtain an acceptable outcome. The reason for this variation in response is, of course, everyone varies at the genetic level. Some people are 'good growers' and others are not. Similarly, the degree of functional correction varies from case to case, but most people can expect some degree of improvement most of the time, if correctly diagnosed. Actually, this mode of correction is the essence of craniofacial epigenetics, which we had defined as the use of a person's natural genes to enhance the teeth, the jaws, the soft tissues, and the functional spaces, painlessly, using biomimetic appliances. Clinically, it's also essential to follow the basic rules of medicine: first, do no harm; second, make no assumptions; and third, be better than placebo. One of the things that professional people like to see is evidence-based practice, and so before we start therapy, it's a good idea to do some research to find out if there is a scientific basis for some of the novel procedures being discussed.

In a study, Banabilh *et al.* (2009) assessed the dental arch morphology in patients who had been diagnosed with obstructive sleep apnea (OSA). The sample consisted of 108 individuals, all of whom had a sleep study done in a university-hospital department. The upper arch was measured and compared to non-OSA controls. It was found that the average upper arch in patients diagnosed with OSA was 7–11% narrower when compared to their matched controls (7% in the canine region and 11% in the molar region). The lower arch findings were very similar: for patients who had been diagnosed with OSA, the lower arch was narrower, by about 10% in the canine region and about 11% in the molar region compared to the matched controls. In fact, similar findings for mandibular retrognathia have been found in many other studies also, but Banabilh *et al.* (2009) also showed the direction in which the changes occurred. Using finite element analysis, we determined the direction of the changes in the upper arch, visualized using a circular pseudocolor scale. Taking the overall findings together, the data indicated a concentric collapse of the upper jaw, associated with mandibular retrognathia. Thus, to address OSA, the idea is to redevelop the upper jaw, reversing the concentric pattern of collapse, and allowing the mandible to occupy a new spatial matrix. This enhancement of functional space represents a biomimetic correction. However, doing scientific studies in the controlled clinical setting of a university hospital environment is all well and good, but is it possible to translate these findings in real life clinical practice? One way of testing the findings is to repeat the studies in different clinical settings. The clinical procedure starts with a comprehensive working diagnosis; there needs to be excellent patient compliance, and the device adjustments have to be implemented correctly by the treating doctor. In those circumstances, there is no reason to suggest why our research findings can't be reproduced. In fact, over the past ten years or so, our experience suggests that as long as the epigenetic-pneumopedic protocol is followed, there's little reason why the research findings can't be replicated and reproduced consistently by independent practitioners with an appropriate degree of training.

The case illustrated in Figure 6 had originally been treated using a standard orthodontic protocol when the patient was a young teenager. Recently this same patient, now in the late 40s, presented to a dental office, but the chief complaint was not about teeth that we noticed had undergone relapse, as discussed previously. The main concern of this patient was the recent diagnosis of OSA. Taking the biomimetic approach, it is notable that premolar teeth were likely extracted (Fig. 6a) as part of the original orthodontic treatment plan to align the remaining teeth. By so doing, however, functional space has likely been lost, and part of the treatment objectives to address the OSA might be to recapture the functional space. Regaining the lost premolar spaces (Fig. 6b) will likely provide sufficient functional space to accommodate the tongue, and then as time goes on, it might be possible to unravel the anterior teeth, especially if they were retracted during the original orthodontic treatment. Taking a biomimetic approach means that as well as looking at the alignment of the teeth, it's important to look at functional spaces. These spaces will, perhaps partially, be recaptured by remodeling the bony architecture of the jaws, and the new shape and size of the jaws ought to permit the soft tissues, for example the tongue, to be accommodated in the palate. In some cases of OSA, the tongue falls back during sleep and causes upper airway obstruction. Therefore, by remodeling the bony architecture and allowing the tongue to sit in the palate, not only might we avoid relapse from reoccurring, but

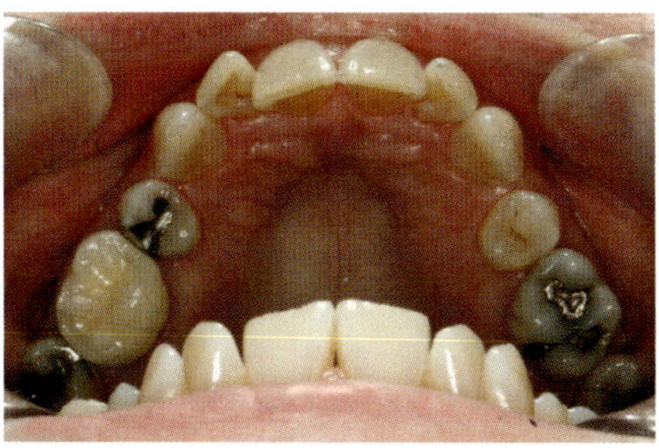

Figure 6a Pre-treatment upper arch with missing first premolars.
Courtesy: Dr Dennis Alleman

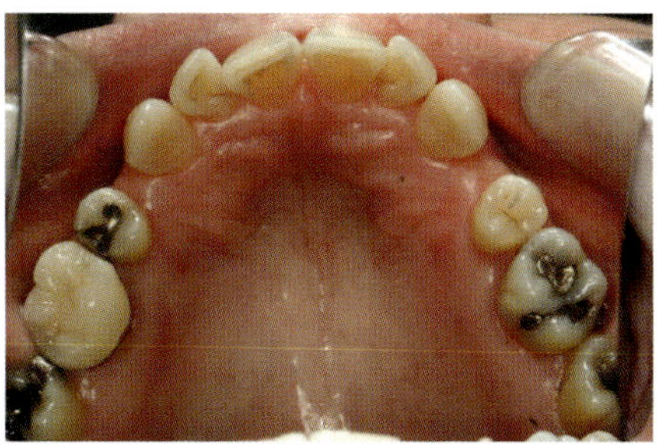

Figure 6b: Mid-treatment upper arch 14 months later with space-recapture in the first premolar regions.

we might also alleviate and possibly eliminate the OSA. This new level of homeostasis will try to avoid relapse from re-occurring as the patient undergoes further ageing, while addressing the current diagnosis of OSA. If this protocol is correct and the predictions made from the spatial matrix hypothesis are true, then bony remodeling of the upper arch should also induce pneumopedic changes of the upper airway. Current technology provides techniques to monitor and assess these particular changes in 3D.

In another case, a cone-beam computerized tomography (CBCT) scan was taken prior to treatment, and then another CBCT scan was taken just after the treatment had been finished. Using the cranial base as a fiducial structure in Figure 7, the mid-sagittal slice of the pre-treatment CBCT going through the midline of the body has been superimposed on to the same slice in the post-treatment CBCT scan. Figure 7 shows that prior to the treatment the minimum retropalatal distance of the upper airway behind the soft palate was 9.6mm, and the retroglossal distance was 8.5mm. Superimposition of the post-treatment scan reveals that the retropalatal distance has increased to 13.6mm and the retroglossal distance has increased to 12.7mm with no device in the mouth when the measurements were taken. This simple analysis indicates an enhanced upper airway behind

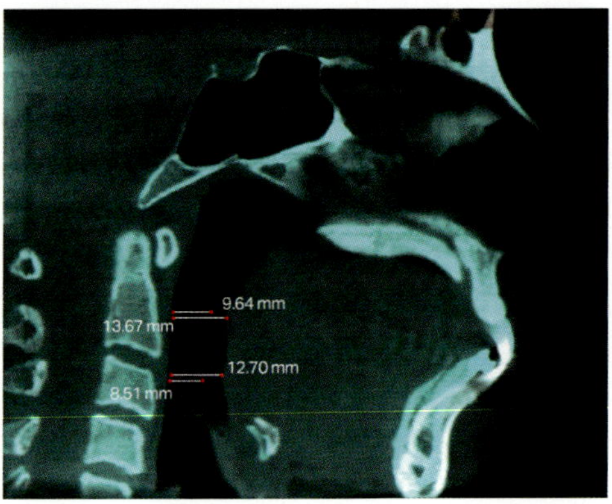

Figure 7: The mid-sagittal slice of the pre-treatment CBCT scan has been superimposed on the same slice mid-treatment. Courtesy: Dr Tammarie Heit

the soft palate and behind the tongue, with the mandible occupying a new spatial matrix. These changes in upper airway morphology can be referred to as pneumopedics.

Medical advances are reliant on evidence-based protocols. In yet another case study (Singh *et al.*, 2011), a 38-year-old adult male had been diagnosed with moderate OSA. The pre- and post-treatment digital study models from the same patient can be compared (Figure 8). Analysis indicated that the transpalatal bone width, measured at the cervical margin of the mesio-palatal cusp of the first permanent molars (McNamara, 2000), increased from 34mm (Fig. 8a) to 39mm after 10 months of treatment (Fig. 8b). Anteriorly, however, there is spacing between the teeth because functional space has been recaptured concentrically, distributed in the anterior segment of the upper arch in this specific case, and not localized to the premolar region where teeth were extracted for orthodontic reasons several years ago, as in the previous case. In order to close those spaces, the treatment plan in this particular case was to use veneers to provide an esthetic finish at the end of the treatment. However, there are other changes that occurred in this specific case.

While the midfacial structures were being remodeled, the response of the mandible was carefully monitored. Figure 9 shows the jaw tracking

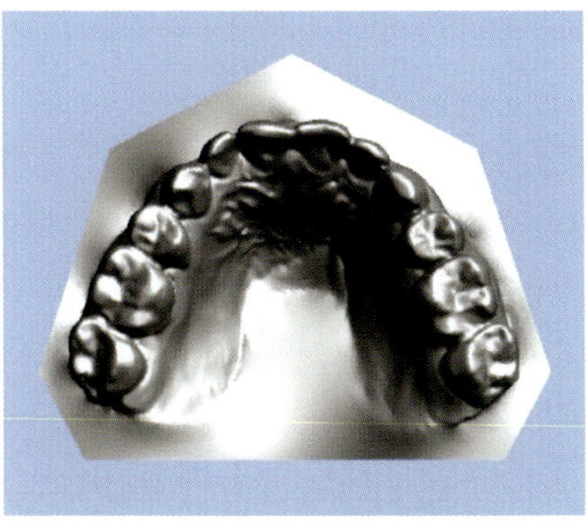

Figure 8a: Pre-treatment transpalatal bone width is 34mm. Courtesy: Dr Sue Wendling

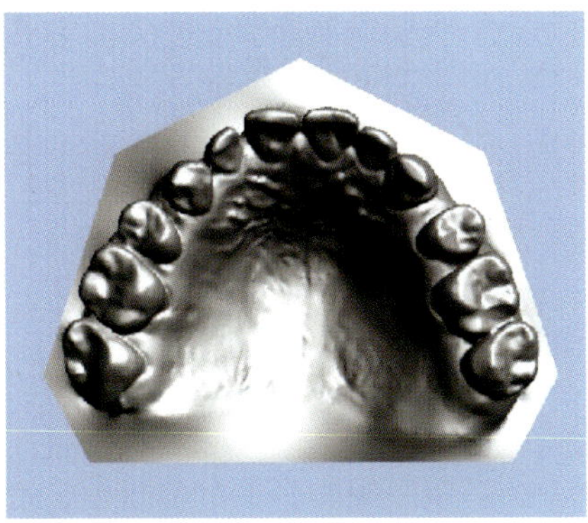

Figure 8b: Post-treatment transpalatal bone width is 39mm.

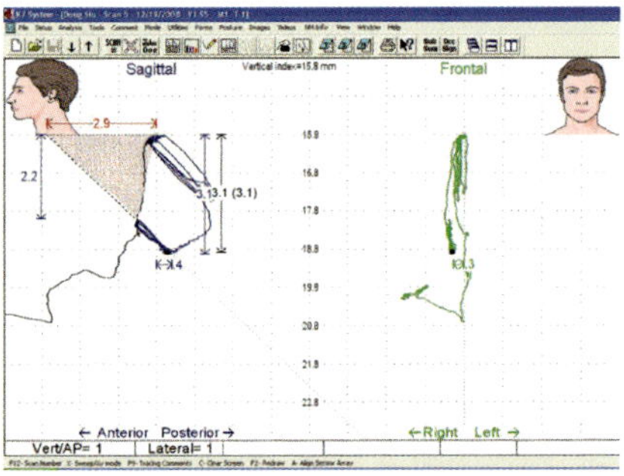

Figure 9a: Pre-treatment the mandible is approx. 3mm behind its physiologic rest position. Courtesy: Dr Sue Wendling

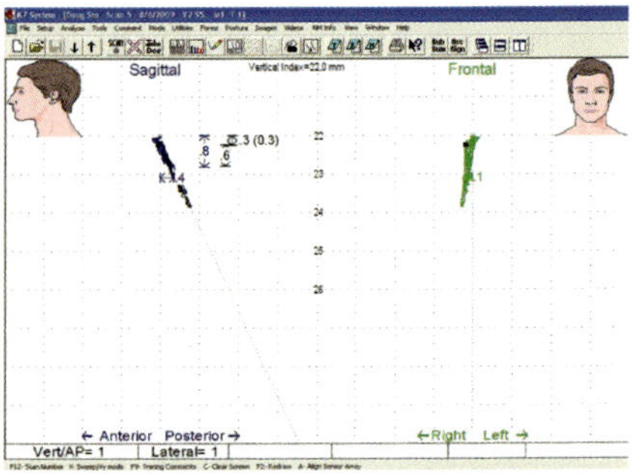

Figure 9b: Mid-treatment the mandible is closer to its physiologic rest position.

data from this case, including the movements of the jaw in the sagittal and frontal planes. The jaw muscles were subjected to transcutaneous electrostimulation (TENS), which enables the jaw muscles to relax and allows the mandible to achieve its physiologic rest position. The blue tracking in Figure 9a shows the new jaw trajectory is almost 3mm in front of its original position after TENS. The green tracking in Figure 9a shows the same jaw movements from the frontal aspect with the jaws opening and closing. Figure 9b shows the same patient after five months of treatment. The blue tracking shows the jaw opening sagittally and the green tracking shows it from the frontal plane. Interestingly, both of these tracings now appear to coincide in both planes, suggesting that the mandible may have achieved its physiologic rest position. These types of data help to illustrate that when the midfacial structures are remodeled, the mandible may also respond to the new spatial matrix. However, in cases where the mandibular response is not sufficient, a lower device is indicated to help re-coordinate the lower arch with changes in the upper arch.

Figure 10 shows the changes in the upper airway using 3D CBCT scans in this case. Figure 10a shows the upper airway of the patient prior to treatment, reconstructed using an edge detection algorithm to show the boundaries of the upper airway. Pre-treatment, the upper airway appeared

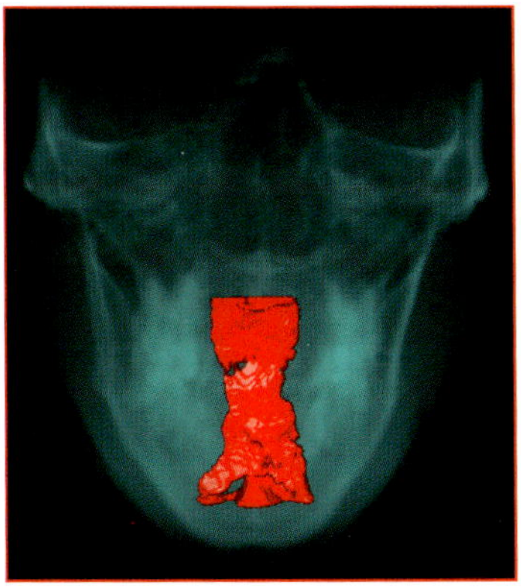

Figure 10a: Pre-treatment the upper airway (red) has a volume of 12.9cm^3.

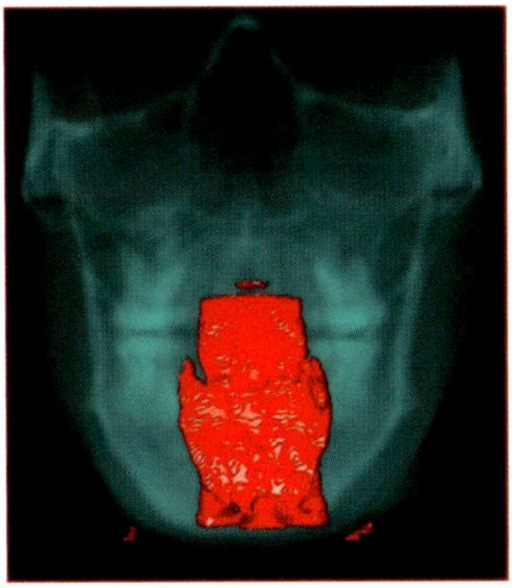

Figure 10b: Post-treatment the upper airway (red) volume has increased to 22.0cm^3.

to be funnel-shaped with a constriction in the midline. Figure 10b shows the same patient 15 months later, indicating that the upper airway has changed in shape, becoming broader and the original constriction has disappeared. Note that this change in the morphology of the upper airway was achieved non-surgically and included an increase in size. Prior to treatment the upper airway volume was about 12.9cm^3 and, according to Schendel *et al.* (2012), that is slightly below the average of 13.5cm^3 for a 36-40yr-old male. In fact, there was a 70% improvement in the upper airway volume in this specific case; the upper airway volume increased to about 22cm^3 after the treatment had been finished. Indeed, there is independent evidence (Alsufyani *et al.*, 2013) that CBCT measured anatomic airway changes are associated with surgery or biomimetic oral device treatment. In fact, there are many studies in the medical literature that describe airway remodeling in pathologic conditions, such as asthma, chronic obstructive pulmonary disease, emphysema, etc. (Singh, 2017). But evidence is emerging that the anatomy of the upper airway can also be changed physiologically by using pneumopedics.

Earlier, the notion that 'form follows function' was mentioned. If the form of the upper airway has been improved, it might be expected that the function or behavior of the upper airway might also be improved. To assess any changes in functional response, sleep studies are required, and these studies can be done either in a sleep lab as a polysomnograph (PSG) or they can be done as a home sleep apnea test (HSAT). In terms of diagnosis, it has been agreed that an apnea hypopnea index (AHI) of < $5hr^{-1}$ (less than 5 events per hour on average) indicates that a patient does not have OSA. Apnea is defined as a period of time during sleep when a patient stops breathing for at least 10 seconds. On the other hand, an episode of hypopnea in simple terms is reduction in airflow of about 50% accompanied by oxygen desaturation of 3–4% of the blood. Thus, if the AHI is > $5hr^{-1}$ but < $15hr^{-1}$, the patient is diagnosed with mild OSA. If the AHI is > $15hr^{-1}$ but < $30hr^{-1}$ then moderate OSA is diagnosed, and an AHI > 30 hr^{-1} represents severe OSA. Current clinical guidelines indicate that a patient with mild to moderate OSA may be treated with oral appliance therapy. In this particular case, an HSAT was performed, and it was found that the AHI was approx. $24hr^{-1}$ prior to treatment. Another sleep study was done on this patient after the treatment being completed some 10 months later. At that time, the AHI had decreased to approx. $3hr^{-1}$ with no device in the patient's mouth while sleeping. Therefore, according to the agreed criteria, we can conclude that this particular patient no longer had OSA after successful pneumopedics and craniofacial epigenetics. However, further studies are needed to verify these initial findings.

Figure 11 shows the clinical photographs of the patient's dentition after the treatment had been completed. In this case, although the midface was redeveloped, the recaptured premolar spaces have been

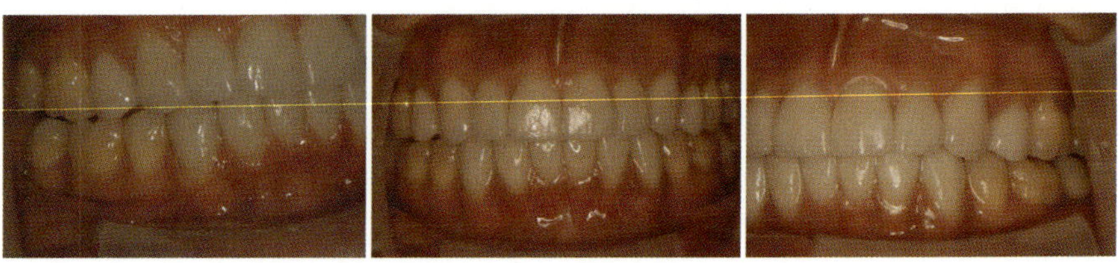

Figure 11: Post-treatment occlusion after restorative reconstruction.
Courtesy: Dr Sue Wendling

closed using techniques from cosmetic dentistry, and the lower jaw has been brought into a harmonious relationship within the new spatial matrix, producing a very reasonable and acceptable occlusion. One of the things mentioned earlier was the notion that the occlusion represents an endpoint of the body with respect to the plantar surfaces of the feet. Hypothetically then, changes in the occlusion and head posture ought to precipitate changes further caudally. One way to assess these putative changes would be to measure the length of the legs of an individual, to investigate the theme of biomimetic effects following epigenetic principles. The findings of one study (Chapman and Singh, 2013) that measured leg lengths prior to any treatment found discrepancy and asymmetries. Next, a biomimetic oral appliance was inserted into the patient's mouth and equilibrated by a dentist. When the leg lengths were re-measured, on average the discrepancy decreased. Next, a chiropractic adjustment was performed to realign the first cervical vertebra (C1), and when the leg lengths were re-measured the asymmetries decreased further, and the findings were statistically significant. Therefore, when a biomimetic oral appliance is used in combination with chiropractic adjustment of the cervical vertebrae, there appears to be a synergistic effect that reduces the leg length discrepancy in adults. This study provides some preliminary data on the concept of the kinetic chain, linking the occlusion with the plantar surfaces of the feet.

In another case study (Singh and Cress, 2013), a patient presented to a dental office with cosmetic concerns. The overall treatment took about 12 months and enhanced symmetry of the face was discernible by the end of treatment. Figure 12a shows a 3D CBCT superimposition prior to and after treatment. The grey color depicts the bony structures before treatment and the light blue coloration represents the same bony structures after the treatment had been finished. The two scans have been superimposed on the cranial base, and on the patient's right side the maxillary region and the mandible show a blue coloration, but less so on

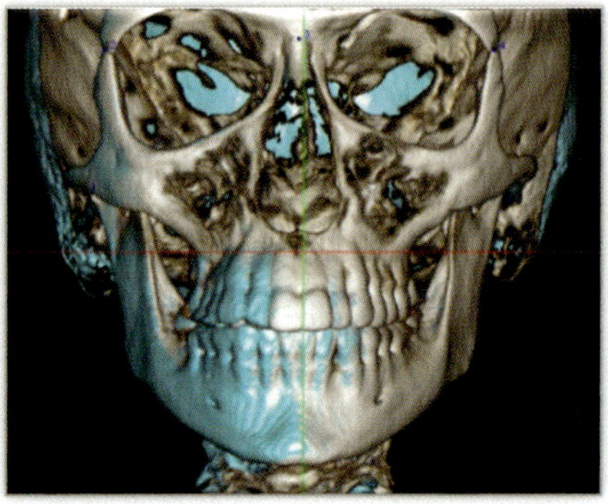

Figure 12a: Pre-treatment (grey) and post-treatment (blue) 3D CBCT superimposition. Courtesy: Dr Sam Cress

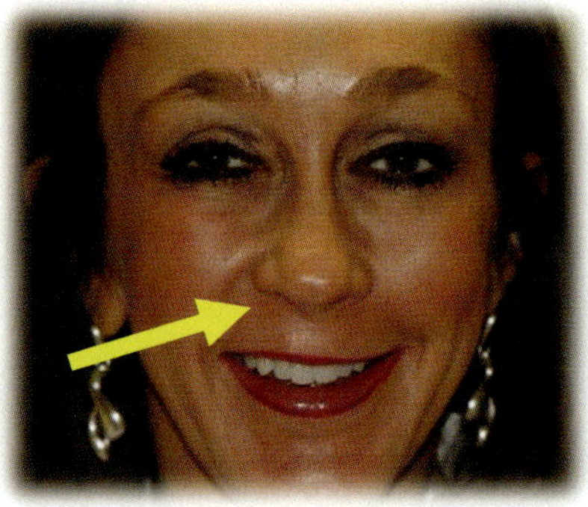

Figure 12b: Pre-treatment facial appearance showing right-sided asymmetry (arrowed).

the left side. In other words, there are asymmetric bony changes after the treatment. This difference is explained by looking at the corresponding soft tissue profile of the patient prior to treatment. In the facial photograph in Figure 12b, there appears to be a deficiency in the midface on the right side. Therefore, during treatment, redevelopment of the bony architecture appears to preferentially remodel the right side, so the maxilla became more symmetric and, therefore, more similar to the left side, in line with its genetic blueprint. However, the mandible behaved differently because although it can undergo remodeling to produce a more symmetric lower arch, it can also move into a new functional space (Fig. 12a). Therefore, the overall changes are complementary to the correction that's required to produce a balanced and symmetric face. Thus, taking a biomimetic approach, there are dental changes, skeletal changes and corresponding soft tissue facial changes; and these changes will impact the upper airway. Figure 13 shows the upper airway analysis for a different patient. The upper airway volume prior to treatment is about 17cm^3 and there is constriction of the upper airway localized to a specific region (Fig. 13a). Reconstructing the upper airway for the same patient after the treatment had been completed, which took about 12 months, Fig. 13b shows that the upper

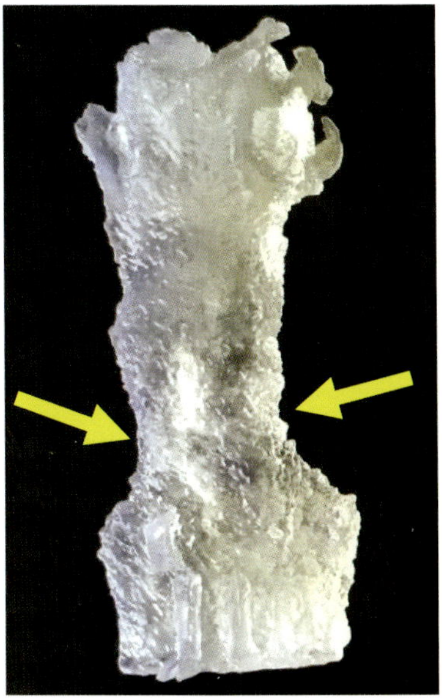

Figure 13a: Pre-treatment upper airway showing constriction in 60-year-old male (arrowed).
Courtesy: Dr Chris Chapman

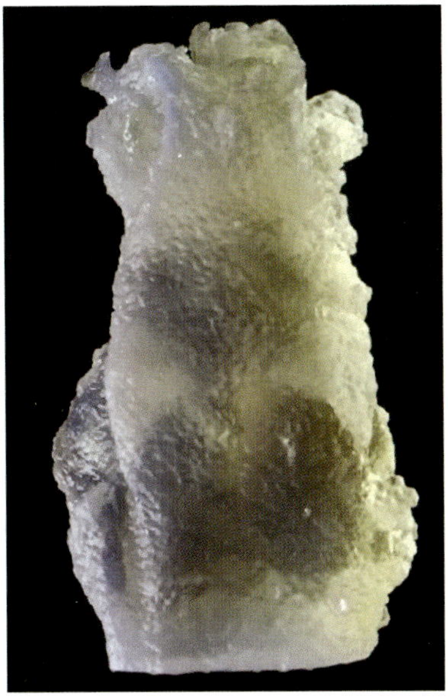

Figure 13b: Post-treatment upper airway showing increased size and shape changes in the same patient after biomimetic oral appliance therapy.

airway volume has increased to from 17cm^3 to 28cm^3 without using drugs, injections, or surgery.

A question that is often asked when this type of remodeling occurs is: Is there an increased transpalatal bone width after biomimetic oral appliance therapy in adults? One way to address this question is by taking skeletal measurements in a sample of patients. In one study (Singh *et al.*, 2014), we were able to measure the minimum transpalatal bone width at the mesio-palatal cusp of the first molar at the cervical margin, as defined by McNamara (2000). This skeletal measurement is preferable over (dental) cusp-to-cusp measurements or fossa-to-fossa measurements since tooth size will have an effect on the transpalatal bone width. Similarly, if the teeth are tipped, it could provide an artificially larger measurement. Therefore, the minimum transpalatal bone width is preferred. In the study sample, the pre-treatment minimum transpalatal bone width was about 33mm.

After a period of about 18 months of the treatment, the minimum width increased to about 35.5mm on average, and that finding was statistically significant. In fact, there are several studies in the orthodontic literature that describe an increase in the transverse width, but they are unable to address the issue of whether any new bone was regenerated. In the study by Singh *et al.* (2014) using 3D reconstruction from CBCT scans, initially the average midfacial bone volume was about 17cm^3, and then 18 months later, the mean bone volume increased to about 19cm^3 in 'non-growing' adults. These findings raised further research questions. For example, is there an increase in the nasal cavity after biomimetic oral appliance therapy in adults and, if so, would there be an increased nasal airway volume? To provide evidence, it's possible to measure volumetric nasal changes, using 3D CBCT scan technology. Singh *et al.* (2014) were able to segment the nasal cavity and measure its volume pre-treatment, and following 18 months of active treatment with a biomimetic oral appliance. Prior to treatment the average nasal airway volume was about 40cm^3 and then after the treatment was finished, it had increased to 42cm^3 without any surgery or drugs, and that change was statistically significant.

Conclusion

The take-home message is that we are finding upper airway changes can be obtained in 'non-growing' adults, and because we can get these changes to occur non-surgically in both children and adults, it suggests that genetically encoded developmental mechanisms may be epigenetically modulated by biomimetic oral devices to enhance the upper airway. Furthermore, if we are able to improve the structure of the upper airway, then these novel findings might help doctors/dentists in the management of patients that have been diagnosed with mild to moderate obstructive sleep apnea, using biomimetic correction, which relies on pneumopedics and craniofacial epigenetics for non-surgical upper airway remodeling.

References

Alsufyani NA, Al-Saleh MA, Major PW. CBCT assessment of upper airway changes and treatment outcomes of obstructive sleep apnoea: A systematic review. *Sleep Breath*. 2013;17(3):911–923.

Ayalon J, Simkin A, Leichter I, Raifmann S. Dynamic bone loading exercises for postmenopausal women: effect on the density of the distal radius. *Arch Phys Med Rehabil*. 1987;68(5 Pt 1):280–283.

Banabilh SM, Suzina AH, Dinsuhaimi S, Samsudin AR, Singh GD. Dental arch morphology in South East Asian adults with obstructive sleep apnoea: Geometric morphometrics. *J Oral Rehab*. 2009;36:184–192.

Ben-Bassat Y, Yitschaky M, Kaplan L, Brin I. Occlusal patterns in patients with idiopathic scoliosis. *Am J Orthod Dentofacial Orthop*. 2006;130(5):629–633.

Borke JL, Yu JC, Isales CM, Wagle N, Do NN, Chen JR, Bollag RJ. Tension-induced reduction in connexin 43 expression in cranial sutures is linked to transcriptional regulation by TBX2. *Ann Plast Surg*. 2003;51(5):499–504.

Burwell RG, Dangerfield PH, Freeman BJ. Concepts on the pathogenesis of adolescent idiopathic scoliosis. Bone growth and mass, vertebral column, spinal cord, brain, skull, extra-spinal left-right skeletal length asymmetries, disproportions and molecular pathogenesis. *Stud Health Technol Inform*. 2008;135:3–52.

Chambers TL, Burnett TR, Raue U, *et al.* Skeletal muscle size, function, and adiposity with lifelong aerobic exercise. *J Appl Physiol*. 2020;128(2):368–378.

Chang CS, Wallace CG, Hsiao YC, Hsieh YJ, Wang YC, Chen NH, Liao YF, Liou EJ, Chen PK, Chen JP, Chen YR. Airway changes after cleft orthognathic surgery evaluated by three-dimensional computed tomography and overnight polysomnographic study. *Sci Rep*. 2017;7(1):12260.

Chaplain MAJ, Singh GD, McLachlan JC (eds). On Growth and Form: Spatio-Temporal Patterning in Biology. England: John Wiley and Sons Publishers, 1999.

Chapman C, Singh GD. Combined effect of a biomimetic oral appliance and atlas orthogonist cervical adjustment on leg lengths in adults. *Annals Vert Sub Res*. 2013;46–50.

Cribbet MR, Carlisle M, Cawthon RM, Uchino BN, Williams PG, Smith TW, Gunn HE, Light KC. Cellular aging and restorative processes: Subjective sleep quality and duration moderate the association between age and telomere length in a sample of middle-aged and older adults. *Sleep*. 2014;37(1):65–70.

D'Attilio M, Filippi MR, Femminella B, Festa F, Tecco S. The influence of an experimentally-induced malocclusion on vertebral alignment in rats: A controlled pilot study. *Cranio*. 2005;23(2):119–29.

Fonder AC. The dental distress syndrome (DDS). *Basal Facts*. 1984;6(1):17–29.

Fuentes MA, Opperman LA, Buschang P, Bellinger LL, Carlson DS, Hinton RJ. Lateral functional shift of the mandible: Part II. Effects on gene expression in condylar cartilage. *Am J Orthod Dentofacial Orthop*. 2003;123(2):160–166.

Harris WG, Singh GD. Resolution of 'gummy smile' and anterior open bite using the DNA appliance™: Case Report. *J Amer Orthod Soc*. 2013;13(4):30–34.

He L, He S, Wu X, Huang Y. Three-dimensional morphological changes of the upper airway in patients with skeletal Class III malocclusion after orthognathic surgery. *J Craniofac Surg*. 2019;30(8):2451–2455.

Hwang H, Hwang C, West J, Singh GD. Changes in pediatric paranasal sinuses following biomimetic oral appliance therapy: 3 case reports. *Cranio*. 2019;2:1–6.

Ilizarov GA, Matveenko VN, Gaĭdamak AN, Irianovlu M. Formation of an organic matrix in the traction method of bone regeneration and characteristics of its mineralization in experimental tibia lengthening. *Vopr Med Khim*. 1982;28(6):27–3. [Article in Russian]

Kaltschmidt B, Kaltschmidt C, Widera D. Adult craniofacial stem cells: sources and relation to the neural crest. *Stem Cell Rev Rep*. 2012;8(3):658–671.

Kambara T. Dentofacial changes produced by extraoral forward force in the Macaca irus. *Am J Orthod*. 1977;71(3):249–277.

Katiyar R, Singh GK, Mehrotra D, Singh A. Surgical-orthodontic treatment of a skeletal class III malocclusion. *Natl J Maxillofac Surg*. 2010;1(2):143–149.

Kent A. Catastrophic occlusion. *Br Dent J*. 2006;201(7):419.

Kim KA, Lee JW, Park JH, Kim BH, Ahn HW, Kim SJ. Targeted presurgical decompensation in patients with yaw-dependent facial asymmetry. *Korean J Orthod*. 2017;47(3):195–206.

Kokich VG. The biology of sutures. In: Cohen MM (ed.) Craniosynostosis. Diagnosis, evaluation, and management. New York: Raven Press, 1986, pp. 81–103.

McNamara JA Jr. Maxillary transverse deficiency. *Am J Orthod Dentofacial Orthop*. 2000;117(5):567–570.

Ng DK, Hui HN, Chan CH, Kwok KL, Chow PY, Cheung JM, Leung SY. Obstructive sleep apnoea in children with Down syndrome. *Singapore Med J*. 2006;47(9):774–779.

Parsons TE, Downey CM, Jirik FR, Hallgrimsson B, Jamniczky HA. Mind the gap: genetic manipulation of basicranial growth within synchondroses modulates calvarial and facial shape in mice through epigenetic interactions. *PLoS One*. 2015;10(2):e0118355.

Pollard KS, Salama SR, King B, Kern AD, Dreszer T, Katzman S, Siepel A, Pedersen JS, Bejerano G, Baertsch R, Rosenbloom KR, Kent J, Haussler D. Forces shaping the fastest evolving regions in the human genome. *PLoS Genet.* 2006;2(10):e168.

Pollard KS, Salama SR, Lambert N, Lambot MA, Coppens S, Pedersen JS, Katzman S, King B, Onodera C, Siepel A, Kern AD, Dehay C, Igel H, Ares M Jr, Vanderhaeghen P, Haussler D. An RNA gene expressed during cortical development evolved rapidly in humans. *Nature.* 2006;443(7108):167–172.

Rai S, Kaur M, Kaur S. Applications of stem cells in interdisciplinary dentistry and beyond: an overview. *Ann Med Health Sci Res.* 2013;3(2):245–254.

Roberts WE, Hartfield JK Jr. Bone development and function: Genetic and environmental mechanisms. *Seminars Orthod.* 2004;10(2):100–122.

Schendel SA, Jacobson R, Khalessi S. Airway growth and development: a computerized 3-dimensional analysis. *J Oral Maxillofac Surg.* 2012;70(9):2174–2183.

Singh GD, Cress SE. Craniofacial enhancement using a biomimetic oral appliance. *Dent Today.* 2013;329(12):92–94.

Singh GD, Heit T, Preble D. Changes in 3D midfacial parameters after biomimetic oral appliance therapy in adults. *J Ind Orthod Soc.* 2014;48(2):104–108.

Singh GD, Krumholtz J. Epigenetic Orthodontics in Adults. Appliance Therapy Group, USA, 2009.

Singh GD, Levy-Bercowski D, Santiago PE. 3-D effects of nasoalveolar molding in patients with orofacial clefts: geometric morphometrics. *Cleft Palate Craniofac J.* 2005;42(4):403–409.

Singh GD, Levy-Bercowski D, Yañez MA, Santiago PE. Three-dimensional facial morphology following surgical repair of unilateral cleft lip and palate in patients after nasoalveolar molding. *Orthod Craniofac Res.* 2007;10(3):161–6.

Singh GD, Lipka G. Case Report: Introducing the Wireframe DNA appliance™. *J Am Acad Gnathol Orthop.* 2009;26(4):8–1.

Singh GD, Maher GJ, Padilla RR. Customized mandibular orthotics in the prevention of concussion/mild traumatic brain injury in football players: A preliminary study. *Dental Traumatol.* 2009;25(5):515–521.

Singh GD, McNamara JA Jr, Lozanoff S. Morphometry of the cranial base in subjects with Class III malocclusion. *J Dent Res.* 1997;76(2):694–703.

Singh GD, Rivera-Robles J, de Jesus-Vinas J. Longitudinal craniofacial growth patterns in patients with orofacial clefts: Geometric morphometrics. *Cleft Palate Craniofac J.* 2004;41(2):136–143.

Singh GD, Wendling S, Chandrashekhar R. Midfacial development in adult obstructive sleep apnea. *Dent Today*. 2011;30(7):124–127.

Singh GD. On Growth and Treatment: The spatial matrix hypothesis. In: McNamara JA Jr (ed.) Growth and treatment: A meeting of the minds. Vol 41, Craniofacial Growth Series, *Ann Arbor*, USA, 2004, pp. 197–239.

Singh GD. Spatial matrix hypothesis. *Brit Dent J*. 2007;202(5):238–239.

Williams DE, Lynch JE, Doshi V, Singh GD, Hargens A. Bruxism and temporal bone hypermobility in patients with multiple sclerosis. *Cranio*. 2011;29(3):1–9.

Woo SL, Kuei SC, Amiel D, Gomez MA, Hayes WC, White FC, Akeson WH. The effect of prolonged physical training on the properties of long bone: a study of Wolff's Law. *J Bone Joint Surg Am*. 1981;63(5):780–787.

Zhao H, Feng J, Ho TV, Grimes W, Urata M, Chai Y. The suture provides a niche for mesenchymal stem cells of craniofacial bones. *Nat Cell Biol*. 2015;17(4):386–396.

Chapter 2 Genetics and Epigenetics of Craniofacial Development

Summary: This chapter introduces the molecular genetics of craniofacial development. It lays the foundation from which clinical craniofacial growth can be more readily understood. In addition, epigenetic factors that affect craniofacial development are presented, and the inter-dependency of gene-environmental interactions is highlighted. Various developmental mechanisms that determine clinical morphology are described and discussed. The concept that growth mechanisms are encoded by the human genome, and that growth outcomes are epigenetically-modulated, is emphasized.

Normal growth and development

The term 'growth' has been used widely throughout the pediatric literature with little agreement on its definition, and perhaps even less emphasis on its meaning. Mao and Nah (2004) opine that growth and development is the net outcome of genetic inheritance and environmental modulation, resulting from cell migration, proliferation, differentiation, and biosynthesis of extracellular matrix in specific, temporo-spatial directions and magnitudes, producing identifiable morphologies. In this book, 'growth' is generally-defined as a quantitative increase in size and/or mass and/or complexity. 'Size' is simply a displacement of two-dimensional or three-dimensional space and can be quantified through measurement. For example, if a child is growing taller, then the increase in height can be measured as a linear increase in length. Similarly, if an adult is becoming obese, then the increase in volume can be estimated by the amount of water displaced if the person is immersed in a bathtub, as in the Archimedes principle. Thus, a linear increase in height is a measure of 2D size, while volume-change indicates 3D size-change. Changes in the morphology and/or position of objects can also be mapped by following identified points (landmarks) in 3D space and their new locations, using x, y, z coordinates. It's important to note that craniofacial growth is non-linear. As the mandible grows longer in the sagittal plane in lateral profile, it may change its transverse arch width and symmetry in the axial plane at the same time. In other words, the jaw is changing also its 'shape' while growing. This phenomenon is possibly the reason why some orthodontic specialists believe it's impossible to grow the mandible using devices; the reliance on 2D cephalometric analyses of a 3D object are deficient (Moyers and Bookstein, 1979), and cannot be relied upon to capture the features of the change completely (Bookstein, 2016). In contrast, 'shape' can be defined as the properties of an object that remain invariant when size information is removed. Thus, while a football and a soccer ball can have the same volume i.e. the same size, they simply differ in shape. Their respective shape characteristics remain constant even if the balls are rotated and translated through space during a game. For human craniofacial structures, size information and shape information are integrated intimately and cannot be disconnected by the naked eye. This integration is so complete that the human eye can often be deceived and optical illusions can occur, such that a patient may appear to have a relatively large nose, while in fact the jaws might actually be small; or the upper incisor teeth may appear to be protruded in a Class II case in which the maxilla is essentially retruded (Lawrence *et al.*, 1985). Facial plastic and cosmetic surgeons sometimes make use of this optical phenomenon, known as facial perception, by placing a chin implant to disguise the prominent appearance of a patient's nose. This integration of size and shape information is summarized by the terms form and/or morphology. In this way, certain facial forms are recognizable clinically, and are sometimes referred to as 'facies'. Thus, most people can recognize a child with Down syndrome, and some studies suggest that these children have macroglossia. However, recent evidence (Silva Jesuino and Valladares-Neto, 2013) suggests that children with Down syndrome may have a cranial base dysmorphology, precipitating midfacial hypoplasia and relative, not absolute, macroglossia.

Due the dynamic nature of developmental processes, growth can also be regressive, leading to a quantitative decrease in size with concomitant changes in shape. An example of regressive changes is physiologic atrophy of the adenoids in the upper airway of adolescents. Taken together, these growth phenomena can be described by the term 'allometry' in that size-related shape-changes occur during normal growth and development. Therefore, the growth potential of the craniofacial system needs to be recognized by the clinician because particular interventions, such as epigenetic orthopedic therapies, amount to growth guidance. In other words, modification of the craniofacial region is possible, especially as a significant amount of growth potential resides in the dentofacial system throughout life, as sub-populations of localized stem cells (Huang and Thesleff, 2013). Yet another feature of growth is its complexity. There are two types of complexity. The first type is structural complexity. For example, an incisor tooth is less structurally complex than a bicuspid tooth. On the other hand, there is also mathematical complexity. For example, the deciduous (primary) dentition consists of 20 teeth, and is thus less complex than the adult combination, which has 32 teeth. Similarly, if two dice are thrown twice, then the second outcome is independent of the first one (unless the dice were loaded), i.e. in a sequence of events a prior event may or may not affect a subsequent event. Similarly, genes encoding for facial features may be independently inherited from the father and mother, and this is how mathematical or statistical complexity is incorporated into the craniofacial system.

Factors affecting growth

Ontogeny is the complete life period of an individual, including ageing. Newborn babies show a rapid rate of growth, which decreases throughout life. At puberty, the rate of growth-decrease decreases, which appears as a relative increased rate of growth, known as the pubertal growth spurt. In other words, growth never ceases during the human lifespan, and the rate of growth varies at different developmental stages. Growth does not even stop in adulthood, as the individual continues to grow older due to the depletion of specific stem cell populations *inter alia*. Ageing is understood to be affected by various factors. For example, premature ageing of the individual (progeria) has been described in the medical literature (Farran-Ridge, 1921). In terms of the mechanism involved, lamin A is a product of the LMNA gene, and is an essential nuclear envelope constituent in most differentiated cells. It is thought that mutations of the LMNA gene, which encodes for the proteins prelamin A and lamin C, gives rise to Hutchinson-Gilford progeria syndrome (HGPS) in children (Yang *et al.*, 2005). Thus, HGPS is caused by progerin, which is the mutant form of lamin A, and these mutations have been linked to premature ageing disorders, which lead to premature death from atherosclerosis (Hamczyk and Andrés, 2019). Similarly, chronic inflammation is thought to accelerate the ageing process. Recently, it's been discovered that the ends of human chromosomes show telomeres. Telomeres are DNA-protein structures that protect the ends of the chromosome from inflammation, oxidative stress and (inappropriate) cellular repair. However, they shorten with age and may be markers of biological ageing. When the telomeres get short enough, the cells no longer divide, and the body stops making those cells. Over time, this leads to senescence, ageing and death. In fact, some studies suggest that people with sleep disordered breathing (SDB) may have shorter telomere lengths (Cribbet *et al.*, 2014). On the other hand, good sleep quality among older adults is associated with telomere lengths similar to those in middle-aged adults, providing evidence for the notion that sleep quality and duration are associated with cellular ageing. Thus, the ageing process may be accelerated by not getting enough quality sleep.

In the dawn of the twenty-first century, about 95% of the human genome had been sequenced by 2003; the first time in human history. During the identification of human genes one thing that became clear by comparing the genomes of different species, was homology. In other words, certain regions of the mammalian genome are highly conserved in, say, mice, monkeys and man. Specifically, homeobox genes encode for facial features, and several of the specific genes involved in craniofacial development have been identified and sequenced. Homeobox genes are expressed in developing facial primordia and are organized in four distinct Hox gene clusters (Hox A, B, C and D). These genes, which all encode for transcription factors, include: Msx-1, Msx-2, Msx-3, LHX-6, LHX-7, LHX-8, Dlx1-6, Barx-1, Goosecoid, Sonic hedgehog (Shh), PRRX-1, PRRX-2 etc. The expression of these genes can be visualized using molecular biology techniques, such as whole mount in situ hybridization. Moreover, disruption of the normal pattern of gene expression can lead to midfacial retrusion (Lozanoff, 1993) or even severe craniofacial defects, such as holoprosencephaly.

In contrast with the previously held beliefs of "the genetic control" of growth, genes are now thought to be intimately associated with the natural processes of growth and development - not in a simple Mendelian fashion as pre-supposed in the 19th and 20th centuries - but rather through a complex cascade of developmental processes, which are surmised by the concept of temporo-spatial patterning (Chaplain *et al.*, 1999). It is now understood that specific genes are expressed at certain times in particular locations to ensure an orderly sequence of developmental events. This developmental mechanism, known as pattern formation (Smith and Wolpert, 1981), is a critical process during the early development of an embryo. For example, it is the process by which the specification of polarity is achieved, including the midline of the body. During this process, the left and right sides of the body are defined, as well as the superior, inferior, ventral and dorsal aspects. In addition, during early development, symmetry and asymmetry are signaled and expressed. Generally speaking, the external features of the human body are symmetric while, internally, specific organ systems, such as the cardio-vascular and digestive systems, are systematically encoded for asymmetry. In limb formation, the importance of the apical ectodermal ridge (Cairns, 1975) has now been established, as well as the role of apoptosis in digit separation (Mori *et al.*, 1995). In another example of temporo-spatial patterning in the craniofacial region, genes responsible for tongue, primary palate (premaxilla) and cheek development are expressed early so that the newborn baby can breast-feed/suckle effectively soon after birth. Similarly, the expression of other genes is modulated; for example, those involved in the development of the respiratory system, as the fetus changes its source of hemoglobin oxygenation from the placenta to the newly aerated lungs and respiratory alveoli. In premature babies, the untimely expression of genes is responsible for deficient biosynthesis of surfactant (Obladen, 1978), which results in neonatal respiratory distress.

Genes, however, do not function in isolation. Rather, they pick up developmental clues from the environment, leading to gene-environmental interactions, a phenomenon that can summarized by the term 'epigenetics' (Wolffe and Matzke, 1999). These epigenetic interactions are numerous, often complex and incompletely understood, although much research is ongoing in this area. One environmental factor of specific interest is nutrition, and a range of developmental anomalies are associated with certain gene-environmental interactions during gestation. For example, excess vitamin A (retinoic acid) during pregnancy can lead to the development of an orofacial cleft in a developing embryo. In fetal alcohol syndrome, a mother's addiction to alcohol can lead to a child being born with mild mental retardation, and the facies associated with this syndrome include hypertelorism. On the other hand, it is now accepted that folate (methyl donor) supplementation of the diet of women of child-bearing age is associated with the prevention of neural tube defects, including spina bifida and cleft lip/palate. Post-natally, malnourishment during early childhood due to dietary deficiencies, for example a lack of vitamin D (1, 25 dihydroxycholecalciferol), leads to rickets with poor bone and joint development. On the other hand, gene-environmental interactions can precipitate childhood obesity, which is occurring more commonly in developed countries than ever before. Although the causes of childhood obesity are still being investigated, it is not inconceivable to suggest that refined, highly processed fast foods are more readily absorbed by a digestive system that evolved during the hunter-gatherer mode of life. This means that a similar volume of ingested food might actually provide many more nutrients in a readily absorbable form, leading to deposition of body stores of fat in genetically determined sites associated with obesity. For example, males tend to store fat around the abdomen and chin/neck regions, whereas females tend to store fat around the buttocks and breasts. Another environmental factor that disrupts the normal working of genes is disease caused by pathogenic organisms. For example, poliomyelitis is a viral infection that can lead to abnormal limb formation in the infected neonate. Similarly, if a developing system is subjected to trauma, the normal developmental pathway is disrupted, leading to deformity. Clinicians are aware that severe trauma to the temporo-mandibular joint (TMJ) during early childhood can lead to ankylosis and mandibular asymmetry in later childhood. However, congenital condylar asymmetries due to gene mutations may be surgically corrected (Santiago *et al.*, 2001) or, in some cases of craniofacial microsomia, non-surgically corrected (Kaplan, 1989), suggesting an epigenetic resolution.

Aside from pathologic influences, possibly the single most important environmental factor interacting with genes in the craniofacial region is function. 'Function' is simply the normal workings of a particular organ system, e.g. swallowing, breathing, feeding etc. This latter function can be described as feeding behavior, in that there are several methods of feeding, which change as a child matures. For example, humans are classified as 'mammals' because the offspring are to be fed primarily from the mammary glands of the mother after the baby is born. Breast-feeding is a feeding behavior that evolved over millennia with concomitant gene expression. However, a busy mother may not spend the time nursing her child and may prefer to bottle-feed the infant instead. This change in feeding behavior may be reflected in changes in craniofacial features, a consequence of altered gene-environmental interactions, producing epigenetic, phenotypic variation (Chen *et al.*, 2016). Similarly, young children that have an active childhood including regular exercise, play etc. tend to be less inclined to develop obesity compared to children that have a more passive or sedentary childhood (Gortmaker *et al.*, 1990). There is no doubt that muscle growth occurs due to gene expression in response to the environmental signals received during function. In fact, research has shown that there may be genetic encoding for a finite number of muscle-producing cells (myoblasts), and that there is a pre-natal propensity for spontaneous muscle firing, which gives rise to random movements during pregnancy. Often, an expectant mother will report that she can feel the baby 'kick'. These random movements are pre-programmed by genes, but the control of final limb morphology is determined by use (function) as the child matures (Del Vecchio *et al.*, 2020). In other words, growth mechanisms, and not growth outcome, are defined by the human genome. As mentioned above, the muscles of facial expression and the tongue are well developed at birth in readiness for suckling (breast-feeding). As the child breast-feeds, muscle mass is increased through growth with an increase in nutritional requirement of the muscles of mastication. This increased functional demand leads to the attraction of new blood vessels (angiogenesis), which provide further nutrients for muscle growth. Thus, new increase in muscle mass leads to increased function (a positive regulatory/feedback cycle), and eventually to a change or deposition of bone to which the new muscle will attach, thus changing the skeletal craniofacial features of the infant. Interestingly, the muscles of mastication, especially the tongue, exert their main influence on craniofacial features in early childhood, another example of temporo-spatial patterning.

Mechanisms of normal growth and development

For a developing system to increase in size and/or mass, the amount of tissue present needs to be increased. One way of achieving these changes is through cell proliferation, so that mitotic cell division results in tissue hyperplasia, resulting in an increased number of cells. In addition, cells can increase in size through hypertrophy so that tissues, such as muscles, get bigger. Another method to increase the tissue mass is through cell migration. It is now clearly established that certain cell populations migrate from one region to another during normal development. For example, neural crest cells originate at the developing neural tube and leave the central nervous system to populate the developing craniofacial regions. This sub-population of cells gives rise to the connective tissues of the head and neck region as well as a number of other tissue lines, such as cardiac cells and autonomic (nerve) ganglia. In addition, cell recruitment is yet another mechanism by which a tissue can grow. Non-committed cells are recruited from local stem cells in the region and undergo differentiation to form specific cell lines. In both cell migration and recruitment, tissue mass is increased following mitotic cell division (proliferation) and/or hypertrophy either prior to or after cell differentiation. Differentiation is the developmental mechanism by which cells change from being non-specific cells to cells that are functionally or morphologically distinguishable. For example, a population of stem cells can proliferate to increase the number of cells by mitosis and maintain their population. From this pool of stem cells, certain members receive signals that induce them to differentiate into a specific cell type. In this way, a population of mesenchymal cells can differentiate to form a host of connective tissues, such as: chondroblasts that form cartilage; osteoblasts that form bone; fibroblasts that produce collagen and extracellular matrix components etc. In each instance, a growth factor and/or cytochemical signals are produced after the expression of the associated gene(s) to induce the process of cell differentiation through signal transduction.

Morphologic determination

There is no doubt that genetics plays a central role in morphologic determination. For example, tall parents tend to have tall children, generally speaking since variation in human height is about 80% heritable through a polygenic mechanism (Yengo *et al.*, 2020). Similarly, inheritance has also a strong influence on facial features through growth. It is well known that malocclusions run in families, such as the Class III appearance associated with the Hapsburg jaw. These phenotypic features are expressed as the children inherit certain genes, which undergo transcription. Having been read, specific protein growth factors are produced from these genes, which act as cytochemical signals. The array of growth factors is large and is increasing as new factors or variants of known growth factors are discovered. These growth factors have names that generally relate to how or where they were first discovered. For example, the term 'growth factor' is a misnomer in the sense that a specific growth factor may not be a determinant of growth, in fact. In this way, fibroblast growth factor 2 (FGF-2), and insulin-like growth factor 1 (IGF-1) were discovered in developing embryos but may be required for normal biologic processes even in a mature individual. Similarly, transforming growth factor alpha (TGF-α) was first described in cells undergoing cancerous change but it is required for normal, healthy cell function. In addition, TGF-β3 is not necessarily involved in tumor formation but, in mice that are TGF-β3 deficient, the palatal shelves fail to fuse during development and these mice are born with cleft palates. In another example, bone morphogenetic protein (BMP) has several variants, some of which are not primarily involved in bone biosynthesis, and it is now known that this series of cytokines belongs to the TGF super-family of growth factors. However, evidence is emerging that the artificial infusion of BMP-2 is associated with new bone formation in fracture non-unions, large bone defects, and spinal fusion. In fact, Hettiaratchi *et al.* (2020) used heparin microparticles to enhance spatial localization of bone regeneration associated with BMP-2 delivery. Thus, growth factors are gene products that play various roles during normal physiology and during development.

In one classic developmental mechanism, known as signal transduction, a growth factor (ligand) undergoes binding at its specific cell surface receptor. Once bound to the cell membrane receptor, signal transduction occurs such that a 'second messenger' is produced within the cell. Following a cascade of events, the genome within the cell's nucleus is activated such that the cell undergoes a specific change, for example, differentiation. In this case, a non-specific stem cell has changed into a specific, identifiable cell type. In other words, the process of cytodifferentiation has been completed. Historically, the first sites of bone formation were described as naturally occurring 'ossification centers' during development. It is now plausible to suggest that stem cells at these sites undergo ligand binding and signal transduction due to temporo-spatial patterning, to produce bone tissue *de novo*. If several different cell lines are produced in an integrated and coordinated fashion, a specific tissue may be produced, such as oral mucosa, the periodontium etc., in a process termed histodifferentiation. The above change in specificity and increase in tissue mass may be visible with the naked eye. For example, during the formation of the human palate, the left and right palatal shelves change their orientation from a vertical to a horizontal position so that they can fuse together in the midline, forming the definitive palate through a process called morphogenesis. The morphogenetic changes are induced by mesenchymal cells within each palatal shelf that undergo differentiation to become embryonic connective tissue cells and produce hyaluronan (hyaluronic acid or hyaluronate), a hydrophilic macromolecule that binds water (Singh *et al.*, 1994). As a result, the extracellular spaces within the shelf undergo expansion, and it is thought that this turgor pressure changes the shelf orientation from a vertical to a horizontal position. Note that this developmental palatal expansion is different from the dento-alveolar effects following clinical 'palatal expansion' treatments. As well, differentiation is highly regulated. For example, similar tissues in very close proximity can undergo different developmental fates, depending on signaling. During palate formation, for example, epithelial cells on the upper (nasal) surface of the hard palate

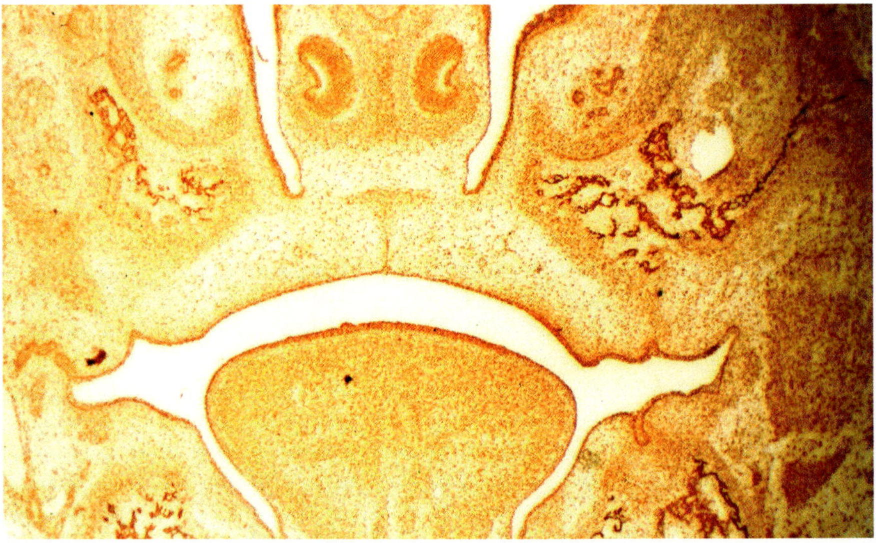

Figure 14: Different developmental fates of embryonic oral epithelium.

differentiate to form respiratory mucosa with ciliated columnar cells and goblet cells (Fig. 14). On the lower (oral) surface, these very same epithelial cells receive a different signal and differentiate to form stratified, keratinized oral mucosa. Even more interesting is that the epithelial cells in the midline are genetically programmed to undergo cell death, through a process called 'apoptosis'.

By removing the midline epithelia, the mesenchyme of the left and right palatal shelves can fuse together to form the definitive palate. In the absence of shelf fusion, a cleft palate is formed (Singh *et al.*, 1997). Thus, even though adjoining cells are separated by distances measured in μm, their developmental fate can be remarkably different (Singh *et al.*, 1998). The developmental mechanism of apoptosis can also be used to explain the persistence of fistulae after cleft palate repair; since the displaced epithelial cells enclosing the fistula are genetically encoded to produce a free, epithelialized surface, a fistula is formed. Moreover, the palatal mesenchymal cells enclosed within the surface epithelia discussed above can differentiate to form bone of the hard palate or muscles of the soft palate, depending on the signals received. In addition, specific sites within the hard palate undergo differential signaling, forming sutures in the midline, which remain as sites where further osteogenesis can occur in later life, as discussed above. Thus, it appears at first sight that gene expression determines the phenotypic outcome, the so-called genomic or genetic thesis.

The genetic thesis

Put simply, the genomic thesis, according to Darwinian thought, asserts that the genotype determines the phenotype. Conversely, the epigenetic antithesis contends that a phenotype can be changed without altering the underlying DNA sequence. It is well known that genetic inheritance has a strong influence on facial features since children look like their parents. Therefore, jaw shape and size can predispose children to malocclusions through growth, and it's known that malocclusions can run in families e.g. the Hapsburg jaw of the Austro-German-Spanish royal families, as noted above. The genes responsible for these features are found in the human genome and contained within 46 XY chromosomes, with the XY combination determining the gender of the individual. Molecular genetics is very sophisticated technology that is used to decipher the genetic code or base pair sequence. Put simply, human DNA is contained within the nucleus of the cell and consists of a double helix sugar-phosphate backbone, containing base pairs joined together by hydrogen bonds. This DNA can undergo replication. In this case, an enzyme (helicase) is used to unwind the double helix. Free nucleotides then base pair to the original polynucleotides since adenine binds with thymine and guanine binds with cytosine. Another enzyme, DNA polymerase, re-joins the sugar-phosphate backbone, producing two new double helices, each containing one of the original polynucleotides. For gene identification, the first step is to collect a sample of messenger RNA (mRNA), which is a single-stranded, complimentary copy of the DNA. Starting with as little as 5ng of mRNA from the experimental sample, the isolated sample is denatured with an enzyme, called DNAase. Next another enzyme called reverse transcriptase is used to generate cDNA (a complimentary copy of the mRNA). The amount of cDNA will also be very small, so the amount needs to be amplified. This amplification is achieved by using a technique called polymerase chain reaction (PCR), which produces sufficient cDNA for gene identification. The cDNA to be amplified is heated to separate the strands and attach primers. Once replication has been completed, the DNA is denatured again, and the procedure is repeated. After 30 cycles, approx. 1 billion identical molecules are produced for gene identification. Using these molecular genetic techniques, approx. 99.9% of human genome has been sequenced to date. In terms of evolutionary history, it is estimated that it took about 7,000-50,000 years for dark-skinned early humans to develop light skin to permit vitamin D metabolism as they migrated away from the equator, according to the 'Out of Africa' theory of human evolution. These genes include candidates such as MC1R, SLC24A5, MFSD12, DDB1, TMEM138, OCA2 and HERC2 (Crawford *et al.*, 2017) although conditions such as vitiligo suggest that the genetic history of skin pigmentation is more complex than previously understood. It is now thought that there are about 25,000 genes in the human genome, and certain regions, which have been highly conserved during evolution are, therefore, homologous. For example, the homeobox genes encode for facial features. Thus, a homeobox gene that produces tooth enamel in a mouse, likely produces enamel in a monkey and also in humans. Table 1 summarizes some genes involved in craniofacial development, including functional gene groupings in skeletal development such as: bone mineralization; cartilage condensation; ossification; osteoclast differentiation; bone mineral metabolism; calcium ion homeostasis; cell growth and differentiation; regulation of the cell cycle, cell proliferation, and cell differentiation. But not all genes function equally, leading to the concept of 'Hub' genes. Inactivation of these highly connected hub genes can enhance phenotypic changes caused by alterations of many different

Gene symbol	Function
CHRDL1 (chordin like 1)	Proposed to modulate the bone morphogenetic protein (BMP) signaling pathway during formation of the neural plate. Chicken CHRDL1 is an antagonist of BMP-4.
POSTN (periostin)	Cell adhesion protein, mediator of TGF-β in new bone formation. Has been shown to be regulated by Twist1.
IL7 (interleukin 7)	IL-7 may act on T-cells to produce RANKL, which leads to increased bone resorption via induced osteoclastogenesis. Plays an essential role in lymphoid cell survival.
COL15A1 (collagen type XV, α1)	Adheres basement membranes to underlying connective tissues.
COL27A1 (collagen type XXVII, α1)	Major structural elements in extracellular matrices of cartilage, skin, and tendon.
PGF (VEGF-related protein)	Placental growth factor (PGF). Paracrine role for mesenchymal stem cell-derived PGF in the angiogenesis and hematopoiesis that accompany BMP-2-induced bone formation.
VEGF (vascular endothelial growth factor, PDGF family)	Involved in vasculogenesis and also hypertrophic cartilage remodeling, ossification and angiogenesis during endochondral bone formation.
THBS1 (Thrombospondin 1)	Adhesive glycoprotein that mediates cell-to-cell and cell-to-matrix interactions. Involved in TGF signaling.
LIF (Leukemia inhibitory factor)	Induces terminal differentiation in leukemic cells, hematopoietic differentiation in normal and myeloid leukemia cells, neuronal cell differentiation, and stimulation of acute-phase protein synthesis in hepatocytes. Involved in TGF signaling.
RUNX3 (Runt-related transcription factor 3)	Drosophila Runt pair rule-related transcription factor 3 homolog, expressed in various lymphoid and myeloid cells, involved in hematopoiesis and osteogenesis. Involved in TGF signaling.
IL8 (Interleukin 8)	Chemoattractant, and potent angiogenic factor. Implicated as a potent activator of the bone destruction common in metastatic bone disease.
CCL20 (Chemokine, C-C motif, ligand 20)	Also known as MIP-3α. MIP-3α has the ability to stimulate odontoblast differentiation in addition to its more traditional role in inflammation.
TNFAIP6 (Tumor necrosis factor, α-induced protein 6)	Secretory protein that contains a hyaluronan-binding domain, known to be involved in extracellular matrix stability and cell migration. Regulated by TNF, associated with inflammation.
IL1RN (Interleukin 1 receptor antagonist)	Inhibits the activities of interleukin 1α and β. Associated with increased risk of osteoporotic fractures and gastric cancer.
IL24 (Interleukin 24)	Induced during terminal differentiation in melanoma cells. Induces apoptosis.

Table 1: Summary of some functional genomics.

pathways and/or mutations of many genes. Hub genes encode chromatin regulators, and their activity appears to be conserved (Lehner *et al.*, 2006).

Basically, the essential role of a gene is to produce a protein. This protein is often part of a complex biochemical pathway, and that pathway is a part of a sophisticated physiologic process, which is, therefore, dependent on proper gene expression. Consider a dormant gene that receives a signal and starts to function. The first step is gene transcription within the nucleus of the cell, leading to the formation of messenger RNA (mRNA). The mRNA leaves the nucleus and, in the cytoplasm of the cell, can lead to the formation of growth factors, which are peptides, polypeptides or proteins that act as cytochemical signals. The study of these vast array of proteins is called proteomics. Note that the original mRNA that left the nucleus requires further processing. The mature form of an RNA molecule is a nucleic acid sequence that is called an exon, after portions of a precursor RNA (introns) have either been removed by cis-splicing or when precursor RNA molecules are ligated by trans-splicing. The growth factors resulting from this exon, for example BMP, EGF, FGF, TGF-1, TGF-β3, etc. attach to specific cell membrane receptors (e.g. FGF-R), referred to as ligand-binding. The (stem) cell then undergoes signal transduction (or the second messenger effect), often leading to cell differentiation and the biosynthesis of new tissues (Maxim *et al.*, 2015). In other words, growth factors bind to cells expressing specific receptors, and through a cascade of intracellular biochemical signaling events, they elicit numerous cellular responses, such as: cell division; cell differentiation; angiogenesis; apoptosis (programmed cell death), and the production of extracellular matrix components, etc. as noted above.

Consider the mechanism of action of BMP-2. This cytokine is sometimes added to surgical sites e.g. dental implants. Here, it acts in a chemotactic manner, attracting mesenchymal stem cells and other bone-forming cells to the site of the implant. It also has a proliferative effect by providing an environment where stem cells multiply prior to differentiation. The mechanism of action of BMP-2 also includes differentiation. In this case, it binds to specific receptors on stem cells causing them to change into osteoblasts, which subsequently results in bone formation. Indeed, osteoblasts respond to local mechanical forces to produce new mineralized tissue, and new blood vessel formation also occurs in addition to remodeling, as the body continues to remodel bone in response to the local environment and mechanical forces. Thus, in BMP signaling, signal transduction occurs whereby BMP first attaches to the cell membrane receptor (BMPR-1). Within the cytoplasm, a second messenger (smad4) forms a complex (with smad1). This smad complex activates the expression of BMP target genes through interactions with transcriptional factors (OAZ). In other words, the smad complex translocates into the nucleus and initiates co-activators (OAZ), which can upregulate target genes (Luo, 2003). The reverse is also possible such that an activated gene can be downregulated or switched off. Ito *et al.* (2002) described negative regulation in TGF-β signaling. Here TGF-β binds to the cell membrane receptor (TBR-1) and within the cytoplasm, a second messenger (smad2) translocates into the nucleus and forms a co-repressor (ski). Thus, the activity of smad complexes can be modulated by interaction with nuclear co-repressors. In turn these complexes act as negative regulators for TGF-β responsive genes. In addition to gene modulation by up- and down-regulation, alternative splicing of a gene (e.g. IGF-1) can produce a different protein signal (e.g. mechano-growth factor; MGF). Alternative splicing is a regulated process during gene expression that results in a single gene coding for multiple proteins. In this process, particular exons of a gene may be included or excluded from the final processed mRNA produced from that gene. Consequently, the proteins translated from alternatively spliced mRNAs will show differences in their amino acid sequence and, often, in their biological functions. Alternative splicing allows the human genome to direct the synthesis of many more proteins than would be expected from its 20,000 protein-coding genes. One way of controlling alternative splicing is through the use of micro-RNA (miRNA). This miRNA is a short, non-protein-coding RNA molecule, which is found in eukaryotic cells.

It functions in RNA silencing and post-transcriptional regulation of gene expression. The human genome may encode over 1000 miRNAs that may, in turn, target about 60% of mammalian genes.

Genetic mutations

In normal genetic inheritance, the usual number of chromosomes is inherited, but there are some rare genetic mutations; abnormalities in the number of chromosomes are known as aneuploidy. For example, in autosomal trisomy, non-disjunction meiosis occurs during gametogenesis (in the father or mother), and the offspring possesses three sets of a particular chromosome. A neonate with Trisomy 13 syndrome has three copies of chromosome 13 with its attendant genes. These additional genes disrupt the normal sequence of temporo-spatial patterning, precipitating bilateral cleft lip/palate, omphalocele and polydactyly in this particular syndrome. Apart from chromosomal abnormalities, specific mutated genes can also be inherited. These genetic mutations include: single-nucleotide polymorphisms; deletions; insertions; amplifications, and translocations. These offspring may be heterozygotes, carrying only one mutated gene from either the father or mother or they may be homozygotes, carrying two copies of the mutated gene for that particular condition. In a group of conditions, called craniosynostoses, the craniofacial sutures are unable to respond to environmental stimuli because the inheritance of a mutated gene renders the cell membrane receptors (e.g. FGF-R) non-functional. This means that signal transduction does not proceed normally, and since the sutures are synostosed (fused) they are unable to produce bone. Abnormalities due to premature fusion of sutures produce specific syndromes e.g. Apert syndrome, Crouzon's syndrome, etc. depending on the specific gene mutation.

In very rare circumstances duplication of craniofacial components, perhaps due to mutation of the Hoxa-2 gene have been reported (Sjamsudin *et al.*, 2001). Gene expression can be investigated using whole mount in situ hybridization. In Fig. 15, 3H1 Br mice were outcrossed to Balb mice to

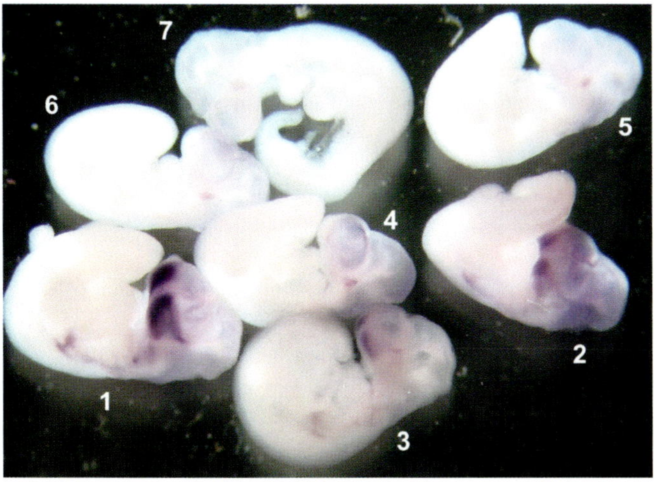

Figure 15: Whole mount in situ hybridization in embryonic mice. The dark-staining (1, 2) indicates the homozygotes for the mutated Br gene; pale-staining (3, 4) indicates heterozygotes, and no staining (5-7) indicates normal littermates. Courtesy: Dr Scott Lozanoff.

facilitate genotyping using D17Mit76. This marker separates 3H1 and Balb alleles based on a 60 base-pair difference, so genotyping is more easily performed using standard PCR methods. The Br gene mutation is associated with the brachyrrhine (short face) phenotype that can predispose to other craniofacial anomalies, such as cleft lip and/or palate. In another clinical example, Frazier-Bowers *et al.* (2010) reported that primary failure of eruption (PFE) of permanent teeth in the absence of mechanical obstruction is also associated with gene mutations. Specifically, PFE segregated with a novel mutation of the PTH1-R gene. A heterozygous c.1353-1 G>A sequence alteration caused a putative splice-site mutation and skipping of exon 15 that segregated with the PFE phenotype. Therefore, a PTH1-R mutation is associated with unerupted, ankylosed teeth and failure of orthodontically-assisted tooth eruption or tooth movement.

Note that the above discussion centered around the natural inheritance of specific genes. Advances in molecular genetic technologies, however, have permitted the modulation of genes being transmitted from one generation to the next. The most well-known example of genetic engineering is transgenics. In this procedure, a gene sequence that has been isolated from one organism is introduced into the genome of a different species, using a vector. For example, an insect gene can be transferred into a plant genome, using a virus as a vector. This non-native segment of DNA may either retain its ability to produce mRNA/proteins in the transgenic organism or alter the normal function of the transgenic organism's genetic code. In this way, the foreign gene may confer additional benefits to the recipient, such as being resistant to certain diseases. Genetic modification can also be accomplished by injecting foreign DNA into the nucleus of a fertilized ovum. This technique is routinely used to introduce human disease-causing genes (e.g. the gene for cystic fibrosis) into laboratory mice to study the function or pathology associated with that particular gene. The 'transgene' requires various components in order to function, such as: a promoter, which is a regulatory sequence that will determine where and when the transgene is active; an exon, a protein-coding sequence, and a stop sequence. These components are typically combined in a bacterial plasmid. Transgenic or genetically modified organisms (GMOs), be they bacteria, viruses or fungi, serve all kinds of purposes. Transgenic plants, fish and mammals have also been bred, some for human consumption. Transgenic (GMO) plants, such as corn and soybean, have even replaced wild strains in some countries (e.g. the United States). Note that GMO crops can escape and thus pose ethical questions, since they may potentially cause biosafety problems either now or at some point in the future.

Yet another technique of gene manipulation is known as CRISPR. CRISPR is an abbreviation for Clustered Regularly Interspaced Short Palindromic Repeats. Originally, CRISPRs were described as segments of prokaryotic DNA containing short, repetitive base sequences. In a palindromic repeat, the sequence of nucleotides is the same in both directions. CRISPR is a family of DNA sequences in bacteria, etc. that contain snippets of DNA from viruses that have attacked the prokaryote. These snippets are used by the prokaryote to detect and destroy DNA from similar viruses during subsequent attacks. Currently, these sequences also form the basis of a genetic technique known as CRISPR/Cas9 that effectively and specifically changes genes within organisms. The RNA harboring the sequence helps Cas (CRISPR-associated) proteins recognize and cut exogenous DNA since Cas is a nuclease (enzyme) that cleaves the chains of nucleotides in nucleic acids. Therefore, the CRISPR/Cas technique can be used for experimental and perhaps therapeutic "gene editing". In fact, a version of the CRISPR/Cas system, CRISPR/Cas9, has been modified to edit human genomes. By delivering the Cas9 nuclease complexed with a synthetic guide RNA (gRNA) into a cell, the cell's genome can be cut at a desired location, allowing existing genes to be deleted and/or new ones inserted. In this way, a mutated gene can be deleted from an individual's genome and the genetic defect can be prevented. In addition, if the mutated gene is deleted from an individual's germline (the cells that pass on genetic material to the progeny through cells that form the future ova, sperm cells, etc.), the defect would be eliminated from being inherited in future generations. Therefore, CRISPR/Cas genome editing techniques have many potential applications, but bioethical concerns have been raised about the prospect of using CRISPR to yield a specific, desired phenotype as well as germline editing.

The epigenetic antithesis

Epigenetics is the study of phenotypic changes that occur via mechanisms that do not change the DNA sequence (Spivakov and Fisher, 2007), unlike the genetic mechanisms discussed above. Epigenetics helps clarify how genomes work; it addresses complex biological systems, such as the plasticity of our genome, and how cells that carry the same genome express different genes at different times. It is now considered that combinations of heritable and environmental factors, including behavior, lead to altered gene expression, which can yield modified structural and functional phenotypes. More specifically, human DNA is wrapped around proteins called histones. Both the DNA and histones are covered with chemical 'tags', and this second layer of the genetic structure is called the epigenome. While the human genome was sequenced in 2003, researchers in molecular genetics are now working on a mapping of the human epigenome (Novik *et al.*, 2002). They are beginning to understand the complex system of switches that regulates gene expression, and these discoveries will likely lead to a better understanding of diseases and novel ways to treat or cure them. It is understood that epigenetic changes are mediated by covalent attachments of chemical groups of the DNA and its associated proteins, histones and chromatin. Indeed, it is now believed that the epigenome shapes the physical structure of the genome and is capable of activating the genome. In effect, reactive genes are exposed and become accessible through epigenetic tags that can respond to various signals from the external environment. Subsequently, the types of epigenetic modification include biochemical reactions, such as methylation, ribosylation, acetylation, phosphorylation, sumoylation and ubiquitination, leading to histone modification, non-coding RNAs (including microRNAs), and RNA editing (Spivakov and Fisher, 2007). For instance, genes can be silenced by the environmental (dietary) addition of methyl groups. This biochemical reaction is called DNA methylation and it is a well-studied molecular epigenetic phenomenon. For example, Weaver *et al.* (2004) studied attentive and inattentive mother mice as they raised their pups. Later, the hippocampus region of the brains of the grown pups were examined. It was found that in pups raised by attentive mothers, the genes were highly methylated. On the other hand, in pups raised by inattentive mothers, the genes were rarely methylated. In the next part of the study, the pups of attentive and inattentive mothers were switched, so that the mothers raised foster pups. Again, the hippocampus region of the brains of the grown foster pups was examined. It was found that the foster pups raised by an attentive mother had genes that were highly methylated; while foster pups raised by an inattentive mother rarely had methylated genes. In the final part of the study, an attentive mother raised her own pups, but these pups were treated with trichostatin A, a drug that removes methyl groups. It was found that the epigenetic changes disappeared, and the genes were rarely methylated. Thus, the biochemical environment of a gene may cause reversible silencing marks or tags on the DNA, and while we cannot easily alter the genome, the epigenome is amenable to changes. In effect, phenotypic variation can occur without altering the genotype, the antithesis of Darwinian thought.

If the above is true, then the same genes can, in effect, produce different outcomes. This idea can be tested clinically in monozygotic (identical) twins. Studies show that varying epigenetic tags makes twins differ, especially as they age. In fact, although identical twins are born with the same DNA, they can become surprisingly different as they grow older. Factors such as stress and nutrition cause this divergence by changing how individual genes behave (Miller, 2012). Thus, epigenetic tags are biochemical mechanisms that can activate or suppress genes by different degrees. Although these tags do not change the DNA, it is thought that tags can be inherited. In addition, random epigenetic shifts may also occur without any external influence. Over a period of time, the variation in epigenetic tags makes the twins more different than they were at the outset. In fact, recent studies suggest that homozygotic twins can be discordant for sleep disordered breathing (SDB) since preliminary imaging studies show morphologic differences of the upper airway. Because of these types of findings, it is now being more widely accepted that environmental influences may change gene expression. In earlier studies, gene-environmental interactions were investigated to understand the epigenetic effects of nutrition. Genetically-identical, pregnant Agouti mice were fed with or without folate. It was found that maternal methyl donor supplementation during pregnancy changed the coat-color of the offspring from yellow to brown, and reduced the incidence of obesity, diabetes and cancer. Therefore, genetically identical mice can produce phenotypic variations through gene-environmental interactions or epigenetic mechanisms (Dolinoy *et al.*, 2006). More recently, Parsons *et al.* (2015) investigated genetic manipulation of cranial base growth

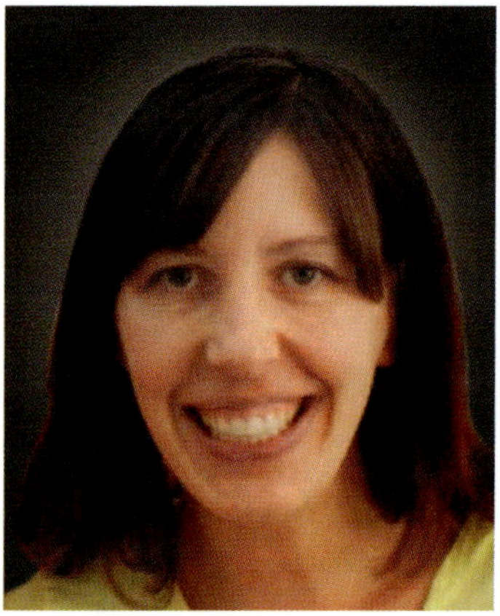

Figure 16a: Adenoid facies persisting in an adult.
Courtesy: Dr Jon Caulfield

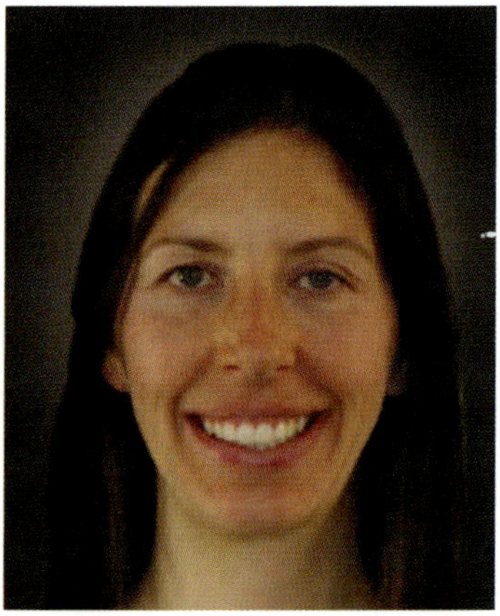

Figure 16b: Post-treatment appearance after biomimetic oral appliance therapy.

and reported that it modulates calvarial and facial shape in mice through epigenetic interactions. In that study, they disturbed the cartilaginous genes of the chondrocranium during development and found that it produced shape changes in the adult calvarium and face in mice, even though those genes were unaffected by the perturbation. Recognizable changes in facial features are sometimes referred to as 'facies'. Most people can recognize the facies of Down syndrome (Trisomy 21), where non-disjunction of chromosome 21 leads to the characteristic facial features, which may in fact represent a cranial base anomaly, as well as mild mental retardation in these cases. Thus, epigenetic changes in facial features have been described in the medical literature, and these include other examples such as fetal alcohol syndrome and 'adenoid facies'. Adenoid facies are sometimes called long face syndrome. Interestingly, these cases typically show no genetic mutations. Instead, features such as mouth-breathing, 'gummy smile' and nasal obstruction are often present (Fig. 16a). Therefore, adenoid facies most likely represent epigenetic changes in childhood facial features that persist through adulthood unless active intervention is provided (Fig. 16b).

It is clear that during pediatric development epigenetic mechanisms are at work through molecular compensations. These molecular compensations can produce recognizable clinical phenotypes or presentations. For example, the perinatal period of childhood development is characterized by the development of the biofilm and the microbiome of the infant. Simultaneously, changes in child-rearing practices may have inadvertently precipitated conditions such as deformational (positional) plagiocephaly. In terms of etiology, it can be considered that current medical advice is to put babies to sleep on the back with nothing in crib in an effort to prevent sudden infant death syndrome (SIDS). While this objective can largely be achieved, it is sometimes at the cost of producing deformational (positional) plagiocephaly. Since the developing cranium represents a spatial matrix, developmental events unfold as epigenetic, gene-environmental interactions proceed. Therefore, these children may show craniofacial developmental compensation, such as deformational plagiocephaly, crowding of the developing teeth, etc. In fact, López del Valle *et al.* (2006) reported an association between child-rearing practices (breastfeeding) and malocclusion in young children. By age 5yrs., nearly 60% of Puerto Rican children who were studied were insufficiently breastfeed and showed signs of malocclusion. The mechanisms of epigenetic phenomena are not always apparent, however. One study investigated benzyl butyl phthalate (BBP) regulation of the mesenchymal stem cell epigenome, and its effect on adipogenesis in neonates. It was found that BBP exposure enhanced lipid accumulation and adipogenesis in a dose-dependent manner compared to controls. Therefore, by simply bottle-feeding babies with plastic bottles, the risk of childhood obesity might be increased by BBP tipping the epigenomic balance towards adipogenesis (Sonkar *et al.*, 2016). On the other hand, breastfeeding duration is related to methylation of the leptin gene that, in turn, plays a role in the child's lifetime risk of obesity. Leptin is an appetite-suppressing hormone, and Obermann-Borst *et al.* (2013) reported that the duration of breastfeeding is associated with methylation of the leptin gene in young children. Therefore, breastfeeding can have a beneficial, epigenetic effect on children above and beyond craniofacial development. But note that another dietary problem associated with obesity is leptin resistance. In this case, increased calorific intake leads to weight gain. This weight gain means that the number and/

or size of fat cells increases, as do leptin levels. However, increased fat stores and whole-body inflammation lead to the development of leptin resistance. Despite the fact that there is abundant stored fat and leptin, the signal to the brain is disrupted and the brain senses low leptin levels, leading to food cravings and overeating; thus, the vicious cycle is repeated. One way to break this cycle of events is to "re-set" leptin sensitivity by finding a nutritional balance that is appropriate for that individual (Masley, 2014; Lin, 2019). On the other hand, an inflammatory diet of fast food/junk food/soda, etc. can lead to food allergies, eczema, nasal obstruction/rhino-sinusitis, adenoidal hypertrophy, asthma, etc. mediated through various mechanisms, including disruption of the microbiome and increased systemic inflammation. Interestingly, some pediatric cases of nasal obstruction/rhino-sinusitis, including adenoidal hypertrophy, appear to respond well to biomimetic oral appliance therapy (Singh *et al.*, 2016; Hwang *et al.*, 2019). Fig. 17a shows maxillary sinus congestion in an 8-year old girl, and Fig. 17b shows clinical changes achieved without any surgical or pharmaceutical interventions.

In view of these findings, additional questions arise, such as: How can (renewed) growth and development be achieved? What are the craniofacial effects in adults following epigenetic treatments? What

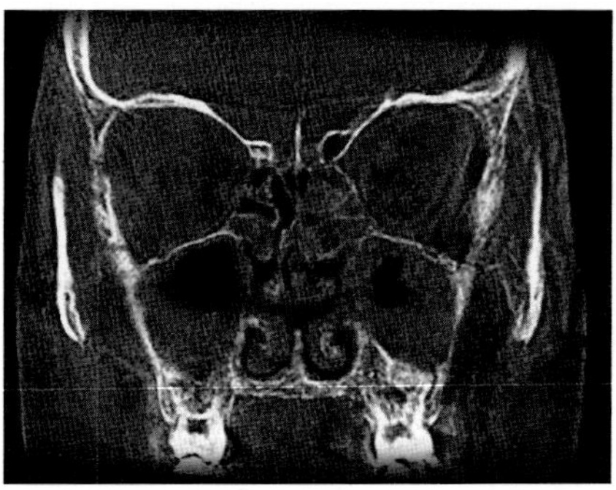

Figure 17a: Pre-treatment appearance showing bilateral congestion of the maxillary sinuses. Courtesy: Dr Hwasub Hwang and Dr Charin Hwang

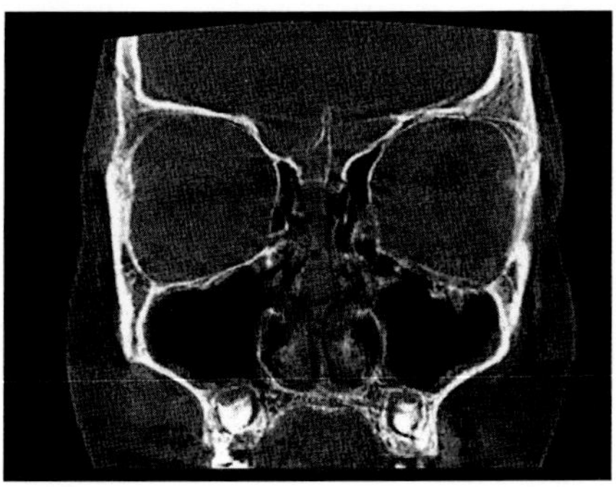

Figure 17b: Post-treatment clinical improvement in maxillary sinus congestion following biomimetic oral appliance therapy in the same patient.

are the underlying developmental mechanisms? Some of the answers come from the work of Fuentes *et al.* (2003). In a study on rats, an oral device was fitted that postured the mandible in lateral excursion. On the protruded and non-protruded sides, gene expression of insulin-like growth factor-1 (Igf-1), fibroblast growth factor-2 (Fgf-2), and their receptors (Igf-1r, Fgfr1, Fgfr2 and Fgfr3) were studied. It was reported that the expression of Igf-1, Fgf-2 and Igf-1r were altered. For example, after three days of wearing the oral device, Igf-1 and Fgf-2 were over-expressed on the protruded side compared to controls, while Fgf-1r was switched off. While no consistent pattern was identified, it was concluded that changing the mandible's spatial position is associated with changes in gene expression. Similarly, biomimetic oral appliances change the spatial relations of the jaws and teeth clinically. In so doing, the altered pattern of gene expression might re-activate the mechanisms of sutural homeostasis, and it is postulated that renewed pneumatization can be achieved. In fact, some preliminary data (Table 2) appears to support this contention.

Since genes are subject to temporo-spatial patterning, by changing the environment (spatial orientation, nutrition, disease, trauma, drugs, function, behavior, exercises, etc.), it may be possible to change a Class I phenotype to a Class III or a Class II phenotype to a Class I clinically. If so, craniofacial epigenetics might prove to be a very powerful technique since it can putatively harness genetic potential without using surgery or pharmaceutical drugs.

Introduction to the spatial matrix hypothesis

Early investigations of the effect of changing spatial relations on craniofacial growth and development were first carried out by Kingsley (1880) who introduced the concept of "jumping the bite" for patients with a retrognathic mandible. Later, Breitner (1930), Häupl and Psansky (1938), Hoffer and Colico (1958), Baume and Derichsweiler (1961), Joho (1968), and Stöckli

	Left		Right	
Subject	**Pre-Tx**	**Post-Tx**	**Pre-Tx**	**Post-Tx**
1	20.99	21.82	21.80	26.73
2	13.89	14.45	12.23	12.58
3	22.09	21.82	20.69	15.89
4	12.54	13.50	12.16	12.19
5	22.50	25.28	21.13	23.16
6	16.35	19.39	17.29	19.07
7	31.38	32.72	31.25	32.66
8	28.24	28.68	22.17	22.53
9	21.39	22.52	23.68	25.83
10	15.27	16.01	17.10	17.04
11	13.19	15.40	15.89	18.16
12	26.64	26.08	22.12	22.43
13	8.56	14.77	8.57	13.31
14	11.77	13.02	13.42	14.76
Mean	**18.8**	**20.1**	**18.5**	**19.7**
Std. Dev	6.5	6.1	5.7	5.8
p value		**0.03**		**0.04**

Table 2: Changes in adult maxillary sinus volume (cm^3) demonstrating enhanced pneumatization after 15.5 months. Pre-Tx = Pre-treatment. Post-Tx = Post-treatment.

and Willert (1971) did similar studies. Most of these experimental studies on 'functional' mandibular protrusion were done on Rhesus macaques, and later McNamara and Carlson (1979) quantified adaptations of the TMJ in mandibular protrusion. McNamara and Bryan (1987) also described long-term mandibular adaptations to protrusion in Rhesus monkeys, which indicated that the mandibular length increased by approx. 7mm in the protrusive group compared to controls after nearly 3 yrs. These findings indicated that the mandible did not grow to a genetically pre-determined length, supporting the spatial matrix hypothesis, and appear to follow the developmental mechanisms reported by Fuentes *et al.* (2013). Earlier, Singh and Clark (2001) localized changes at the condylar cartilage after mandibular advancement device use in children and teenagers. In pubertal boys, we found a 28% increase in condylar length, similar to the reports of studies on Rhesus macaques. These types of findings lead me to suggest that 'functional' appliances may actually be 'formational appliances' (Singh, 2009), in the sense that bone and other tissues are being formed in response to the change in spatial relations of the jaws and teeth. Moreover, these correlations of form and function are also supported by the work of Williams and Murphy (2008), although Singh (2004) first captured the concept of how spatial changes might invoke gene expression. According to the Spatial Matrix Hypothesis (Singh, 2004), changing the bite affects the spatial relations of the teeth, which lose their normal occlusal contacts and thus are no longer in homeostasis. These spatial changes are detected by mechanoreceptors in the periodontium and periosteal cells. Consequently, remodeling occurs due to signal transduction, as predicted by the Spatial Matrix Hypothesis (Singh, 2004; Singh, 2007; Singh and Krumholtz, 2009) in an effort to regain (sutural) homeostasis.

Systemic examples of homeostasis include blood pressure maintenance, body temperature regulation, etc. These systems are subject to physiologic control through sophisticated feedback loops. Similarly, the craniofacial region is under spatial and functional regulation. However, the craniofacial region is also subject to developmental compensation, which differs quantitatively and qualitatively according to genomic variation from patient to patient. Because of complexity, therefore, patients may present with a range of clinical signs and symptoms associated with developmental compensation, such as: TMD, UARS/OSA, malocclusions, facial asymmetry, tooth wear/bruxism, headaches, orofacial pain, etc. even though the underlying etiology may be similar in most cases, most of the time. Since craniofacial epigenetics is aimed at the overall health of the craniofacial region, appropriate treatment protocols must be provided that address the underlying etiology of the signs and symptoms of these conditions. Therefore, despite these phenotypic variations, the outcomes of all of these epigenetic processes require clinical decompensation prior to final correction. This decompensation is often achieved surgically but can also be addressed through appropriate spatial signaling, which can help re-establish (genomic) pattern formation for optimal form and function (Singh, 2004, 2007; Singh and Krumholtz, 2009). Thus, craniofacial epigenetics deploys a person's natural genes to correct the jaws, teeth, soft tissues and functional spaces, painlessly, using biomimetic oral appliances.

The Spatial Matrix Hypothesis differs from Moss' old Functional Matrix Hypothesis, which taught that the facial skeleton (maxilla and mandible) is formed mainly by ossification within genic membranes (such as osteogenic periostea and osteogenic perichondria). Moss argued that its form was largely secondary and adaptive to surrounding soft tissues and functional spaces. Here is the first point of divergence from the Spatial Matrix Hypothesis (Singh, 2004) since dental tissues (teeth) have been omitted from the old Functional Matrix Hypothesis. I contend that a spatial matrix is an arena in which development events unfold as gene-environmental interactions proceed e.g. the developmental dynamics of the orofacial complex. The old Functional Matrix Hypothesis was based on functional changes to some extent. For example, if a tooth is lost (through extraction) then loss of alveolar bone ensues since local bone is no longer required to accommodate that tooth in the jaw. While this example holds true in clinical practice, it does not comprehensively describe how the craniofacial region attains homeostasis thereafter. Consider loss of an upper molar tooth, say second or third maxillary molar. In these cases, it is often noted that the maxillary air sinus expands into the alveolar region (Fig. 18a). Sometimes, an opposing tooth (over)erupts into the vacated space (Fig. 18b), and the tongue learns to avoid those new occlusal contacts to avoid trauma during function. In other words, the Spatial Matrix hypothesis takes all four craniofacial components (hard tissues, bone: soft tissues, muscle: dental tissues, teeth; and functional spaces, sinuses) into account with a unifying principle; craniofacial homeostasis.

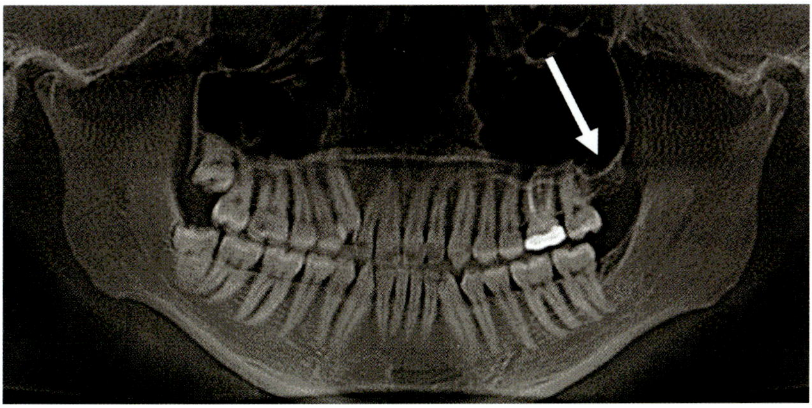

Figure 18a: Maxillary air sinus has pneumatized into extraction space of upper left third molar (arrow).

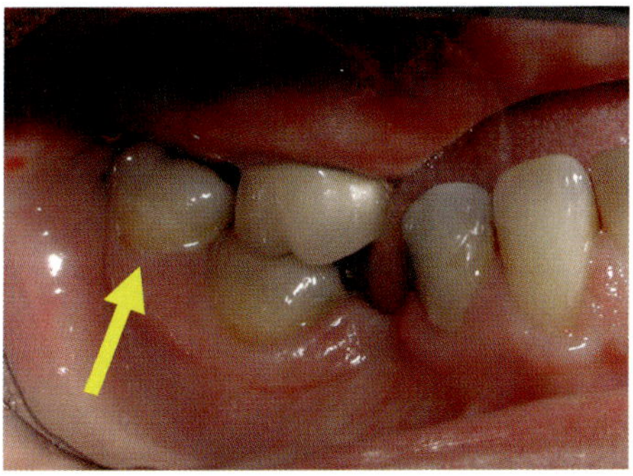

Figure 18b: Lower second molar supra-erupted into extraction space of upper second molar, leading to a new level of homeostasis.

On the other hand, the old Functional Matrix Hypothesis simply stated that during growth, spatial and functional alignment of skeletal elements (maxilla and mandible) is maintained through remodeling of bony surfaces (cortical bone remodeling). This statement omits the dental tissues (teeth) that are intimately and uniquely associated with the maxilla and mandible. Conversely, the Spatial Matrix Hypothesis teaches that sutural homeostasis is a craniofacial requirement, and this may be associated with pneumatization of (new) functional spaces (Fig. 18a). The Functional Matrix Hypothesis also taught that 'ossification centers' arise during growth but at the time of its formulation (Moss and Young, 1960) there was little or no information on how they arise. It is now known that these ossification centers are, in fact, sites of signal transduction, based on temporo-spatial patterning. In other words, according to the genetic blueprint, certain genes will be expressed at certain sites during development. On receiving an appropriate signal, the local (stem) cells will undergo signal transduction and differentiate into osteoblasts that will lay down new (woven) bone (Williams and Murphy, 2008). Thus, ossification centers arise during development *de novo* and represent sites of signal transduction due to temporo-spatial patterning of genes within stem cell populations. In other words, during growth and development, the craniofacial sutures are gently stretched, sometimes beyond 250–400μm, which is thought to represent a biologic boundary of mammalian sutural homeostasis (Kambara, 1977), resulting in osteogenesis. The FMH correctly described how 'new' bones e.g. the calvaria, are displaced by soft tissue expansion (e.g. brain development) and the subsequent enlarged functional spaces. In this way, sutures are formed when the boundaries of two adjacent bones come into close proximity. In other words, two plates of bone meet at sutures as they grow by deposition of bone (precursor) at the sutural boundaries — but one question remained unanswered: How do they know when to stop bone formation? The most likely answer is the mechanism of sutural homeostasis; when continued bone deposition results in a sutural width of, say 100–250μm, this genetically encoded functional space results in a cessation of osteogenesis. Therefore, similar to other functional spaces in the body (e.g. synapses), the craniofacial sutures, including the periodontium, are subject to functional and spatial regulation.

Another important difference between the FMH and the Spatial Matrix Hypothesis is that during growth, spatial and functional alignment of the maxilla and mandible is maintained through remodeling of bony surfaces, including the periodontium, to permit function. Here, using the Spatial Matrix Hypothesis, dental tissues are included in the equation, perhaps for the first time. Teeth are important craniofacial structures in many regards. While their spatial arrangement permits activities such as mastication, speech and swallowing, they may have other functions, such as load distribution to protect the large and fragile human brain from (micro)trauma. While the calavaria adapt to house the expanding brain, as discussed above, the teeth erupt through the bone and their final positions are dictated, to a greater of lesser extent, by a combination sutural homeostasis and cusp-fossa relationships. During this eruptive phase, the maxillary teeth determine the extent of nasomaxillary pneumatization, and this part of the upper airway provides essential components for gas exchange and oxygenation of the tissues further distally in the lower airway. Specifically, the pneumocytes that line the paranasal air sinus produce nitric oxide (NO) (Lundberg *et al.*, 1995) and NO is a small vessel dilator *inter alia*. Proximal to the pulmonary alveoli, smooth muscle relaxation can help with vasodilation, gas exchange and oxygenation. Therefore, perturbation of normal craniofacial development, including maxillary molar tooth eruption, can impact both the upper airway directly and the distal airway indirectly.

According to the Spatial Matrix Hypothesis, environmentally induced changes in early morphologic relationship precipitate new solutions (phenotypic variation), as depicted in Waddington's epigenetic landscape (Townsend *et al.*, 2009). Clinically, consider a child with a Class I genotype who becomes a habitual digit-sucker. Instead of have having a normal Class I occlusion, the overjet and/or overbite change to yield a Class II phenotype. In effect, there has been a departure away from the genetically encoded developmental program. Because of complexity the later clinical outcome in this particular case might be e.g. Class II malocclusion in a teenager, TMD as a young person, or OSA as an older adult. In other words, developmental compensation occurs to permit compromised function. The teeth are not well-aligned but the teenager can still eat food; the young adult can chew but gets jaw pain or headaches; the older adult can breathe but is snoring or has episodes of apnea at night. These three examples represent developmental compensation. Therefore, decompensation is required through treatment, and this is largely achieved through appropriate signaling by using a biomimetic device clinically. For example, the device is used to reposition a mandible that is retrognathic and/or increase the vertical dimension if the jaws are over-closed. Simultaneously, the device is used to widen a maxilla that is too narrow, representing a change in spatial relations, including the teeth.

During wear, biomimetic oral devices also exert ultra-light, prolonged, intermittent forces/signals on the periodontium of the associated teeth during rest and during function (such as swallowing during sleep). These ultra-light forces are detected by mechanoreceptors on the cell surfaces of the periodontal and periosteal cells. Due to signal transduction, a cascade of events is initiated, resulting in gene transcription and mRNA biosynthesis. In this way, current thought is that mechanical loading can change bony architecture by evoking bone remodeling through the action of a various molecules. Yang *et al.* (2004) noted that mechanical stress plays an essential role in bone remodeling during growth, involving matrix metalloproteinases (MMPs) such as MMP-13. In vitro, when stress was applied to osteoblasts, enzymatic activities of MMP-13 were increased significantly. Overall, it was concluded that mechanical stress induces MMP-13 expression to regulate mechanical adaptation. In addition, it appears that osteopontin plays a critical role in bone remodeling in response to mechanical loading (Fujihara *et al.*, 2006) in mice. Clinically, the midpalatal suture would be gently stretched, activating stretch-sensitive genes in the local stem cells. In turn, these stem cells would undergo signal transduction (mechanotransduction) and differentiate into osteoblasts that would lay down new bone. Hameed *et al.* (2004) studied the expression of mechano-growth factor (MGF), which is an isoform of insulin-like growth factor-I (IGF-I) in elderly men. After 5 weeks of resistance training the mRNA expression of MGF increased by approx. 160%, and when training was combined with growth hormone treatment, the MGF-mRNA increased by approx. 450%. These findings suggest that mechanical loading with or without growth hormone supplementation, can enhance MGF-mRNA levels, which likely reflect up-regulation in transcription of the IGF-I gene prior to alternative splicing. In patients, this type of response may result in remodeling (widening) of the hard palate. Thus, *de novo* bone regeneration or formation of new craniofacial tissues may offer a potential solution for diseases such as sleep disordered breathing (Maxim *et al.*, 2015), providing a basis for the spatial matrix hypothesis.

References

Baume LJ, Derichsweiler H. Is the condylar growth center responsive to orthodontic therapy? An experimental study in Macaca mulatta. *Oral Surg Oral Med Oral Pathol.* 1961;14:347–362.

Bookstein FL. Reconsidering "The inappropriateness of conventional cephalometrics". *Am J Orthod Dentofacial Orthop*. 2016;149(6):784–797.

Breitner C. Experimental change of the mesio-distal relations of the dental arches. *Angle Orthod*. 1930;67–76.

Cairns JM. The function of the ectodermal apical ridge and distinctive characteristics of adjacent distal mesoderm in the avian wing-bud. *J Embryol Exp Morphol.* 1975;34(1):155–169.

Chaplain MAJ, Singh GD, McLachlan JC (eds.). On Growth and Form: Spatio-Temporal Patterning in Biology. England: John Wiley and Sons Publishers, 1999.

Chen XX, Xia B, Ge LH, Yuan JW. Effects of breast-feeding duration, bottle-feeding duration and oral habits on the occlusal characteristics of primary dentition. Beijing Da Xue Xue Bao Yi Xue Ban. 2016;48(6):1060–1066. [Article in Chinese]

Crawford NG, Kelly DE, Hansen MEB, Beltrame MH, Fan S, Bowman SL, Jewett E, Ranciaro A, *et al.* Loci associated with skin pigmentation identified in African populations. *Science*. 2017;358(6365):eaan8433

Cribbet MR, Carlisle M, Cawthon RM, Uchino BN, Williams PG, Smith TW, Gunn HE, Light KC. Cellular aging and restorative processes: subjective sleep quality and duration moderate the association between age and telomere length in a sample of middle-aged and older adults. *Sleep*. 2014;37(1):65–70.

Dolinoy DC, Weidman JR, Waterland RA, Jirtle RL. Maternal genistein alters coat color and protects Avy mouse offspring from obesity by modifying the fetal epigenome. *Environ Health Perspect.* 2006;114(4):567–572.

Farran-Ridge C. Note on a case of premature senility (progeria). J Neurol Psychopathol. 1921;2(7):254–258.

Frazier-Bowers SA, Simmons D, Wright JT, Proffit WR, Ackerman JL. Primary failure of eruption and PTH1R: the importance of a genetic diagnosis for orthodontic treatment planning. *Am J Orthod Dentofacial Orthop.* 2010;137(2):160–161.

Fuentes MA, Opperman LA, Buschang P, Bellinger LL, Carlson DS, Hinton RJ. Lateral functional shift of the mandible: Part II. Effects on gene expression in condylar cartilage. *Am J Orthod Dentofacial Orthop.* 2003;123(2):160–166.

Fujihara S, Yokozeki M, Oba Y, Higashibata Y, Nomura S, Moriyama K. Function and regulation of osteopontin in response to mechanical stress. *J Bone Miner Res.* 2006;21(6):956–964.

Gortmaker SL, Dietz WH Jr, Cheung LW. Inactivity, diet, and the fattening of America. *J Am Diet Assoc.* 1990;90(9):1247–1252, 1255.

Del Vecchio A, Sylos-Labini F, Mondì V, Paolillo P, Ivanenko Y, Lacquaniti F, Farina D. Spinal motoneurons of the human newborn are highly synchronized during leg movements. *Science Advances* 2020; 6(47):eabc3916

Hamczyk MR, Andrés V. Vascular smooth muscle cell loss underpins the accelerated atherosclerosis in Hutchinson-Gilford progeria syndrome. *Nucleus.* 2019;10(1):28–34.

Hameed M, Lange KH, Andersen JL, Schjerling P, Kjaer M, Harridge SD, Goldspink G. The effect of recombinant human growth hormone and resistance training on IGF-I mRNA expression in the muscles of elderly men. *J Physiol.* 2004;555(1):231–240.

Häupl K, Psansky R. Histological studies on the mode of operation of the devices used in functional orthodontics. Deutsch Zahn, mund und kieferheilkunde. 1938;19;641–648.

Hettiaratchi MH, Krishnan L, Rouse T, Chou C, McDevitt TC, Guldberg RE. Heparin-mediated delivery of bone morphogenetic protein-2 improves spatial localization of bone regeneration. *Sci Adv.* 2020;6(1):eaay1240.

Hoffer O, *Colico* GL. The modifications of the TMJ consequent to mesial displacement of the jaw. *Rass Internaz Stomatol Prat. 1958*;9:27.

Huang GTJ, Thesleff (eds). Stem cells in craniofacial development and regeneration. Wiley-Blackwell, 2013.

Hwang H, Hwang C, West J, Singh GD. Changes in pediatric paranasal sinuses following biomimetic oral appliance therapy: 3 case reports. *Cranio*. 2019;2:1–6.

Ito Y, Bringas P Jr, Mogharei A, Zhao J, Deng C, Chai Y. Receptor-regulated and inhibitory Smads are critical in regulating transforming growth factor beta-mediated Meckel's cartilage development. Dev Dyn. 2002;224(1):69–78.

Joho JP. Changes in form and size of the mandible in the orthopaedically treated Macacus Irus (an experimental study). *Rep Congr Eur Orthod Soc*. 1968;44:161–173.

Kambara T. Dentofacial changes produced by extraoral forward force in the Macaca irus. *Am J Orthod.* 1977;71(3):249–277.

Kaplan RG. Induced condylar growth in a patient with hemifacial microsomia. *Angle Orthod*. 1989;59(2):85–90.

Kingsley NW. A Treatise on oral deformities as a branch of mechanical surgery. New York, 1880.

Lawrence TN, Ellis E, McNamara JA Jr. The frequency and distribution of skeletal and dental components in Class II orthognathic surgery patients. *J Oral Maxillofac Surg*. 1985;43(1):24–34.

Lehner B, Crombie C, Tischler J, Fortunato A, Fraser AG. Systematic mapping of genetic interactions in Caenorhabditis elegans identifies common modifiers of diverse signaling pathways. *Nat Genet.* 2006;38(8):896–903.

Lin S. The Dental Diet: The surprising link between your teeth, real food, and life-changing natural health. Hay House UK Limited: 2019; ISBN 978–1-7818–0930-3.

López del Valle LM, Singh GD, Feliciano N, Machuca Mdel C. Associations between a history of breast feeding, malocclusion and parafunctional habits in Puerto Rican children. *PR Health Sci J*. 2006;25(1):31–34.

Lozanoff S. Midfacial retrusion in adult brachyrrhine mice. *Acta Anat (Basel).* 1993;147(2):125–132.

Lundberg JO, Farkas-Szallasi T, Weitzberg E, Rinder J, Lidholm J, Anggåard A, Hökfelt T, Lundberg JM, Alving K. High nitric oxide production in human paranasal sinuses. *Nat Med.* 1995;1(4):370–373.

Luo K. Negative regulation of BMP signaling by the ski oncoprotein. *J Bone Joint Surg Am.* 2003;85-A Suppl 3:39–43.

Mao JJ, Nah HD. Growth and development: hereditary and mechanical modulations. *Am J Orthod Dentofacial Orthop*. 2004;125(6):676–689.

Masley S. The 30-Day Heart Tune-Up: A breakthrough medical plan to prevent and reverse heart disease. Hachette/Center Street: 2014; ISBN 978-1-4555-4713-5.

Maxim MA, Soritau O, Baciut M, Bran S, Baciut G. The role of dental stem cells in regeneration. *Clujul Med.* 2015;88(4):479–482.

McNamara JA Jr, Bryan FA. Long-term mandibular adaptations to protrusive function: an experimental study in *Macaca mulatta*. *Am J Orthod Dentofac Orthop.* 1987;92:98–108.

McNamara JA Jr, Carlson DS. Quantitative analysis of temporomandibular joint adaptations to protrusive function. *Am J Orthod.* 1979;76:593–611.

Miller P. Twins alike but not alike. *Nat Geo.* 2012;39–65.

Mori C, Nakamura N, Kimura S, Irie H, Takigawa T, Shiota K. Programmed cell death in the interdigital tissue of the fetal mouse limb is apoptosis with DNA fragmentation. *Anat Rec.* 1995;242(1):103–110.

Moss ML, Young RW. A functional approach to craniology. *Am J Phys Anthropol.* 1960;18(4):281–292.

Moyers RE, Bookstein FL. The inappropriateness of conventional cephalometrics. *Am J Orthod.* 1979;75(6):599–617.

Novik KL, Nimmrich I, Genc B, Maier S, Piepenbrock C, Olek A, Beck S. Epigenomics: genome-wide study of methylation phenomena. *Curr Issues Mol Biol.* 2002;4(4):111–28.

Obermann-Borst SA, Eilers PH, Tobi EW, de Jong FH, Slagboom PE, Heijmans BT, Steegers-Theunissen RP. Duration of breastfeeding and gender are associated with methylation of the LEPTIN gene in very young children. *Pediatr Res.* 2013;74(3):344–349.

Obladen M. Factors influencing surfactant composition in the newborn infant. *Eur J Pediatr.* 1978;128(3):129–143.

Parsons TE, Downey CM, Jirik FR, Hallgrimsson B, Jamniczky HA. Mind the gap: genetic manipulation of basicranial growth within synchondroses modulates calvarial and facial shape in mice through epigenetic interactions. *PLoS One.* 2015;10(2):e0118355.

Santiago PE, Singh GD, Yáñez MA, Dietrich RA, García P, Grayson BH, McCarthy, JG. Restitution of the temporomandibular joint in patients with craniofacial microsomia after multiplanar mandibular distraction: Assessment by magnetic resonance imaging. *Seminars Orthod.* 2011;17(3):186–196.

Silva Jesuino FA, Valladares-Neto J. Craniofacial morphological differences between Down syndrome and maxillary deficiency children. *Eur J Orthod.* 2013;35(1):124–130.

Singh GD, Clark WJ. Localization of mandibular changes in patients with class II division 1 malocclusions treated with twin-block appliances: finite element scaling analysis. *Am J Orthod Dentofacial Orthop.* 2001;119(4):419–425.

Singh GD, Johnston J, Ma W, Lozanoff S. Cleft palate formation in fetal Br mice with midfacial retrusion: tenascin, fibronectin, laminin, and type IV collagen immunolocalization. *Cleft Palate Craniofac J.* 1998;35(1):219–241.

Singh GD, Jung SC, Chandrashekhar R. Resolution of pediatric chronic rhinitis using biomimetic oral appliance therapy: a case report. *Open J Clin Med Case Rep.* 2016;2(4)1082:1–6.

Singh GD, Krumholtz J. Epigenetic Orthodontics in Adults, Appliance Therapy Group, USA, 2009; ISBN: 9780984054701.

Singh GD, Moxham BJ, Langley MS, Embery G. Glycosaminoglycan biosynthesis during 5-fluoro-2-deoxyuridine-induced palatal clefts in the rat. *Arch. Oral Biol.* 1997;42(5):355–363.

Singh GD, Moxham BJ, Langley MS, Waddington RJ, Embery G. Changes in the composition of glycosaminoglycans during normal palatogenesis in the rat. *Arch Oral Biol.* 1994;39(5):401–407.

Singh GD. Epigenetic orthodontics: Developmental mechanisms of functional (formational) orthodontic appliances. *J Amer Orthod Soc.* 2010;10(6):16–26.

Singh GD. On Growth and Treatment: The spatial matrix hypothesis. In: McNamara JA Jr (ed.) Growth and treatment: A meeting of the minds. Vol 41, Craniofacial Growth Series. *Ann Arbor, USA,* 2004, pp. 197–239.

Singh GD. Spatial matrix hypothesis. Brit Dent J. 2007;202(5):238–239.

Sjamsudin J, David DJ, Singh GD. An Indonesian child with orofacial duplication and neurocristopathy anomalies: Case Report. *J Craniomaxillofac Surg.* 2001;29(4):195–197.

Smith JC, Wolpert L. Pattern formation along the anteroposterior axis of the chick wing: the increase in width following a polarizing region graft and the effect of X-irradiation. *J Embryol Exp Morphol.* 1981;63:127–144.

Sonkar R, Powell CA, Choudhury M. Benzyl butyl phthalate induces epigenetic stress to enhance adipogenesis in mesenchymal stem cells. *Mol Cell Endocrinol.* 2016;431;109–122.

Spivakov M, Fisher AG. Epigenetic signatures of stem-cell identity. *Nat Rev Genet.* 2007;8(4):263–271.

Stöckli PW, Willert HG. Tissue reactions in the temporomandibular joint resulting from anterior displacement of the mandible in the monkey. *Am J Orthod.* 1971;60(2):142–155.

Townsend G, Hughes T, Bockmann M, Smith R, Brook A. How studies of twins can inform our understanding of dental morphology. *Front Oral Biol.* 2009;13:136–141.

Weaver IC, Cervoni N, Champagne FA, D'Alessio AC, Sharma S, Seckl JR, Dymov S, Szyf M, Meaney MJ. Epigenetic programming by maternal behavior. *Nat Neurosci.* 2004;7(8):847–854.

Williams MO, Murphy NC. Beyond the Ligament: A Whole-Bone Periodontal View of Dentofacial Orthopedics and Falsification of Universal Alveolar Immutability. *Semin Orthod.* 2008;14(4):246–259.

Wolffe AP, Matzke MA. Epigenetics: regulation through repression. *Science.* 1999;286(5439):481–486.

Yang CM, Chien CS, Yao CC, Hsiao LD, Huang YC, Wu CB. Mechanical strain induces collagenase-3 (MMP-13) expression in MC3T3-E1 osteoblastic cells. *J Biol Chem.* 2004;279(21):22158–22165.

Yang SH, Bergo MO, Toth JI, Qiao X, Hu Y, Sandoval S, Meta M, Bendale P, Gelb MH, Young SG, Fong LG. Blocking protein farnesyltransferase improves nuclear blebbing in mouse fibroblasts with a targeted Hutchinson-Gilford progeria syndrome mutation. *Proc Natl Acad Sci USA*. 2005;102(29):10291–10296.

Yengo L, Wood AR, Vedantam S, Marouli E, Sidorenko J, Sakaue S, Raghavan S, Lettre G, Okada Y, Hirschhorn JN, Visscher PM. A meta-analysis of height in 4.1 million European-ancestry individuals identifies ~10,000 SNPs accounting for nearly all heritability attributable to common variants. https://www.abstractsonline.com/pp8/#!/9070/presentation/1956

Chapter 3

Growth and Developmental Compensation of the Craniofacial Complex: Spatial Matrix Hypothesis

Synopsis: In this chapter, early postnatal craniofacial development, and the functional changes that occur at birth are discussed. The development of the craniofacial system at the organ level is described and early influences on craniofacial development are also explored, leading to definitive spatial matrices. Clinical identification of spatial perturbations is noted in the hard tissues, soft tissues, and dental tissues; and the importance of functional spaces, such as the upper airway, is emphasized. The concepts outlined here are re-integrated as the spatial matrix hypothesis that predicts how craniofacial developmental compensations produce functional compromise as illustrated by clinical findings observed in children and adults, such as malocclusions, temporomandibular dysfunction, and sleep disordered breathing.

At fertilization, the full complement of genes is established, the sex of the individual is determined, and metabolic activation through mitochondrial DNA of the zygote proceeds. The first 8 weeks of life are referred to as the embryonic period, but bone development begins at about 8 weeks *in utero*, which represents the beginning of the fetal period of life. During these stages, precocious growth and development of the brain, spinal cord, and neurocranium is evident. The developing craniofacial components can be classified in various ways. For example, the neurocranium consists of a series of cranial base cartilages, which are often referred to as the chondrocranium. The developing brain rests on the chondrocranium, through which the cranial nerves emanate. The chondrocranium gives rise to most of the occipital bone; the petrous part of the temporal bone, including the mastoid process; the sphenoid bone (except its greater wing); the ethmoid bone; and the cartilaginous nasal septum. Anteriorly, the prechordal cartilage gives rise to the nasal capsule, which forms the ethmoid bone, the nasal septum, and the inferior concha. The inferior concha migrates inferiorly during development from the cranial base and ends up in the inferior meatus of the nose, as the inferior turbinate. In addition, during cranial base development: the presphenoid cartilage forms the body of the sphenoid bone anteriorly; the optic capsule, including the orbito-sphenoid cartilage, forms the lesser wing of the sphenoid bone; the alisphenoid cartilage contributes to the greater wing of the sphenoid bone; while the hypophyseal and post-sphenoid cartilages ossify as the body of the sphenoid and sella turcica. Posteriorly, the otic capsule gives rise to the petrous part of the temporal bone and the mastoid process, and the parachordal cartilage forms the basilar part of the occipital bone. One feature on the basilar part of the occipital bone is the pharyngeal tubercle. This is the point of attachment of the pharyngeal raphe, which itself provides the insertion of the pharyngeal constrictors that form the upper airway, the development of which is discussed later in this chapter. In any case, cranial base development proceeds in an orderly cranio-caudal fashion, according to temporo-spatial patterning.

As the above cranial base cartilages ossify, they border on adjacent ones, which are also undergoing signal transduction, converting the cartilage templates into bone through a physiologic process called endochondral ossification. Adjacent sites of cartilaginous growth form synchondroses: a synchondrosis is a joint formed between two bones that undergo endochondral ossification, the antithesis of a suture. For example, the spheno-ethmoidal synchondrosis is located anteriorly in the cranial base between the ethmoid bone anteriorly and the body of the sphenoid bone posteriorly. Since the maxilla articulates with the ethmoid bone in the midline, anterior translation of the midface (up to age of about 10 yrs) is largely dependent on antero-posterior elongation of the anterior cranial base via cartilaginous proliferation at the spheno-ethmoidal synchondrosis. Singh *et al.* (1999) studied cranial base allometry in various ethnic groups. We reported both size- and shape differences in Asian (Korean) children when compared to their Caucasian (American) counterparts. Specifically, the Asian children had a shorter anterior cranial base phenotype. Empirically, this feature would clinically predispose an individual to a concave facial profile with a Class III skeletal pattern (Fig. 19a). In fact, some studies suggest that the Class III presentation of adult Korean orthognathic cases is associated with a shorter anterior cranial base, a shorter maxilla, as well as mandibular prognathism (Baik *et al.*, 2000). Therefore, deficient anterior cranial base growth may yield a skeletal Class III malocclusion. However, using traditional cephalometric analyses, a short anterior cranial

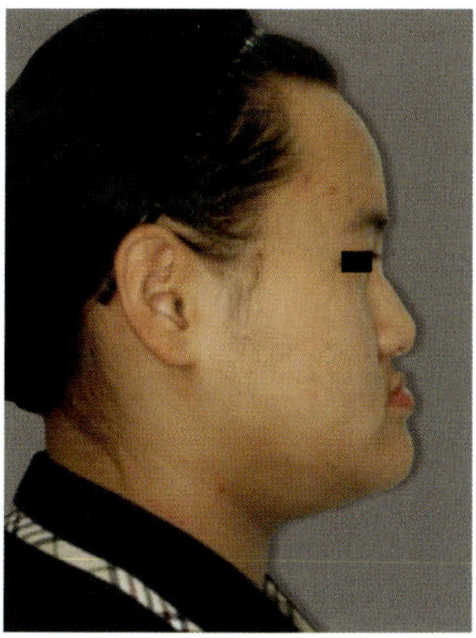

Figure 19a: Pre-treatment appearance showing concave facial profile. Courtesy: Dr Kwangyeon Kim

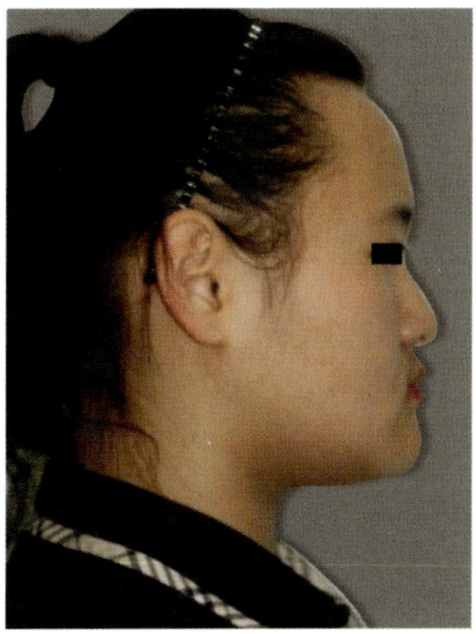

Figure 19b: Post-treatment appearance after biomimetic oral appliance therapy.

base would likely be described as 'maxillary retrusion' since the midface would appear to be deficient secondary to cranial base morphology. In addition, if mandibular prognathism is also present, this may result in a severe Class III malocclusion, which might necessitate orthognathic surgery unless epigenetic alternatives are explored (Fig. 19b). On the other hand, a long anterior cranial base phenotype can be associated with an aquiline facial convexity. Allied with mandibular retrognathia clinically, a severe Class II malocclusion may be produced in these types of cases.

Further posteriorly in the cranial base lies the spheno-occipital synchondrosis, between the body of the sphenoid bone anteriorly and the basilar part of the occipital bone posteriorly. Some mistakenly refer to it as the 'spheno-basilar symphysis', but a symphysis is a joint which crosses the midline, uniting two halves of a particular bone. There are only two symphyses in the human body: the mandibular symphysis and the pubic symphysis. Regardless, the spheno-occipital synchondrosis is responsible for the antero-posterior elongation of the cranial base in humans up to the age of approx. 16-20yrs. The condyles of the mandible articulate with the temporal bones at the glenoid fossae, which lie below the middle cranial fossa. This arrangement means that changes in posterior cranial base morphology can largely determine the positioning of the mandible. In fact, for the assessment of facial features, the cranial base was established as a refence plane, known as the Frankfurt plane, following an anthropologic conference held in Frankfurt, Germany (Ranke, 1884). At that time, neither radiography nor cephalometry were available. Thus, it was decided to use a line connecting the highest point on the external auditory meatus (Porion) and the lowest point infra-orbital foramen (Orbitale) as the Frankfurt plane. Later, radiology was introduced and, in combination with the cephalostat (Broadbent, 1931), orthodontic assessment shifted its focus away from the face, relying predominantly on 2D cephalometric analyses instead. Thus, despite the advantages of the Frankfurt plane, the sella-nasion plane became the preferred, standard reference plane in orthodontic cephalometrics. Sella (S) is defined as the center of the sella turcica, and nasion (N) is the frontonasal suture as seen in cephalometric radiographs. In addition, another cephalometric landmark was introduced, known as Basion (Ba), which is the antero-inferior-most point of the foramen magnum on the occipital bone. These three landmarks on a lateral cephalograph provide additional information. First, the S-N length represents the length of the anterior cranial base. Therefore, a simple linear measurement, either on a 2D cephalograph or more preferably on the mid-sagittal slice of a 3D cone-beam CT scan, will determine whether an individual has a long or short cranial base phenotype. On 3D CBCT scans, the average length of the anterior cranial base appears to be approx. 65mm (Fig. 20a). Variation from this value can be found in patients with a short anterior cranial base (Class III) phenotype (Fig. 20b). Note that patients vary in size (some people can be very tall or short), and this variation is not taken into account during the measurement protocol. Thus, the assessments are taken under the conditions of parsimony and clinical judgement needs to be applied. In fact, Moyers and Bookstein (1979) and Bookstein (2016) consider 2D cephalometric analyses to be entirely inappropriate. Nevertheless, the posterior cranial base length can also be determined by measuring the linear

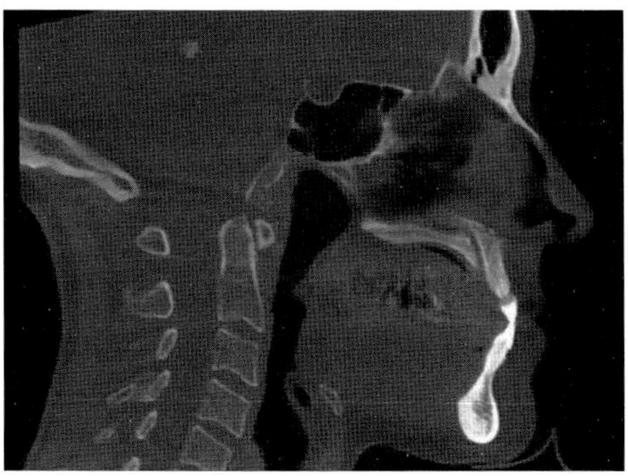

Figure 20a: CBCT scan of a Caucasian case showing a Class I cranial base phenotype.

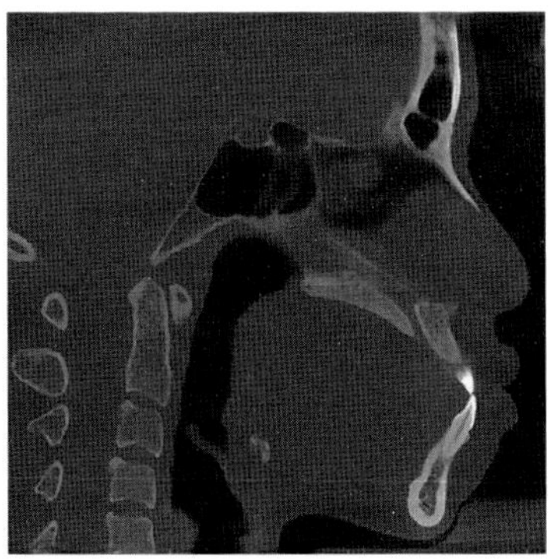

Figure 20b: CBCT scan of an Asian case showing a short (Class III) cranial base phenotype.

distance between Sella and Basion. The average S-Ba distance is approx. 45mm. Moreover, the angle enclosed by N-S-Ba, sometimes referred to as the 'saddle angle' can also be calculated. In a typical Class I case (Fig. 20a), the average cranial base angle is around 130°. Variation from this norm can be found in patients with a Class III phenotype. In some of these cases, the cranial base angle is relatively acute (i.e. < 130°). This change in the saddle angle has the effect of displacing the glenoid fossae further anteriorly, perhaps contributing to mandibular prognathism, thus increasing the severity of a Class III facial profile. The above 'bending' of the cranial base is a component of klinorhynchy (the cranial adaptations for speech; Davidson, 2003). It is also thought that 'unbending' or orthocephalization (straightening) of the cranial base occurs during life. Therefore, deficient orthocephalization can also precipitate a Class III appearance (Singh *et al.*, 1997). Moreover, using cephalometric parameters, the heritability of craniofacial traits can be estimated (Table 3). It is thought that cranial base components, such as S-N and N-S-Ba, have a high degree of inheritance (Table 3), which will impact facial appearance. In addition, the inheritance of mutated genes can also impact craniofacial outcomes. One of the most commonly studied is the gene associated with achondroplasia (dwarfism). In this condition there is a failure of chondroblastic proliferation — the

Craniofacial Traits	Heritability	Standard Error
Basion-sella	0.34	0.08
Basion-nasion	0.53	0.07
Sella-nasion	0.71	0.06
Sella-sphenoethmoidale	0.55	0.07
Sella-vertex (ectocranial)	0.65	0.07
Posterior-anterior	0.45	0.08
Cranial thickness	0.48	0.09
Ba-S-N angle	0.60	0.07
S-N-pt. a angle	0.54	0.09
N-S-PNS angle	0.41	0.07

Table 3: Heritability of craniofacial traits after Sherwood *et al.* (2008).

cartilage cells fail to grow adequately. Typically, this disruption affects the long bones, producing individuals of short stature. In addition, however, cartilaginous proliferation of the cranial base can also be affected. In these cases, the cranial base fails to elongate sufficiently and, as a consequence, the midface fails to translate anteriorly. Clinically, a Class III phenotype can be produced with an anterior and/or posterior crossbite. Another less commonly studied condition is brachyrrhine (short face). This brachyrrhine mutant gene is found in bulldogs, pugs, boxers, etc. and produces a short-face phenotype. Although the mandible appears to be large or normal in these breeds, the cranial base dysmorphology can impact the maxilla significantly, producing midfacial hypoplasia, which has its own sequelae, such as nasal obstruction and difficulties with breathing. Lozanoff (1993) studied this condition in mice. He noticed that brachyrrhine mice have midfacial retrusion with the lower incisors erupting ahead of the upper ones — a mouse with a malocclusion! More importantly, these mice also have an increased disposition for cleft lip and/or palate (Singh *et al.*, 1998). In addition, an anterior cranial base dysmorphology is suspected in these mice, and this cranial base contribution affects the facial profile both genetically and epigenetically. Parsons *et al.* (2015) reported that genetic manipulation of the synchondroses within the growing cranial base cartilages can modulate both the calvarial and facial shape in mice on an epigenetic basis. In humans, cranial base dysmorphology is suspected in conditions such as Trisomy 21 and fetal alcohol syndrome since characteristic facies are identifiable. These clinical changes likely represent an epigenetic phenomenon. The facies associated with Down syndrome have also been discussed earlier as another epigenetic change, but this phenotypic deviation has other craniofacial consequences on the upper airway since these children have a significantly higher incidence of sleep disordered breathing. Finally, it is suggested by some researchers that the cartilaginous nasal capsule is responsible for anterior translation of midface. Findings in animal studies, such as resection of the nasal septum in chimpanzee (Siegel *et al.*, 1990) produced midfacial deficiencies, leading to the septal traction hypothesis. However, in humans, given that the anterior aspect of the midface is a resorptive surface (Enlow and Hans, 1996), it's unlikely that the nasal septum elongates significantly to pull the midface forward, since humans do not develop a snout or muzzle. Therefore, in terms of craniofacial development, it can be surmised that "the cranial base sets the pace for the rest of the face".

Early postnatal cranial development

Surrounding and protecting the developing brain is the cranial vault, often referred to as the calvaria. Each calvarium represents flat, intramembranous bones that form the dermatocranium. Articulating with the cranial base inferiorly is the facial skeleton, which consists of the developing maxilla and mandible. The facial skeleton is essentially a part of the dermatocranium since it undergoes intramembranous ossification. However, the condyles of the mandible are formed from secondary cartilages (the condylar cartilages), which are not primary cartilages, unlike the cranial base cartilages that arise earlier during development. In fact, there are several transient, primary cartilages that give rise to specific parts of various craniofacial bones. For example, Meckel's cartilage provides an anlage of the mandible but undergoes programmed cell death with only a few remnants persisting postnatally, such as: the spine of the sphenoid, the pterygomandibular raphe (perichondrium), the lingula of the mandible, and the mental ossicles. Put simply, the viscerocranium is a term used to describe skeletal craniofacial components derived from the primary (branchial arch) cartilages, and these components include: the greater wing of the sphenoid, the ear ossicles (malleus, stapes and incus), the styloid process, etc.

At birth, the metopic suture divides the two halves of the developing frontal bone, and the cranial vault has a greater degree of curvature due partly to frontal and parietal tuberosities, which represent their early ossification centers, respectively. Ossification centers have been widely described in the early literature. It is now understood that these centers represent the nascent sites of signal transduction, where specific cytokines such as platelet-derived growth factor (PDGF) and insulin-like growth factor-2 (IGF-2) can bind to cell surface receptors and induce a cascade of events that leads to differentiation of identifiable connective tissues from undifferentiated mesenchymal cells, e.g. bone. Other examples of molecules involved in signal transduction networks regulating craniofacial development include the extracellular signaling molecule sonic hedgehog (SHH), fibroblast growth factor receptors (FGF-R), and transcription factors GLI3, MSX2, and TWIST. Thus, during the first postnatal year, the osteogenic cells of the metopic suture undergo signal transduction and differentiation (i.e. synostosis) so that frontal bone becomes a single bone in the majority of cases. Early in postnatal development also, the glabella and superciliary arches are relatively flat, as the frontal air sinuses do not develop until the age of about two years. In the anterior cranial base, only the labyrinths of the ethmoid bone are ossified, as the ethmoidal air sinuses are identifiable at birth. In contrast, the perpendicular and cribriform plates of the ethmoid unite by endochondral ossification with the lateral labyrinths to form the single ethmoid bone by about two years of age. Thus, even at the earliest stage of perinatal life, spatial considerations in the developing nasopharynx have been reserved, compatible with neotenous function, i.e. nasal breathing. Indeed, it is now thought that one of the functions of the paranasal sinuses is to produce nitric oxide (NO), the function of which is to modulate pulmonary function. Specifically, NO is thought to play a role in the adaptation of the respiratory system to postnatal life.

Further posteriorly, the temporal bone has a rudimentary mastoid process, as neck movements via the sternocleidomastoid muscle are not yet possible; the stylo-mastoid foramen is superficial (and the facial nerve emerging from it is vulnerable in forceps delivery). The three parts of the temporal bone — squamous, tympanic, and petrous — and the styloid process, are usually ossified by the first year. The tip of the styloid process, however, does not fuse completely with the rest of the temporal bone until around puberty, although the perichondrium (of Riechert's cartilage) surrounding the styloid process may ossify throughout life to form a stylohyoid chain, extending to the hyoid bone in some rare instances (Eagle's syndrome; Jackson, 1974). Nevertheless, the cartilaginous apex of the petrous part of temporal bone (the foramen lacerum) remains as cartilage from birth till death in the majority of humans. This little recognized fact of human temporo-spatial patterning may help explain the role of the cranial base in both the etiology and correction of malocclusions. On the squamous part of the temporal bone, the mandibular fossa is flat and there is no articular tubercle as mandibular movements are not yet developed fully.

For the posterior cranial base, the occipital bone is divided into its constituent four parts; squamous, basilar, and lateral, which unite by ossification by the age of about six years. The basilar part of occipital bone is separated from the basilar part of the sphenoid bone by the spheno-occipital synchondrosis. The central portion of the sphenoid bone (the body and lesser wings) is in cartilaginous continuity with its bilateral portions (the greater wings and the pterygoid processes). Signal transduction and differentiation ensure that these three components unite by ossification in the first postnatal year. Conspicuously, the sphenoidal sinus within the body of the sphenoid is identifiable at birth. This pattern of temporo-spatial organization may reserve space for the developing nasopharyngeal airway but may impact also on the relation of the anterior and posterior parts of the cranial base, with which the maxilla and mandible articulate, respectively. Thus, it is stated often that during growth of the cranial base, the glenoid fossae are transported somewhat backward and downward so that 'forward growth' of the mandible is required to attain a normal occlusion. The pharyngo-basilar fascia and pharyngeal raphe are attached also to the inferior surface of the cranial base. Their lateral extensions include the superior constrictor muscle of the pharynx, which forms part of the upper airway. As well, at birth, the mandibular body has no mental protuberance, the chin is divided by the mandibular symphysis, and the articular eminence of the temporal bone only attains its form after the establishment of the deciduous dentition. Similarly, the maxilla is small, as the maxillary air sinus is rudimentary at birth and the palate is shallow, in accord with the individual's genome. Thus, a rudimentary craniofacial template of skeletal support for developing soft tissues is present at birth and in the early postnatal period.

Development of the midface

The proportions of the neurocranium and the facial skeleton, above and below Frankfurt plane respectively, can be compared. In the neonate, the neurocranium dominates in an approx. 8:1 ratio when compared to the facial skeleton. However, the maxilla reaches adult size by about 9-10yrs of age while the mandibular growth spurt occurs at around 12-13yrs. Therefore, in adults the ratio of the neurocranium to the facial skeleton decreases to about 3:1 due to postnatal facial growth. Development of the human face begins at about 4–6 weeks *in utero*. Initially, the facial primordia, such as the maxillary and mandibular processes, consist of undifferentiated mesenchymal stem cells. These cells later differentiate in a site-specific manner into osteoblasts, myoblasts, fibroblasts, etc. to form tissues such as bone, muscle, and other connective tissues. As mentioned previously, stem cell differentiation due to temporo-spatial patterning results in the formation of maxillary and mandibular ossification centers due to signal transduction. The ossification of the maxilla proceeds in various directions from the ossification center, which is located near the infra-orbital foramen. The ossification center extends upward to form the frontal process of the maxilla, which articulates with the frontal bone and nasal bone at the fronto-maxillary and naso-maxillary sutures, respectively. The initial ossification center also extends posteriorly, forming the zygomatic process of the maxilla, which articulates with the zygoma at the zygomatico-maxillary suture. In addition, the ossification center extends medially as the palatal process of the maxilla, meeting its counterpart in the midline at the midpalatal suture. In addition, the ossification center extends inferiorly, enclosing the buds of the developing teeth. These bony extensions form the medial and lateral alveolar plates, which eventually form the tooth sockets for individual deciduous and permanent teeth. Finally, the ossification center spreads outward, forming the facial process of the maxilla anteriorly, as well as the primary palate, which articulates with the palatal process of the maxilla at the premaxillary-maxillary suture.

Continued maxillary size-related shape-change (allometry) is an interesting phenomenon. As the maxilla grows there are distinct changes in size and shape but there is also anisotropy; the changes show directionality. Significantly, the anterior aspect of the maxilla is a resorptive surface (Enlow and Hans, 1996). In other words, osteoclastic activity predominates, and **the anterior aspect of the human face appears to grow downward — not forward**. This downward growth is checked by the tongue, which if properly seated in the palate, gives an upward and outward expansion of the midface so the zygomas become more prominent. However, if the tongue has a low posture, residing in the floor of the mouth, the downward vector of growth is unchecked and the patient develops vertical maxillary excess, often presenting as a 'gummy smile' clinically (Fig. 21a). Anterior maxillary remodeling due to osteoclastic activity also produces specific morphologic features, such as 'A point' or subspinale. Note that this same phenomenon (anterior maxillary remodeling) might be harnessed for the clinical correction of a 'gummy smile' (Fig. 21b). In addition, the maxilla appears to elongate backward and downward during growth. While this distal elongation is required for the development, eruption, and accommodation of the molar teeth, there is a risk of upper airway compromise. During early postnatal development, neural crest migration occurs in a postero-anterior direction with the anterior teeth forming first, close to the midline. From there, the dental lamina extends distally with the development of the posterior tooth buds. As long as the maxilla grows back sufficiently, the posterior elongation of the dental lamina will be accommodated, but deficient maxillary growth might 'buckle' the

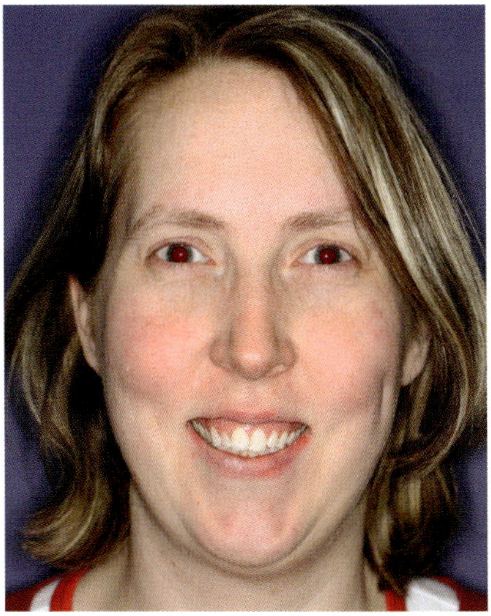

Figure 21a: Pre-treatment adult case showing 'gummy smile' esthetics. Courtesy: Dr Tammarie Heit

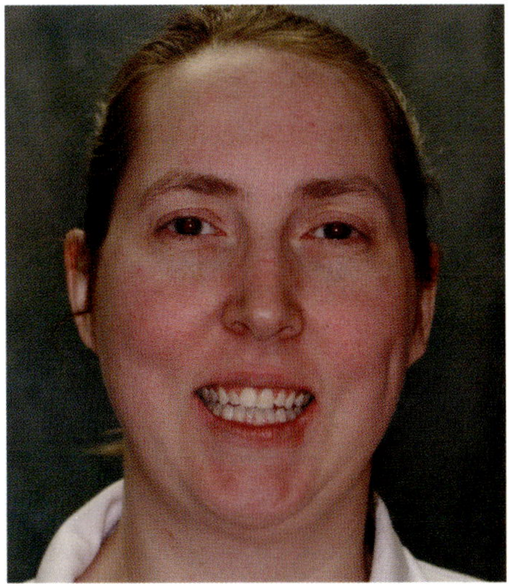

Figure 21b: Post-treatment after biomimetic oral appliance therapy showing resolution of 'gummy smile'.

dental lamina with the subsequent displacement and/or impaction of the third molar buds. Therefore, a developmental mechanism is required to translate the maxilla forward during growth to provide sufficient space for its distally directed development. This mechanism is found in the anterior cranial base, as discussed above. In addition, anterior translation of the midface would prevent upper airway obstruction by anisotropic maxillary growth, especially if the adenoids are hypertrophied.

Maxillary allometry includes the integration of the dento-alveolar spatial matrix. Put simply, the sequential eruption of the deciduous and permanent teeth increases vertical maxillary height due to alveolar bone deposition to house the tooth roots and periodontium. Simultaneously, within the body of the maxilla, the functional space of the maxillary sinuses is formed. This well-known phenomenon has been referred to as pneumatization for over a century (e.g. Tremble, 1934). Here the space vacated by the tooth crowns is replaced not by bony tissues but by an epithelial-lined cavity within the bone filled with air. Interestingly, these epithelial cells, which are referred to as pneumocytes, produce nitric oxide (NO). It is known that NO is a potent small vessel dilator *inter alia* (e.g. Gruetter *et al.*, 1979) and, if transported distally during nasal breathing into the lower airway, will enhance gas exchange in the pulmonary alveoli. In this way, the paranasal air sinuses can be viewed as representing the proximal-most part of the upper airway, indicating the functional relationship and clinical behavior of the jaws with respect to the upper airway. Specifically, during naso-maxillary and palatal growth, the palatal complex remodels inferiorly (Fig. 22a) so that the nasal cavity increases in volume (Singh *et al.*, 2016; Singh and Kim, 2020). Simultaneously, the maxillary air sinuses increase in volume as well (Singh and Kim, 2020). This palatal remodeling may be induced to change the 3D palatal morphology even in adults, using clinical protocols that mimic the natural phenomenon. In fact, palatal shape changes can be modeled from 3D digital study models using sophisticated geometric morphometric techniques such as principal components analysis (Fig. 22b). Therefore, the morphology of the maxilla is determined by temporo-spatial patterning, while other membranous bones, such as the frontal bones, the zygomas, the (squamous part of the) temporal bones, the parietal bones, and most of the mandible are ossifying at about the same time.

From the above brief overview, it's clear that the maxilla does not develop in isolation, and the events are coordinated such that the maxilla is

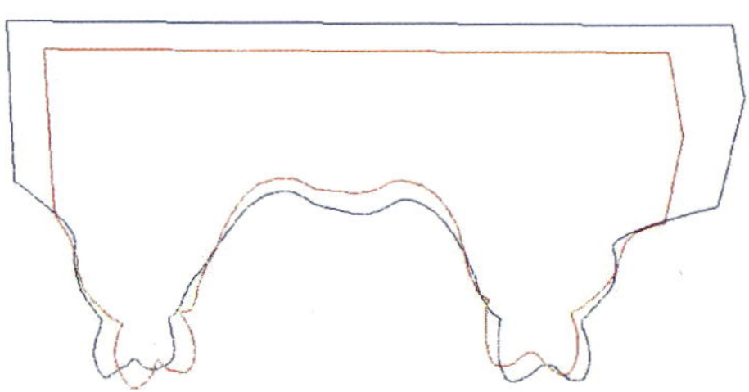

Figure 22a: The pre-treatment palatal outline in red and the post-treatment palatal outline in blue show the palatal level is lower after biomimetic oral appliance treatment.

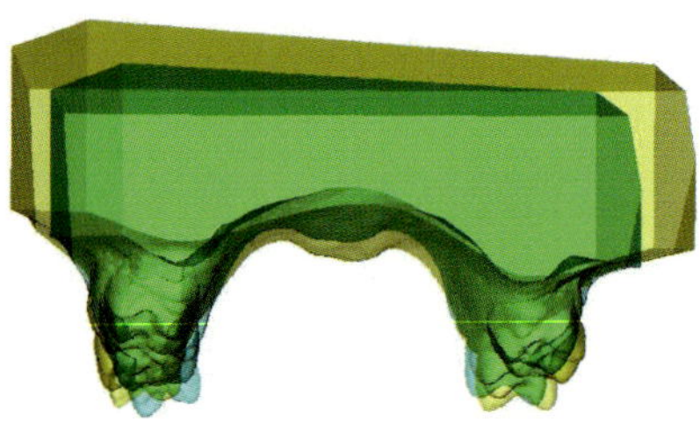

Figure 22b: The pre-treatment digital study model (blue) is overlapped by the post-treatment study model (yellow), with green showing common areas.

surrounded by a system of circum-maxillary sutures. These sutures provide a developmental mechanism for midfacial morphogenesis compliant with functional forces that gently stretch the sutures, e.g. suckling, swallowing, mastication, etc. In other words, while the skeletal components are ossifying, functional demands and influences help to determine the final phenotypic outcome. For example, humans have palatal rugae that are almost as unique as fingerprints. These rugae are folds of mucosa that increase the surface area of the primary palate and are used to grip the areolar of the nipple during breast-feeding. Note that in some mammals, the rugae are used entirely differently during feeding. In baleen whales, the rugae extend from the palate to the floor of the mouth, forming baleen plates for filter-feeding. In humans, it is thought that breast-feeding leads to the development of good swallowing patterns with the tongue moving upward and backward during swallowing, sometimes associated with a peristaltic wave within the tongue. Conversely, a lack of breast-feeding duration is thought to be associated with an 'infantile' or 'perverse' swallow with the tongue protruding to form an oral seal with active circumoral musculature. Since adequate breast-feeding is associated with good orofacial development, nursing or suckling is thought to prevent orofacial problems such as malocclusions. However, not all babies are competent at breast-feeding.

One common finding in modern newborns is tongue-tie, tongue-restriction, or ankyloglossia. In this condition, the anterior two-thirds of the tongue is restricted in its movements or tethered by a prominent lingual frenum. Recall that during development, the tongue arises from the floor of the mouth. In order to be free to move, the epithelial cells in the floor of the mouth need to undergo apoptosis or programmed cell death. This process proceeds from the lateral aspects of the tongue towards the midline. In terms of phylogeny, it's likely that there were three frenae attaching the mammalian tongue to the floor of the mouth. Two of these frenae undergo complete apoptosis in humans, leaving the frenulated folds on the ventral surface of the tongue (Fig. 23a). With insufficient apoptosis,

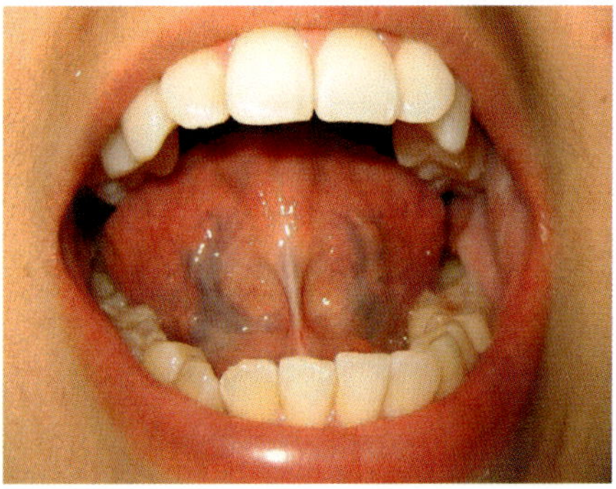

Figure 23a: Pre-treatment tongue restriction is evident with a short, thick blanched lingual frenum. Courtesy: Dr Payam Ataii

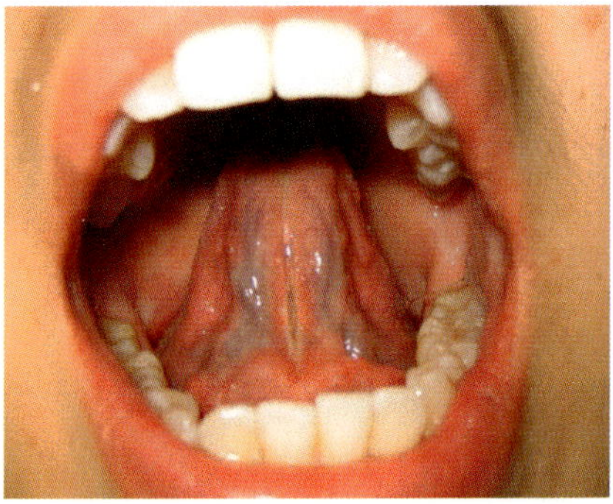

Figure 23b: Post-frenectomy, notice the change in size, shape, and position of the tongue.

however, a short midline frenum may persist (Fig. 23a) and restrict tongue movements so that the baby can't latch during breast-feeding. This makes breast-feeding difficult for the baby and painful for the mother. Parents-to-be need to be informed and educated about this possibility. Soon after birth the neonate should be screened for tongue-tie. If tongue-restriction is diagnosed, a frenectomy needs to be performed in conjunction with lactation support for the mother, if needed. Note that tongue-restriction may persist in childhood, adolescence, or adulthood. Patients need to be screened for tongue-tie by asking: Is the frenum long or short? Is the frenum thick or thin? Is the frenum blanched or not when the tongue is raised to the roof of the mouth with the mouth wide open? Depending on the responses to these questions, oral myofunctional therapy may be indicated with or without frenectomy (Fig. 23b). Note that similar questions can be asked for the midline and buccal frenae in both the upper and lower vestibules as well.

During breast-feeding, functional forces from the tongue mold the palate and gently stretch the circum-maxillary sutures. This sutural system includes: the fronto-maxillary, naso-maxillary, lacrimo-maxillary, zygomatico-maxillary, palatine-maxillary sutures, and the ethmo-maxillary joint. While these sutures undergo growth and development during infancy and childhood, according to Kokich (1986) some of these sutures may not synostose even during adulthood and remain viable while conforming to the principle of sutural homeostasis. Because of this adaptive capacity, exercises such as the 'zygoma lift' can be used to stretch the zygomatico-maxillary and zygomatico-temporal sutures in an attempt to enhance midfacial development. In addition to the circum-maxillary sutures, within the midface lies a sophisticated palatal suture system responsive to changes in postnatal functional requirements of the maxilla. For example, in terms of the transition from the deciduous dentition to the permanent dentition, there is a need for an increase in width of the anterior segment of the upper arch. The alveolar process in this region needs to become wider to accommodate larger permanent anterior teeth. In addition, there needs to be a longer arch length. This posterior elongation of the alveolar process is needed to accommodate an additional two permanent molar teeth, which are much larger mesio-distally than the two deciduous molars. There also needs to be an increase in vertical arch height due to the eruption of bigger permanent teeth and their longer roots. In other words, a new spatial matrix is required to account for postnatal functional requirements of the maxillary arch. To permit these adaptations, in the midline there is a sagittal maxillary suture system formed by the vomer articulating with the maxilla at the vomero-maxillary suture. It is thought that growth disturbance at this site is associated with a decreased facial height in children with cleft palate. Further anteriorly is the short septo-premaxillary joint where the septal cartilage articulates with the anterior-most part of the maxilla, including the anterior nasal spine. It was once thought that cartilaginous growth of the nasal septum somehow pulled the entire midface forward during growth (Siegel *et al.*, 1990). While this idea may have some applicability in mammals, human conditions, such as Binder's syndrome and some midfacial cleft cases that show deficient nasal septum growth, appear to exhibit acceptable midfacial growth. It is also unlikely that the smaller, bilateral naso-maxillary and lacrimo-maxillary sutures are sufficiently stretched during function to provide enough momentum for forward midfacial growth. Therefore, the trajectory for forward midfacial translation in humans must reside in sites external to the midfacial complex. As alluded to above, in the midline, the maxilla articulates with the anterior cranial base at the ethmo-maxillary joint. Thus, elongation of the anterior cranial base at the spheno-ethmoidal synchondrosis is most likely responsible for forward translation of the midfacial complex. In addition, growth and development of the midfacial structures at other sites results in an increase in the size of the bony architecture of the midface with concomitant pneumatization.

Some people suggest that the 'premaxillary-maxillary suture' may also be responsible for forward midfacial growth. This region represents the rugae-bearing primary palate. *In utero*, the primary palate develops from the frontonasal process embryologically, while the secondary palate develops from the medial aspects of the maxillary processes. It is now thought that modern humans do not possess a separate 'premaxilla' postnatally. In other words, ossification centers are found in the 'premaxilla' in the pre-natal period but these merge with the maxillary ossification centers so that the 'premaxillary-maxillary suture' does not persist into late childhood, but instead undergoes synostosis in the deciduous dentition. This temporo-spatial patterning might explain why upper anterior crowding is prevalent, especially in children with an insufficient history of breast-feeding. Note that the 'premaxilla' represents the predominant structure seen in bilateral cleft lip and primary palate cases. Regardless, the midfacial palatal suture system extends intra-orally in the midline as various named sutures. The two hemi-maxillae articulate on the facial aspect in the midline at the inter-maxillary suture (Fig. 24a), which continues onto the hard palate as the midpalatal suture (Fig. 24b) that finishes at the posterior nasal spine (Fig. 25a). This suture has been the target of rapid palatal expansion (RPE). Historically, the first physician to describe palatal expansion in children appears to be White (1860). Later, Schwartz (1966) developed a double-plated palatal expander and since that time numerous devices have been used for RPE. Classically, this technique splits the midpalatal suture and, as

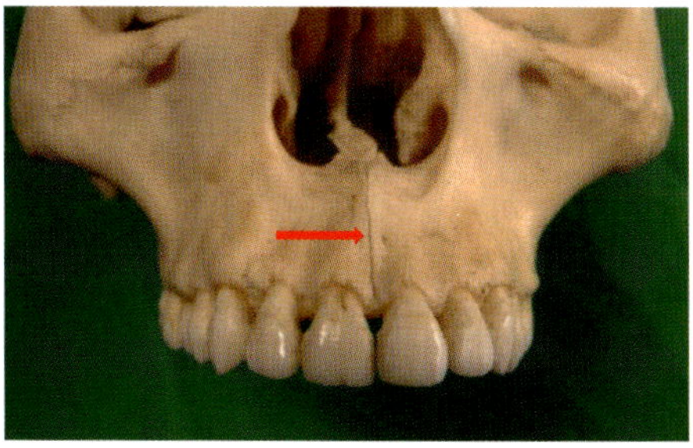

Figure 24a: The inter-maxillary suture is a continuation of the midpalatal suture on the facial aspect of the maxilla.

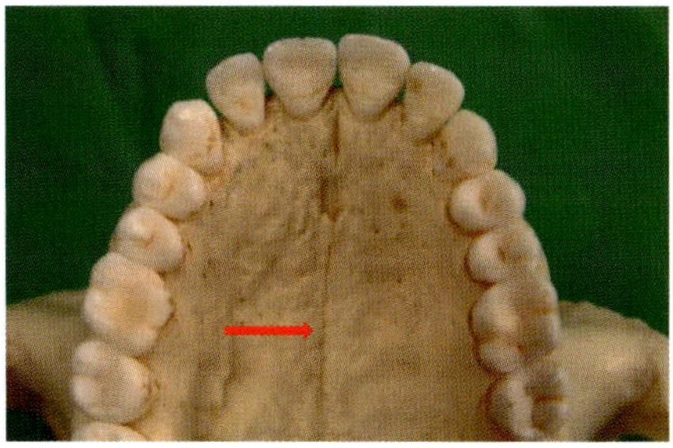

Figure 24b: The midpalatal suture uniting the right and left palatine processes of the maxilla (arrowed).

a consequence, a midline diastema is often precipitated between the two maxillary central incisors. In effect, a bone fracture has been induced with hematoma formation. Thus, the wound healing process is initiated, and the fracture heals through deposition of bone so that the sutural width returns to within normal limits, in accord with the principle of sutural homeostasis. There are numerous studies on this technique using either tooth-borne or tissue-borne appliances. However, a recent case study (Bressane *et al.*, 2016) suggests that some children do not show a good healing response and may suffer from dehiscence and fenestrations that predispose to periodontal bone loss in adult life. Therefore, the rationale of RPE remains uncertain, and a biomimetic approach that gently stretches sutures might be preferable, as it mimics the tension of natural growth and development.

Further posteriorly, the transverse palatine suture marks the articulation between the maxilla and the palatine bone, forming the hard palate. It is interesting to consider why two bones are required to make one hard palate? Ostensibly, the answer likely relates to two disparate functions. The primary function of the maxilla is to accommodate the teeth, while the primary function of the palatine bone is likely to keep the posterior nasal (airway) aperture patent. The horizontal plates of the palatine bone meet in the midline anteriorly at the midpalatal suture, forming a cruciform sutural complex, while posteriorly they form the posterior nasal spine (Fig. 25a). The functional space above this site is the posterior nasal

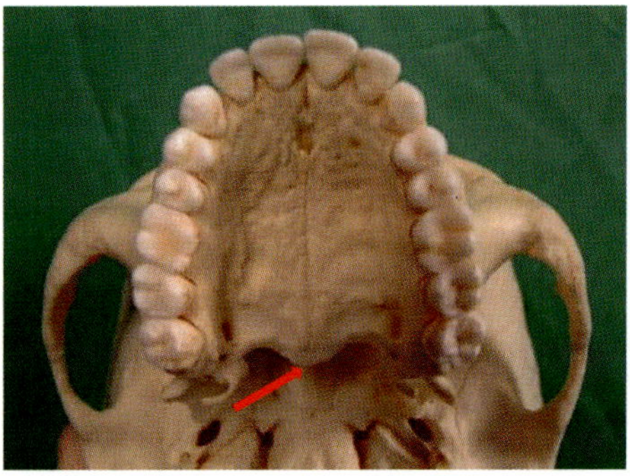

Figure 25a: The posterior nasal spine is formed at the termination of the midpalatal suture uniting the right and left horizontal plates of the palatine bone.

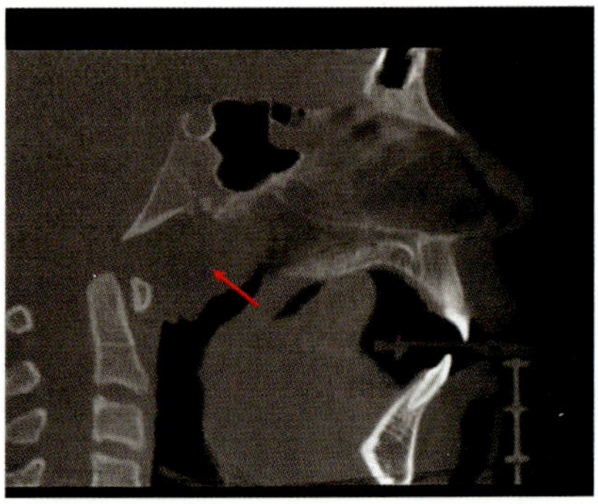

Figure 25b: Obstruction of the posterior nasal aperture secondary to gross adenoidal hypertrophy identified by the red arrow on a CBCT scan of a child.

aperture or choanae, and obstruction at this site increases the resistance to nasal airflow. Typically, patients with good facial development have wider choanal openings, whereas patients with underdeveloped faces can have narrow posterior nasal apertures associated with an obstructed nasal airway. Commonly, obstruction of the posterior nasal aperture is secondary to adenoidal hypertrophy in children (Fig. 25b).

On the other hand, it has been reported that palatal expansion permits the posterior nasal spine to remodel inferiorly (e.g. Ramoglu and Sari, 2010), so the height of the posterior nasal aperture is increased. This increase in height represents an increase in the radius of the posterior nasal aperture and, according to Poiseuille's equation, the resistance to laminar airflow will be decreased exponentially in this region, as it is inversely proportional to the radius of the structure to the fourth power (Singh and Chandrashekhar, 2009). As airflow is directly proportional to the pressure difference that exists between the nose and the pulmonary alveoli in the lung, the flow (Q) is directly proportional to the pressure difference (ΔP) divided by the resistance (πr^4). In standard fluid dynamics notation:

$$\Delta P = \frac{8 \mu L Q}{\pi r^4}$$

where ΔP is the pressure difference, L is the length of the tube, μ is the dynamic viscosity, Q is the volumetric flow rate, r is the radius and π is a mathematical constant. Put simply, a small change in the posterior nasal aperture will have a dramatic effect on resistance to airflow. Lateral to the confluence of the midpalatal and transverse palatine sutures are the second permanent maxillary molars. Indeed, the position of the second molars with respect to the first molars may indicate the extent of maxillary hypoplasia since their developmental positions are better maintained by other structures adjacent to the transverse palatine suture. Specifically, the pyramidal process of palatine bone may help maintain the developmental positions of the second maxillary molars as they are wedge-shaped pieces of dense bone through which the greater and lesser palatine nerves emanate. Indeed, it is thought that the sutural complex behind the maxillary tuberosity involving the pyramidal process of the palatine bone is involved in increasing midfacial height. In fact, in cleft palate cases, the palatine bone does not form correctly and may suppress the increase in height of the midface, i.e. account for a decrease in vertical height of the midface. Therefore, the posterior maxillary region is functionally diverse with consequences on the upper (nasal) airway.

Studies suggest that craniofacial changes are associated with OSA (Johns *et al.*, 1998; Sakakibara *et al.*, 1999). Specifically, the upper arch morphology in adults with OSA differs from control, non-OSA individuals, being 7–11% narrower on average (Banabilh *et al.*, 2009). If midfacial development is still possible in adults, then would there be any therapeutic effect on the upper airway? Genetic potential suggests that midfacial re-development should be achievable, and any clinical changes elicited could be gauged by simply measuring the transpalatal bone width, assuming that a minimum intermolar or transpalatal bone width of 38mm is within normal limits (McNamara, 2000). However, physiologic limits to midface expansion are currently unknown and the notion of 'overexpansion' has to be considered. Whilst a preliminary discussion on sutural homeostasis has been presented, it is important to recall that the entire midface is enclosed within an osteogenic periosteum. In cases of trauma or surgery, specific stem cell populations differentiate to biosynthesize new bone in the subsequent healing process. Conversely, violation of biologic limits might result in buccal dehiscence and/or fenestrations. Since the maxilla articulates with the anterior cranial base, a general rule of thumb is that the midfacial width must not exceed the anterior cranial base width. However, it is known that the cranial base phenotype can vary according to ethnicity, thus palatal width needs to be assessed on a case by case basis. In one study, Nada *et al.* (2012) undertook a prospective evaluation of surgically-assisted rapid maxillary expansion (SARME) in adults. They reported that while there were increases in the posterior alveolar segments of the maxilla indicating lateral expansion, there were also negative distances or posterior displacement of the anterior maxillary region. In contrast, Singh *et al.* (2014) found that both transpalatal bone width and midfacial bone volume increased after biomimetic oral appliance therapy in adults. In another study, Nada *et al.* (2013) assessed volumetric changes in the nasal airway using a surgical procedure, consisting of Le Fort I osteotomy, midline osteotomy and pterygomaxillary disjunction. Following this intervention, the patients wore a fixed palatal expander for 24hrs/day for 22 months. This protocol increased the nasal volume by approx. 9.5%. On the other hand, Singh *et al.* (2016) found that the nasal airway volume increased by approx. 5.5% in adults over a period of 18 months who followed a non-surgical, biomimetic protocol, wearing the device for up to 16hrs/day. Therefore, midfacial changes in non-growing adults are achievable both surgically and non-surgically, and this suggests that genetically-encoded developmental mechanisms can be epigenetically modulated by biomimetic oral appliances to enhance the midface in adults. In another study, Singh and Krumholtz (2009) took pre- and post-treatment lateral cephalographs of about 100 adults (mean age: approx. 43 years; mean treatment time: 21 months). The average pre- and post-treatment upper airway configurations were computed using Procrustes superimposition, and analyzed using finite-element analysis (FEA). Using pseudo-colored FEA, a relative 22% increase in nasopharyngeal airway area was found above and behind the soft palate. As well, a 16% increase in oropharyngeal airway area was located behind the base of the tongue with a 13% increase in hypopharyngeal area near the level of the hyoid bone. These upper airway changes in non-growing adults are similar to those of actively-growing children undergoing dentofacial orthopedic corrections (Singh *et al.*, 2007), and support the notion that genetic developmental mechanisms can be epigenetically modified by biomimetic oral appliances to improve the upper airway in both adults and children.

Development of the upper airway

It is interesting to study the development of the human upper airway in children, which starts early on in the embryonic period. A distinct developmental event is the migration of neural crest cells from the forming neural tube into the developing head and neck region. This unique population of cells gives rise to a 'fourth' embryonic tissue, known as mesenchyme, which produces the embryonic connective tissues of the head and neck region, as well as other tissues such as the dorsal root ganglia, various endocrine gland components, and pigment cells (melanocytes). In the craniofacial region specifically, distinct swellings covered by epithelium and composed of mesenchyme arise. These prominences are known as the frontonasal process in the midline with bilateral maxillary processes more laterally. Below these two swellings are the mandibular processes, which together constitute the first pharyngeal or branchial arch. After about 28 days *in utero*, other sequential pharyngeal swellings arise, known as the second, third, fourth, and sixth pharyngeal or branchial arches (the fifth arch is rudimentary in humans). Note that deficient neural crest cell migration into the developing branchial arches is known as neurocristopathy and is characterized by congenital absence or malformations of structures derived from this region (Sjamsudin *et al.*, 2001). It is interesting to speculate that as a consequence of neurocristopathy, deficient upper airway development may result in a smaller upper airway with an increased risk of obstructive sleep apnea. In fact, OSA is disproportionately more common in preterm infants compared to babies born at term. One study (Smitthimedhin *et al.*, 2018) measured the volume of the upper airway from brain MRI scans in preterm and term infants. They reported that term infants showed significantly larger naso- and oropharyngeal volumes than preterm babies (independent of weight, sex, and ethnicity). To avoid such possible sequelae, women of child-bearing age are encouraged to add a folate supplement to their diet prior to and during pregnancy in an effort to mitigate the chances of precipitating a neural tube defect and associated conditions, such as spina bifida and cleft lip and/or palate (Kappen, 2013).

At 4 weeks *in utero*, bilateral thickenings of ectoderm are discernible on the frontonasal process. These sites are known as the nasal placodes and as they deepen into the underlying mesenchyme, they form nasal pits, which are the precursors of the nares and nostrils. As the deepening nasal pits approach the underlying primitive oral cavity, they are separated by a thinning membrane, known as the oronasal membrane. This membrane undergoes rupture (apoptosis; programmed cell death) so that the newly formed primitive nasal cavity is in communication with the oral cavity below it. Meanwhile, the tissue between the frontonasal process and the mandibular processes on the surface (the stomadeum) also undergoes apoptosis so that the opening of the primitive oral cavity is formed. Inside this cavity and arising from its floor is the developing tongue. It's likely that apoptosis in the floor of the mouth leads to the formation of the lingual frenum, during the development of the tongue from the first and third pharyngeal arches. By about 8 weeks *in utero*, vertical palatal shelves on either side of the developing tongue undergo elevation to form the secondary palate (Singh and Moxham, 1994), which separates the nasal cavity from the oral cavity. Failure of these shelves to re-orientate from the vertical to the horizontal axis can lead to cleft palate formation (Singh and Moxham, 1996).

The third branchial arch mesenchyme undergoes differentiation with its stem cells forming pharyngeal muscle tissue from myoblasts. Specifically, the third branchial arch mesenchyme forms the stylopharyngeus muscle exclusively. Further down, the fourth arch mesenchyme gives rise to the superior, middle and inferior constrictors of pharynx, which largely form the oropharyngeal region of the upper airway. In the midline posteriorly, the overlapping pharyngeal constrictors are attached to the pharyngeal hilum, which itself originates at the pharyngeal tubercle on the basilar part of the occipital bone. It is interesting to note that historically, the pharyngeal muscles are referred to as constrictors. This terminology suggests that activation of these muscles closes and narrows the lumen of the upper airway. In contrast, for the aperture of the pupil, there are both constrictors and dilators. Thus, sphincter pupillae make the pupils smaller (for example, when a light is shone into the pupils), while dilator pupillae make the pupils larger (for example, during darkness). In contrast, there appears to be no direct mechanism for the pharyngeal muscles to dilate, except by relaxation of muscle tone. Moreover, this mechanism may predispose certain individuals to an increased risk of obstructive sleep apnea. Consider an individual sleeping in the supine position. If the upper airway is narrow there is an increased risk of airway collapse since the upper airway during normal sleep is characterized by a relatively negative critical collapsing pressure (Pcrit), and airway obstruction may be induced when nasal pressure is decreased below Pcrit (Schwartz, 1985). In these cases, airway dilation is necessary to avoid obstruction/collapse and subsequent apnea. However, relaxation of the pharyngeal muscles in an attempt to open the airway in the supine position will be futile because of the effects of gravity. If this situation goes unchecked and airflow ceases for 10 seconds, an episode of apnea would be recorded during a sleep study. Thus, the dynamics of maintaining a patent upper airway in adults are complex, still not fully understood, and differ from those of a newborn or young child.

At birth, several dramatic changes occur as the neonate transitions from the placental circulation to external oxygenation by breathing atmospheric air. These changes include: closure of the umbilical artery, which becomes the medial umbilical ligament; closure of the ductus venosus, which becomes the ligamentum venosum; closure of the ductus arteriosus, which becomes the ligamentum arteriosum; and closure of the foramen ovale in the heart, which becomes the fossa ovalis. Thus, the two-arm circulation of venous (deoxygenated) and arterial (oxygenated) blood flow is established in the child. Looking at a sagittal section through the head of a newborn, differences in the morphology of the upper airway are also noticeable when compared to an adult. First, the epiglottis is in contact with the soft palate in the neonate, and second, the larynx in the newborn and infant is positioned considerably higher than in the adult. The position of the epiglottis means that a newborn baby can suckle and breathe simultaneously. Later, a descent of the larynx occurs, so that older individuals can either breathe or feed but not simultaneously, as noted above. Note that this descent of the larynx may be associated with Sudden Infant Death Syndrome (SIDS). Because of this issue, current medical advice is to put a baby to sleep lying on the back with nothing else in the crib. This practice has led to a significant reduction in the incidence of SIDS but may precipitate positional or deformational plagiocephaly as discussed earlier. However, in Asian and other cultures, co-sleeping is the norm with the baby sleeping in the same bed as the parent, and this practice is associated with a lower incidence of SIDS (Balarajan *et al.*, 1989) although Mossey *et al.* (1999) suggest that a more extensive craniofacial analysis is needed when predisposing factors of SIDS are being considered.

Postnatally, the upper airway undergoes growth and development like other systems of the body. Gonçalves *et al.* (2011) and Schendel *et al.* (2012) described upper airway developmental changes between the ages of 6yrs and 60yrs (Fig. 26). Briefly, the upper airway shows incremental growth between 6yrs and 16yrs, increasing in volume from about 7cm^3 to 15cm^3. A growth plateau occurs between the ages of 6yrs and 9yrs with a volume of approx. 7cm^3–8cm^3, which is followed by a period of growth acceleration from 9yrs to 16yrs when the volume increases from 8cm^3

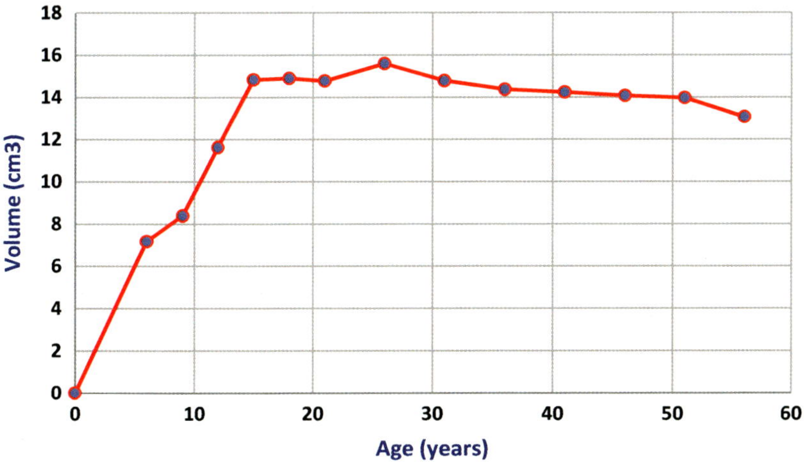

Figure 26: Airway volume change with age. After Gonçalves *et al.* (2011) and Schendel *et al.* (2012).

to 15cm^3 approx. Thereafter, another plateau between the ages of 16yrs and 21yrs occurs (with an average volume of approx. 15cm^3) followed by a slow decline at around 30yrs, when it starts to decrease to a volume of 13cm^3 or less. Note that volumetric measurements are dependent on the landmarks that are chosen to represent the boundaries of the upper airway. In our assessments, the adult upper airway when measured from the posterior nasal spine to the inferior border of the vertebral body of C3/superior border of C4 varies at around 15cm^3–25cm^3. And, our preliminary data appear to suggest that epigenetic protocols may not only enhance the upper airway but might be able to inhibit the upper airway atrophy associated with the ageing process (Singh and Liao, 2019). While the above discussion focuses on the development of the upper airway under normal circumstances, in a preliminary study, Au and Li (2015) studied cephalometric parameters and the severity of OSA in children and young adults aged between 6 and 18yrs. They noted a lower position of the hyoid bone in both pediatric and adult male subjects but not in females. The lower position of the hyoid bone was associated with OSA in both men and boys. However, while the length of soft palate and mandibular angle correlated with the AHI in adult males, this was not the case in pediatric males. In addition, a retrognathic mandible was associated with the AHI in pediatric females and in adult males. These initial cephalometric findings support the notion that there is a clear interaction between craniofacial morphology and upper airway adequacy (Guilleminault and Stoohs, 1990). Therefore, it's worth reviewing other anatomical factors that influence upper airway structure and function.

In children, the pattern of craniofacial lymphatic development needs to be considered. Between the ages of about 6 and 16yrs there is dramatic development of lymphoid tissues throughout the body. In the region of the oropharynx, Waldeyer's lymphatic ring provides an interrupted circle of protective lymphoid tissues at the upper end of the respiratory tract. This ring includes: the adenoids, the tubal tonsils, the palatine tonsils, and the lingual tonsils. Most tonsils usually regress by age 16yrs approx. but allergic hypertrophy can cause snoring or upper airway obstruction in children. In these cases, adenoidectomy, tonsillectomy, or partial tonsillotomy may be indicated. The function of tonsillar tissues is to remove inhaled/ingested toxic products and protect the upper airway and pharynx, partly by initiating an immune response. For example, nasal lymph vessels drain to local lymph nodes that initiate immune responses, such as helper CD4+ T cells, CD8+ T cells, etc. (Braun *et al.*, 2020; Singh, 2020). Histology of the tonsillar tissues reveals non-encapsulated lymphoid tissue in the lamina propria, which contains lymphocytes organized as lymphatic nodules with (stem-cell containing) germinal centers. These structures in the connective tissue of the lamina propria are covered by a stratified, squamous epithelium.

The adenoids (or pharyngeal tonsils) are located in the midline in the upper nasopharynx. They are found behind the uvula on the posterior pharyngeal wall and often clearly seen on lateral cephalographs taken for orthodontic reasons. However, the adenoids can also be viewed directly using nasoendoscopy during a retropalatal exam. In this location, hypertrophy of the adenoids, associated with nasal obstruction and mouth breathing, can lead to obstruction of the upper airway in the region of the posterior nasal apertures (Fig. 25b). On the other hand, nitric oxide (NO) production in the paranasal sinuses may help to reduce the size of the adenoids, although the mechanism of this regression is not fully understood. Further laterally in the nasopharynx are the tubal tonsils, which are best viewed using nasoendoscopy or 3D CBCT scans (Fig. 27). These are small amounts of lymphoid tissues located around the openings of the pharyngo-tympanic (Eustachian or auditory) tubes and may have some significance in the development of sleep bruxism in children with allergies. At first, the pharyngo-tympanic tubes are somewhat horizontally orientated in children, and then become more vertical during adulthood. This means that infection is more likely to track to the middle ear from the pharynx in children. Second, it is thought that allergic edema of the mucous membrane of the tympanic cavities can cause intermittent blockage of Eustachian tubes (Marks, 1980). However, the mucosae of the tympanic cavity and tympanic membrane are only a few cells in thickness, so it's unlikely that these thin tissues can cause significant blockage. On the other

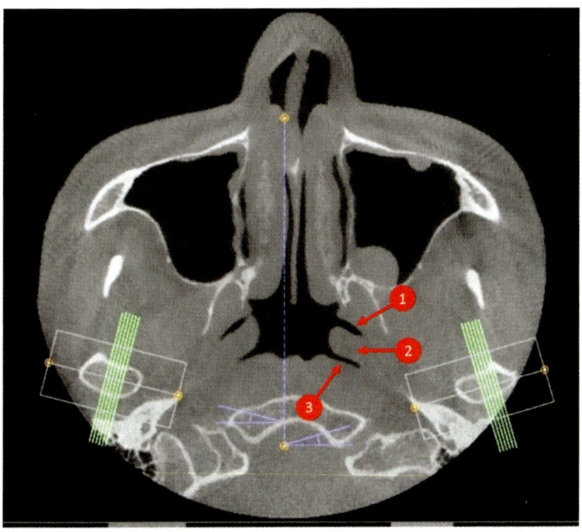

Figure 27: Arrow 1. Opening of Eustachian tube; Arrow 2. Torus tubaris; Arrow 3. Fossa of Rosenmuller.
Courtesy: Dr Dania Tamimi

hand, hypertrophy of the tubal tonsils, which surround the openings of the auditory tubes, is a more likely candidate.

The function of the pharyngo-tympanic tubes is to equalize the pressure in the nasopharynx and middle ear to permit vibration of the ear ossicles and sound conduction. At high altitudes, for example on an airline flight, the ears might 'pop' as pressure equalization occurs. This equalization is often enhanced by chewing gum or jaw movements since various muscles of the palate open the Eustachian tube. For example, tensor veli palatini tenses the soft palate and opens the auditory tube, while levator veli palatini is attached to the auditory tube and elevates the soft palate. On the other hand, palatopharyngeus, salpingopharyngeus (which lies deep to the salpingopharyngeal fold), and stylopharyngeus muscles elevate the pharynx and larynx. Consider a child with allergic hypertrophy of the tubal tonsils. To open the Eustachian tubes, the child starts chewing movements due to the pressure differential. In fact, during upper airway collapse, pressure differentials are detected by mechanoreceptors in the pharyngeal walls (Marks, 1980). In pediatric cases of sleep disordered breathing, upper airway obstruction during sleep may initiate chewing movements due to the pressure differential, and this learned behavior may present clinically as sleep bruxism in children with or without allergies. The hypertrophied tubal tonsils can be viewed directly as the torus tubaris endoscopically. Nasopharyngeal lymphoid hyperplasia with peritubular hypertrophy of the tubal tonsil may extend into the salpingopharyngeal fold and, with lateral pharyngeal wall collapse, possibly cause OSA (Agrawal, 2015). On a 3D CBCT scan, the opening of the Eustachian tube in relation to the torus tubaris (and the fossa of Rosenmuller) can sometimes be clearly seen (Fig. 27), which leads to my novel hypothesis: Does a child learn bruxing behavior to open the Eustachian tube — and then use this behavior reflexly as an adult when a pressure drop occurs in the upper airway during a respiratory effort related arousal (RERA) or OSA?

The palatine tonsils are located on either side of the oropharynx, between the anterior and posterior pillars of the fauces. They contain fused lymphatic nodules with (stem-cell containing) germinal centers and superficially they show 10-12 epithelial invaginations. These folds produce tonsillar crypts that increase the surface area of the tonsils and can entrap inhaled/ingested particles. Hypertrophy of the palatine tonsils is common and is graded on the Friedman scale from 0-IV. Grade 0 means that no tonsils are seen intra-orally. Grade I tonsils are visible in the tonsillar fossa, while grade II tonsils are visible beyond the anterior pillars of the fauces. Grade III tonsils extend halfway to the midline, and grade IV tonsils contact in the midline ('kissing tonsils'), causing obstruction of the upper airway. In addition, the back of the mouth is the location of the lingual tonsils. These tonsils are buried under the mucosa of the posterior one-third of the tongue, consisting of diffuse lymphoid tissue with germinal centers. Less commonly, hypertrophy of the lingual tonsils can also cause upper airway obstruction.

Clinical visualization of the upper airway can be achieved using nasendoscopy during speech. In addition, in video-fluoroscopy the narrowest part of the upper airway (the velopharyngeal isthmus) and the posterior pharyngeal wall can be viewed from above. Other methods for upper airway imaging and visualization include CBCT scans. This technique revealed that the predominant effect of mandibular appliances on upper airway structure is enlargement of the velopharyngeal (retropalatal) airway space, mediated via an increase in lateral diameter in those patients who respond well to this type of treatment. However, non-responders did not show these changes (Sutherland and Cistulli, 2011). In fact, in one study, 80% of patients had a smaller upper airway aperture when mandibular advancement was increased from 2mm-7mm of protrusion, while 18% showed no difference. These conflicting results can be explained based on the findings of Witzel and Posnick (1989) who investigated patterns of velopharyngeal closure in children with cleft palate. That study indicated 4 patterns of behavior: some children showed an antero-posterior (AP) pattern of airway opening/closing; some showed a medio-lateral (ML) behavior; some showed a concentric or sphincter pattern of opening/

closing; while some children used their adenoids to form a velopharyngeal seal of the upper airway to prevent the nasal escape of air during speech. It follows, therefore, that patients with an AP pattern of airway opening will likely respond well to a mandibular advancement device (MAD). Those with a ML pattern of opening will likely not benefit from therapy with a MAD, while patients with a concentric/sphincteric pattern will probably benefit to a certain amount. Therefore, upper airway behavior as well as its structure needs to be assessed for effective oral appliance therapy.

In a preliminary study, Liu *et al.* (2015) used MRI imaging to assess the growth and development of upper airway in children. Their initial analysis revealed that the cross-sectional area and sagittal dimensions of the laryngopharynx increased significantly with age. They also noted that during the peak period of growth in children, the development of the upper airway mainly demonstrated an increase in its transverse dimension. The volume of the tongue and the volume the soft palate also increased with age. However, it is unclear whether the presence of OSA in parents affects the occurrence of OSA in children. Au *et al.* (2015) investigated familial aggregation of OSA in children without tonsillar hypertrophy. Their study investigated the notion that OSA in either parent is a risk factor for pediatric OSA independent of tonsillar size. They found that tonsillar hypertrophy is a major cause of pediatric OSA and, if present, masked the effect of family history. In contrast, the presence of OSA in parents may indicate a higher risk for OSA in children without tonsillar hypertrophy. Therefore, these children should be identified for early screening for SDB. However, as discussed earlier, inherited genetic anomalies can result in abnormal craniofacial morphology. Abnormal development of the maxilla and/or mandible can lead to a narrow upper airway early in life and contribute to the development of OSA. Guilleminault *et al.* (2015) studied children and adults with hypodontia and OSA. Their initial findings suggest that there is progressive and significant increase in the AHI with ageing in dental conditions that exhibit a congenital absence of teeth, such as hypodontia and oligodontia. These findings led to the conclusion that conditions such as hypodontia and oligodontia (due to genetic mutations) affects facial development and lead to the development of OSA in later life. In addition, since alveolar bone growth is dependent on the development and eruption of teeth, children with a history of tooth extraction might develop a smaller oral cavity, which is thought to predispose to upper airway collapse during sleep, and these individuals may present with OSA in later life (Guilleminault *et al.*, 2016). Bearing in mind the preliminary findings of these studies, the routine extraction of healthy teeth such as premolar and wisdom teeth for orthodontic reasons appears to be untenable.

Mandibular growth

The three ear ossicles (malleus, incus, and stapes) of the middle ear form a chain of bones that vibrate, and sound is conducted to the cochlea where it is transmitted by the vestibulo-cochlear nerve (VIII cranial nerve) to the central nervous system for processing. Interestingly, the malleus (hammer) represents the primordial lower jaw (equivalent to the human mandible), and the malleolar-anvil joint is the original or primary jaw joint (equivalent to the human temporo-mandibular joint). Thus, the lower jaw of a crocodile or alligator is homologous with the tiny malleus in the human middle ear. Over the course of evolution, humans developed a secondary jaw joint for mastication, speech, and swallowing, while the original jaw joint was transferred to the middle ear for sound conduction. This secondary, human jaw joint relies on the formation and maturation of a secondary cartilage, the condylar cartilage, which undergoes endochondral ossification to become the condyle. The condylar cartilage is a 'secondary' cartilage relative to the 'primary' cartilages of the cranial base. As such, it appears much later both in terms of phylogeny during the course of evolution, and in ontogeny, during the course of human development. The head of the condyle is largely ossified but a layer of fibrocartilage is found on its articular surface, and in the underlying 'intermediate cell layer' it's likely that a population of undifferentiated mesenchymal stem cells persists. The stem cells of this intermediate cell layer are subject to temporo-spatial patterning. In this way, some stem cells close to the joint surface differentiate into fibroblasts that contribute to the formation of the fibrocartilage characteristic of the head of the condyle. Similarly, stem cells further away from the joint surface differentiate into chondroblasts that undergo endochondral ossification in the neck of the condyle.

Clinical evidence for the assertion of the existence of a condylar sub-population of stem cells comes from patients that have a rudimentary or congenital absence of the TMJ due to genetic mutations found in syndromes, such as (hemifacial) craniofacial microsomia. These children exhibit facial asymmetry secondary to mandibular maldevelopment, usually unilaterally. In these cases, the TMJ may be hypoplastic or non-functional and surgical procedures, such as distraction osteogenesis, may be deployed in the correction of craniofacial microsomia. After surgical correction, changes are seen both indirectly on the soft tissue facial surface (Cerajewska and Singh, 2001) as well as directly, in relation to the skeletal changes procured in mandibular morphology (Singh and Hay, 1999; Hay and Singh, 2000; Hay *et al.*, 2000). Surprisingly perhaps, concomitant changes are also seen in TMJ morphology after distraction osteogenesis. In one study (Santiago *et al.*, 2011) we found that prior to mandibular distraction osteogenesis, the condyle and glenoid fossa appear to be rudimentary or absent in these cases (Fig. 28a). Post-distraction, a well-defined condylar head was seen, which articulated in a newly formed glenoid fossa of the temporal bone (Fig. 28b).

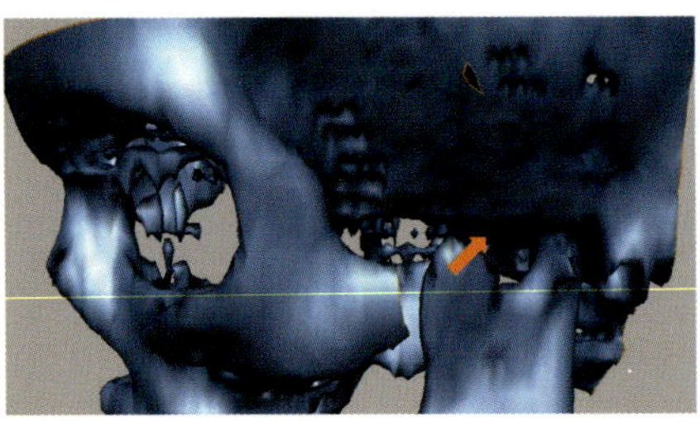

Figure 28a: Pre-treatment, the glenoid fossa is flat and the articular eminence is absent (arrowed).

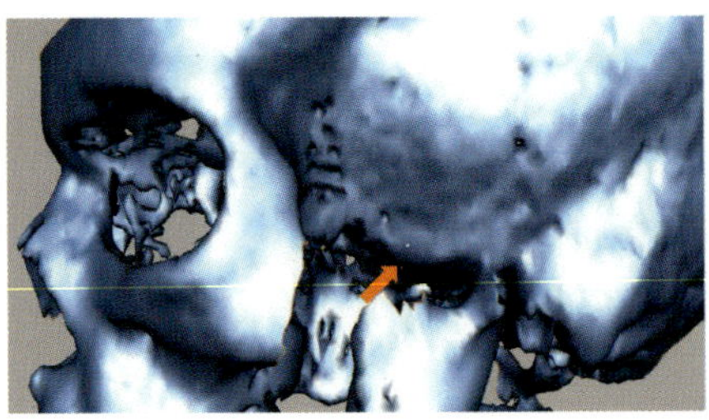

Figure 28b: Post-treatment, the contours of the glenoid fossa and the articular eminence (arrowed) are identifiable.

Note that in the distraction osteogenesis procedure, no attempt was made to modify or sculpt the temporal bone of the cranial base, yet a complete temporo-mandibular joint was formed with an improvement in TMJ function post-distraction. This example highlights the concept of temporo-spatial patterning in the light of epigenetic interactions. Put simply, genes encoding for normal TMJ morphogenesis were likely activated by surgically changing the spatial relations between the temporal bone of the cranial base and the condyle of the mandible. Refinement of TMJ function was probably achieved through functional stimuli once the spatial relations were within normal limits. Presumably, distraction osteogenesis involves the modulation or switching on of 'stretch-sensitive genes' due to the physical tension (stretching of the callus), resulting in deposition of cartilage similar to the epiphyseal plate of a long bone. In addition, growth hormones are likely secreted, which give rise to a multi-tissue response including muscle hypertrophy, epithelial hyperplasia (of the overlying skin) as well as cartilage deposition, following mesenchymal stem cell differentiation, which is converted into bone. Alternatively, stem cell differentiation could result in bone deposition in a process similar to the healing mechanism in bone fractures since osteotomy is the initial phase of the mandibular distraction osteogenesis procedure. In any case, this integrated tissue response is likely to produce a more stable outcome with less relapse due to a physiologic solution being reached by a complex, adaptive system attaining an enhanced level of homeostasis.

In addition, it is likely that conventional orthognathic surgery of the mandible (such as sagittal split osteotomy) produces esthetic changes predominantly, whereas distraction osteogenesis appears to produce size-, shape-, and positional changes that could mimic allometric growth of the mandible. Further evidence for this notion comes from orthodontic-orthopedic corrections of skeletal Class II malocclusions using Twin Block removal appliances (Singh and Clark, 2001). Even though many orthodontists do not believe it is possible to renew the growth of the mandible, experience with mandibular advancements devices in adults diagnosed with OSA has precipitated unwanted mandibular prognathism and Class III malocclusions (Korngut, 2010), presumably due to inappropriate stem cell activation. Despite this unwanted side effect, mandibular advancement devices are considered to be the first line of treatment in mild to moderate cases of OSA (ADA Policy, 2017). The mode of action of these appliances is that they protrude the mandible while being worn, and this new spatial matrix mechanically enlarges the upper airway (Sutherland and Cistulli, 2011). Therefore, comprehension of the natural growth and development of the mandible and its response to environmental stimuli is necessary in the practice of craniofacial sleep medicine.

Some studies suggest that changing the spatial cranio-mandibular relationship can affect other functional outcomes as well. For example, in a preliminary study, Singh *et al.* (2009) reported that a customized mandibular orthotic decreased the incidence of concussion and mild traumatic brain injury (MTBI) in young athletes. A possible mode of action of these types of devices is that they change the craniofacial architecture while being worn, increasing the distance between the (thinnest part of the) temporal bone and the head of the condyle. These new spatial relations appear to help prevent concussions and brain injuries, by avoiding atypical temporal lobe and corpus callosum activation, which is thought to precipitate concussions and MTBIs. Thus, the routine extraction of healthy, symptomless third molars, which dissipate forces by providing an increased surface area, must be viewed with some skepticism. But it has long been argued that human evolution is associated with a decreased jaw size resulting in the inability to accommodate 32 teeth. However, during this same evolutionary time period, the 'big bang' theory (Mithen, 1996) implies that human brains developed disproportionately rapidly, analogous to a hurricane hitting a scrapyard and building a Chevvy, according to the thoughts of Crick (who deciphered the structure of DNA along with Watson). In fact, modern humans develop enough dental tissues (32 teeth) to last a lifetime. In contrast, sheep and other herbivores lack upper anterior teeth and have a diastema instead. This pad is used to grip grass, which is cut using the lower incisors. If these lower incisors are lost through 'broken mouth disease' (Spence *et al.*, 1980), the sheep eventually die since they are no longer able to feed. In contrast, omnivorous humans have developed sufficient enamel on both the anterior and posterior teeth to last a lifetime; specifically, the thickness of enamel has been increasing in our posterior teeth over the course of human evolution (Beynon and Wood, 1986), suggesting that *Homo sapiens* need more dental tissues, not less. Elephants also show an interesting phenomenon in that they erupt each molar one at a time. The successive molar replaces the previous molar once it's worn out. But, if the third molar wears out, the elephant is no longer able to feed and eventually dies, having a lifespan roughly equivalent to that of a human. The pattern of tooth morphology evolution is also interesting. The earliest teeth in cartilaginous and bony fish were conical, and later bicuspid tooth morphology with two cusps emerged. Later still, evolutionary biologists described the trigone (Korenhof, 1978), which is a three-cusped tooth (component) and the talon (Whitney and Sidor, 2019), which gave the tooth a four-cusp arrangement. However, modern humans have a five-cusped tooth morphology (the Dryopithecus pattern; Jørgensen, 1955), and more recently still, the evolution of a sixth cusp, Carabelli's tubercle, has been described. Therefore, the notion that modern *Homo sapiens* need smaller jaws for less teeth does not appear to be supported by current evidence. The question can also be posed, what do teeth and sleep have in common? An answer to the brain-tooth relationship lies in the etiology of oral tori and their clinical significance in sleep disordered breathing.

Consider the aortic and carotid bodies that possess chemoreceptors that are able to detect oxygen desaturation and hypercapnia of the blood. If detected, afferent nerves carry signals back from the carotid and aortic bodies to the brainstem, which responds by increasing ventilation since astrocytes detect increased CO_2 levels centrally and increase respiration efficiency through a variety of peripheral actions and interactions. In addition, there is also neuromuscular accommodation in that cervical repositioning can change the head posture to maintain the airway. In effect, a negative feedback loop is triggered since the body makes postural changes (postural compensation) via the musculoskeletal, cardio-respiratory and sympathetic nervous system to optimize gas exchange. While the forward head posture opens the upper airway, it also increases the spinal moment arm (which is the perpendicular distance from a pivot to a point undergoing torque). Thus, forward head posture, while opening the upper airway, increases the loading on the anterior segments of the spine and intervertebral disks, compresses the thoracic cavity and causes the spine to deviate from its optimal sagittal posture. As a result, pathological remodeling ensues. In other words, bone remodels in response to changes in posture/spatial relations. Unfortunately, tooth enamel prevents optimal positioning of the jaw bones, so that the vicious cycle of aortic/carotid bodies detecting O_2 desaturation/hypercapnia is re-triggered and subtle, 'retrusive' (daytime) bruxism ensues in an attempt to maintain the patency of the upper airway.

Atypical maxillo-mandibular development

Epigenetic modulations result in various manifestations of phenotypic plasticity, including changes in maxillo-mandibular morphology. Here, I posit the notion that sleep bruxism might represent a developmental mechanism for oral torus formation. Nearly all researchers agree that the underlying cause of oral torus development remains unresolved. Thus, the aim of this review is to provide a mechanism for the formation of maxillary and mandibular tori, including buccal exostoses (Fig. 29). In an unpublished study, 99 cases suspected of having SDB were reviewed for the presence of maxillary and mandibular tori, including buccal exostoses. The results indicated that 10 of these 99 cases (≈10%) exhibited maxillary and/or mandibular tori. Tori maybe the missing link in the triad: malocclusion-TMD-SDB. This triad of conditions may present as a diagnosis of craniofacial underdevelopment. In this condition, the jaws may be 'retrusive' with dental wear patterns suggestive of sleep bruxism. In fact, OSA is the most

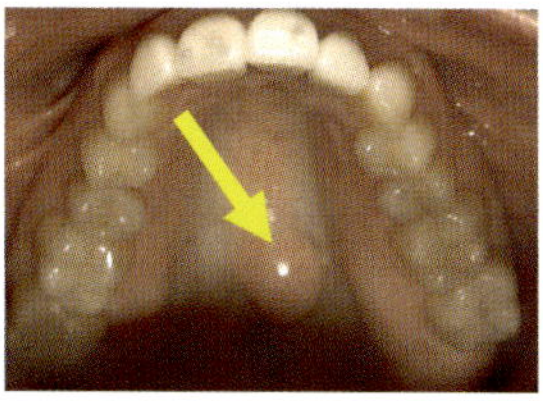

Figure 29a: Torus palatinus localized near midline of the palatal vault (arrowed). Courtesy: Dr Sue Wendling

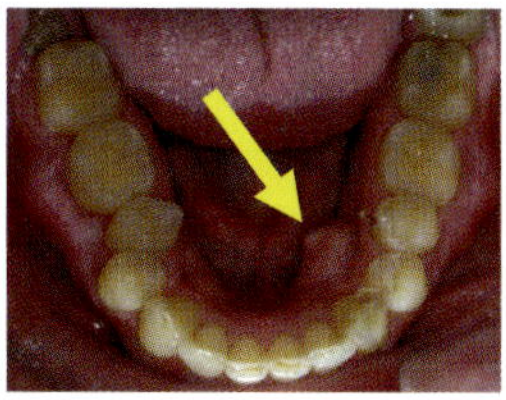

Figure 29b: An unilateral torus mandibularis (arrowed). Courtesy: Dr Edna Santos

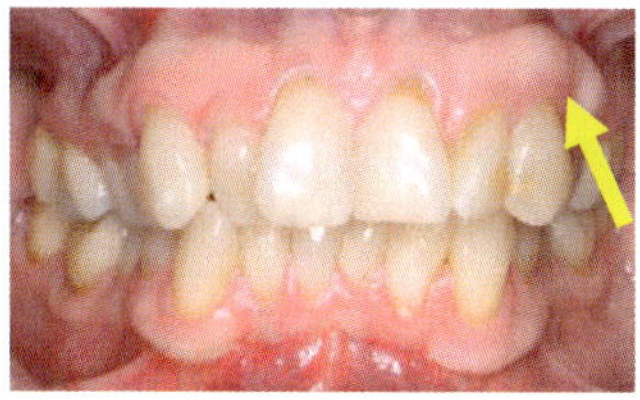

Figure 29c: Buccal exostoses (arrowed) on the left side. Courtesy: Dr Mike Safranek

common risk factor for nocturnal bruxism (Ohayon *et al.*, 2001) since a flattened wear pattern of the teeth is associated with bruxism, and sleep bruxism is more common in patients with OSA. Indeed, some are of the opinion that bruxism may be an airway protective reflex (Simmons and Prehn, 2008 and 2009) that occurs following respiratory events (Hosoya *et al.*, 2014).

Sleep bruxism (SB) is a movement disorder associated with sleep arousals and characterized by a rise in sympathetic-cardiac activity, rhythmic masticatory muscle activity (RMMA) and tooth grinding (Khoury *et al.*, 2008). Before the RMMA, the amplitude of respiration is also increased, producing a classic respiratory effort related arousal (RERA). Esophageal pressure sensors show the increasing respiratory effort and the electroencephalograph (EEG) shows arousal. Thus, bruxism is preceded by an obstructive respiratory event (Hosoya *et al.*, 2014). It has also been noted that there is decreased masseteric muscle activity prior to the RERA (Khoury *et al.* 2008), while a discrete RERA triggers increased masseteric muscle activity. Simmons and Prehn (2008 and 2009) suggest that this increased masseter activity "brings the mandible forward" as an airway protective reflex to keep the airway open. That this is not the case is supported by the fact that the mandible is a jaw elevator muscle; it does not protrude the mandible but results instead in periodic jaw movements (RMMA). Singh (2007) had earlier suggested that tooth-grinding and muscle-clenching activities may be ineffectual attempts to relieve airway compromise in that the muscles of mastication may be acting antagonistically to the constrictors of the pharynx.

For example, in the natural predator-prey life cycle, after the chase the predator is exhausted and needs thorough oxygenation for recovery. However, with the prey clenched within the jaws, the predator must rely on nasal breathing exclusively. To accentuate nasal airflow, the pressure differential needs to be increased with respect to the distal airway. Here I hypothesize that a novel/undetermined mammalian reflex is brought into play with the muscles of mastication acting as antagonists to the pharyngeal constrictors (Singh, 2007). By increasing muscle tension in one set of muscles, the antagonists relax, thereby increasing upper airway volume, decreasing the distal airway pressure and promoting proximal-distal airflow. Note that professional weight-lifting athletes sometimes use a mouthpiece and clench the jaws during athletic performance, such as the clean and jerk. More commonly it is known that, during labor, women were sometimes given a bite cloth or wooden utensil to bite on to assist in parturition. Both examples presumably implicate a novel or as yet undetermined mammalian reflex. Note that Singh and Olmos (2007) demonstrated a 15% increase in the residual volume of the airway during treatment for TMD using a phonetic bite registration. To illustrate this phenomenon further, consider the muscles of mastication during wakefulness. After chewing food, the next stage is swallowing, which necessitates relaxation of the oropharynx to accept the bolus. This means that the upper airway muscles are also relaxed and protected by the epiglottis to prevent food inhalation. Note that food entering the airway during swallowing elicits the gag and/or cough reflex. Now consider the events during sleep. Nocturnal airway collapse requires airway dilation and, therefore, relaxation of the pharyngeal constrictors. In some cases, the individual begins to tooth grind or muscle clench during sleep, leading to nocturnal or sleep bruxism in an ineffectual attempt to open the airway, which has collapsed partly because of the effects of gravity and partly due to oropharyngeal muscle relaxation. Further support for this mechanism of bruxism, with the muscles of mastication acting as antagonists to the pharyngeal constrictors, comes from the gag reflex. Foreign objects entering the oropharynx elicit the gag reflex via the glossopharyngeal nerve. Here, the upper airway constricts, and the mouth opens in an effort to expel the foreign object. Now consider further a case of lockjaw or temporo-mandibular joint spasm. In this case, the muscles of mastication have contracted, and jaw movements/mouth opening are difficult. One clinical way of relieving this muscle spasm is to elicit the gag reflex by placing fingers or some other suitable object into the person's oropharynx. In this situation, the pharyngeal constrictors will be activated during the gag reflex, while the muscles of mastication will relax antagonistically, thus relieving the TMJ spasm. Thus, the muscles of mastication may be antagonistic to the constrictors of the pharynx.

Singh (2010) considers that RMMA plays a critical role in ectopic bone formation and the etiology of oral tori such as torus palatinus, torus mandibularis and buccal exostoses. Note that García-García *et al.* (2010) suggest that there is a hereditary component to torus formation, that they tend to appear more frequently in middle age, and that particular ethnic groups are more likely to develop them. However, most agree that the underlying cause of torus formation remains unresolved. Here, I discuss predictions that emanate from the spatial matrix hypothesis (Singh, 2004; Singh, 2007; Singh and Krumholtz, 2009). First, put simply, the spatial matrix hypothesis suggests that gene-environmental interactions proceed as developmental events unfold even in a perturbed functional space (a matrix that has departed from the ideal temporo-spatial pattern encoded at the genomic level). Second, the spatial matrix hypothesis might explain the occurrence of the symptoms of TMD, which often include clenching, bruxism, tooth grinding, and tooth wear (facets). These parafunctional habits are thought to be secondary or in some way compensatory for a compromised upper airway (Singh and Olmos, 2007), and may provide a possible mechanism for the formation of maxillary and mandibular tori, including buccal exostoses. During clenching/tooth grinding/bruxism, muscular forces are applied periodically to the dentition, which present as tooth wear (facets) over a period of time, but bone deformation also occurs concurrently during bruxing. Note that heavy forces of short duration (< 50kg <1 second) occur during mastication but are largely absorbed by the periodontium. This process results in no orthodontic tooth movement but bending of the collagen and alveolar bone can elicit a piezoelectric effect. Therefore, I posited that during parafunctional activities both the maxilla and mandible undergo similar forces (approx. 200mmHg; 0.27kg/ cm^2), resulting in bone deformation, and the ensuing stress and stretch of the osteogenic periosteum eventually leads to bone formation in the form of tori in a site-specific fashion, according to distribution of force vectors (Singh, 2010). Similarly, Morrison and Tamimi (2013) suggest that there is an increased likelihood of oral tori associated with local abnormal mechanical stress that leads to ectopic bone formation. For example, a typical torus palatinus (Fig. 29a) does not extend beyond transverse palatine suture, while the midpalatal suture likely remains patent until at least age 30yrs (Kokich, 1994) and probably beyond, permitting repetitive, compressive stresses leading to buckling of the maxilla about the midline. The osteogenic periosteum covering the palatal vault and midpalatal suture would be stretched, and this tension leads to new bone formation localized to the midline, being the epicenter of force distribution, thereby precipitating a torus palatinus. However, if the vectors of force distribution are changed, acting medially instead of laterally in the coronal plane, buccal exostoses may be formed with the osteogenic periosteum of the buccal plate depositing new bone in focal areas of force dissemination. In fact, recently, Valigi and Logozzo (2019) demonstrated how maxillary exostosis formation correlates with mechanical stress and load distribution, concluding that exostoses arise as the bone responds to parafunctions such as bruxing.

On the other hand, mandibular tori may be present even in the absence of a palatal torus, and these bilateral mandibular tori are most often found in the premolar region on the medial aspect of the mandible. This finding can be explained using the bone deformation or osteogenic-periosteal stretch hypothesis. First, the morphology of the mandible permits its body to bend, especially in the mental foramen region, which has a low bone volume due to the neurovascular bundle passing through it. The body of the mandible further posteriorly has an additional robust, supporting structure, the mylohyoid ridge, that prevents the corpus from flexing. The same can be said of the ramus, which is enclosed by the muscles of mastication. However, it is understood that parafunctional activity can lead to hypertrophy both of the masseter and its bony attachment, the angle of the mandible. But this mechanism cannot easily explain the preferential location of mandibular tori in the mental region. According to the bone deformation osteogenic-periosteal stretch hypothesis, however, the chin is prevented from undergoing excessive deformation due to the mental process. Humans lack the simian shelf but have instead developed a chin to strengthen the weakest part of mandible. Thus, the morphology of the mandible localizes tori formation to the premolar region as the mandibular body buckles medially due to a combination of muscular compression, localized low bone volume and tooth orientation. Note that with the teeth in occlusion, the buccal overjet will ensure that mandibular dentition is bent medially inward. In addition, if teeth are missing or extracted there would be less force available and should produce smaller deformation and smaller tori or no tori on the tooth deficient side. Therefore, if the magnitude of vectors is changed sufficiently, a unilateral mandibular torus may be formed (Fig. 29b). Indeed, Singh (2010) was the first to report the finding of a unilateral mandibular torus. Similarly, during parafunctional activities, the lateral pterygoid muscle stretches the osteogenic perichondrium surrounding the condyle, leading to bone formation in a site-specific fashion, recognized as epiphyte formation or 'beaking', according to local stem cell differentiation. In any case, clinically, children should be screened for wear facets and developing tori, which can sometimes be palpated. If observed, referral to a sleep physician should be considered to rule out covert or overt sleep disordered breathing. Cases of sleep bruxism can be treated with biomimetic oral appliance therapy (Liao and Singh, 2015) but tori are best managed by surgical reduction, especially in the case of extensive bilateral torus mandibularis (Singh *et al.*, 2012). The surgical technique requires appropriate pre-operative preparation, good clinical skills (akin to removing an impacted lower third molar) and post-operative care to prevent any healing complications. On the other hand, non-surgical reduction in the size of some mandibular tori and buccal exostoses following biomimetic oral appliance therapy has been observed (Singh *et al.*, 2019).

The spatial matrix hypothesis

My spatial matrix hypothesis was first presented at the Moyer's Symposium (2003) and published in the Craniofacial Growth Series (Singh, 2004). Later, it was reproduced in a slightly edited form in the first version of this book (Singh and Krumholtz, 2009). A report on a second symposium reads, "*With our increasing understanding of temporo-spatial patterning, the challenge is to further integrate the functional matrix theory so that the spatial relations of the functional spaces that sanction orthodontic treatments, such as the periodontal space, upper and lower temporo-mandibular joint spaces, nasal airway, maxillary sinus and posterior pharyngeal airway space, as well as the oral cavity, are clinically-optimized to prevent disease, maintain health, ameliorate dysfunction and treat disease, to improve the oral and systemic health of patients*" (Singh, 2004). The reason for the derivation of the spatial matrix hypothesis was based on the realization that reconciliation of the effects produced by treatment and the natural growth that occurs during that time has thwarted the orthodontic profession for many years. There are several reasons for this perhaps, and one might include amongst these the reliance upon lateral cephalometric analysis. While cephalographs initially provided dental clinicians with a valuable diagnostic tool, the modulation of a three-dimensional craniofacial system in space over time warrants questions about the applicability of 2D cephalometry (Moyers and Bookstein, 1979). In cephalometric analyses historically, there was a tacit implication that the craniofacial complex consists of a co-assemblage of a series of components of genetically predetermined form. While this assumption is largely true for the crowns of teeth, treatment-induced changes of their surrounding biologically active structures may be perceived erroneously and was reported often as differential 'movements' of various components. Given inherent, phenotypic variation, increases in size with time can obscure treatment-induced form-changes; but the net results need to be consistent with the biologic mechanisms underlying the perceived clinical changes. Thus, former conceptual limitations did not permit the dynamic, biologic behavior of the craniofacial structures to be taken into account as fully as one might hope. Paraphrasing Williams and Murphy (2008), *"as old as it is new, this new biology is articulated well within the intelligent and compelling perspectives posited by Singh's spatial matrix hypothesis, which points out that tissues constantly regress to homeostasis"*. Therefore, the arena for these clinical gene-environmental interactions is discussed here as the spatial matrix hypothesis.

Several attempts have been made to derive a single theory that encapsulates the biologic behavior of the craniofacial system during its development and during its therapeutic manipulation. One such theory was the old functional matrix hypothesis (FMH; Moss, 1997). The FMH had been successful in explaining some biologic craniofacial phenomena but failed to make testable predictions. For example, the periodontium that supports the roots of teeth represents a functional matrix. As long as the tooth remains in function, e.g. in occlusal contact during mastication, alveolar bone will be deposited, remodeled and maintained to sustain that function. In contrast, if the tooth is extracted, the supporting alveolar bone will be resorbed due an absence of function. This effect is somewhat analogous to a professional athlete; as long as an exercise routine is maintained, the physique will remain in good shape but, when the exercise regimen is halted, muscle tone will be lost. However, if a tooth is lost, the (occlusally) opposing tooth may erupt into the vacated space until its occlusal surface contacts the mucosa of the opposite jaw or some other steric hindrance (Fig. 18b). This clinically observed phenomenon cannot be explained on the basis of the FMH alone but, noting that during this supra-eruptive phase supporting alveolar bone will be deposited, exploitation of this phenomenon can be utilized in non-surgical treatments. For example,

Salama and Salama (1993) described a method of orthodontic extrusive remodeling of bone that can be used to support an implant for later tooth replacement if the supra-erupting tooth is of poor quality or has a dubious prognostic potential. Orthodontic extrusion, which utilizes light eruptive forces, enhances the slow eruption of teeth as the entire attachment apparatus relocates coronally with the crown of the tooth. Consequently, decomposition of the observed clinical changes into growth effects and treatment effects is not possible. This very same eruptive phenomenon, however, when applied to the whole of the periodontium surrounding the tooth roots in the maxillary arch, will be commensurate with a clinical increase in (vertical) anterior facial height (vertical drift), which is a known feature of ageing (Thompson and Kendrick, 1964). This effect is less easy to account for using the FMH alone. As well, vertical downward growth of the human face, especially noticeable in the alveolar processes, is associated with a lack of space and an increasing frequency of crowding (Bishara *et al.*, 1994). Thus, measurable, physical changes may be integrated with the associated biologic response so intimately that resolution of treatment-induced- and natural-change may not be possible.

Introduction to functional spaces: The upper airway

The human body is essentially a tube inside a tube inside another tube. The outermost tube is the ectodermally-derived skin; the innermost tube is the endodermally derived endothelium of the viscera; and, in between these two tubes, are the mesodermally derived connectives tissues. An important craniofacial functional space is the upper airway. This dynamic complex space is roofed by the nasopharynx anteriorly and contains the tubal tonsils (just above the opening of the pharyngo-tympanic tubes). The nasopharynx is continuous with the oropharynx, which houses the palatine tonsils (in the tonsillar fossae), the adenoids (in the posterior pharyngeal wall), and the lingual tonsils (in the posterior one-third of the tongue). The oropharynx extends into the hypopharynx in the supraglottic region, where the glottis is located. This latter region is the laryngopharynx, which is itself continuous with the trachea, bronchi, and lungs. Due to the complexity of its components, the function of this upper airway space is manifold. First, as noted above, it is intimately involved in nasal respiration and lower down, mouth-breathing can augment the nasal air passages during exertion, such as exercise, and during emergency situations of fight or flight. Postnatally, neonates are obligate nasal breathers and most babies sleep with the mouth closed while breathing through the nose (Fig. 30). The closed-mouth posture may have inferred a benefit during the course of human evolution, but more importantly perhaps, is the fact that a baby can breathe and feed simultaneously. For example, during breast-feeding, the laryngeal inlet is protected by the soft palate contacting the epiglottis, so that the mother's milk is directed laterally into the esophagus while respiration continues unimpeded.

In the adult, respiration is momentarily halted with the soft palate in contact with the posterior pharyngeal wall so that food or fluids are prevented from entering the nasal cavity by the velopharyngeal seal, with the epiglottis guarding the laryngeal inlet while swallowing occurs. In cases of velopharyngeal insufficiency, such as children with a repaired cleft palate, nasal escape may occur with air or fluids entering the nasal cavities during speech or swallowing. Similarly, foreign particles entering

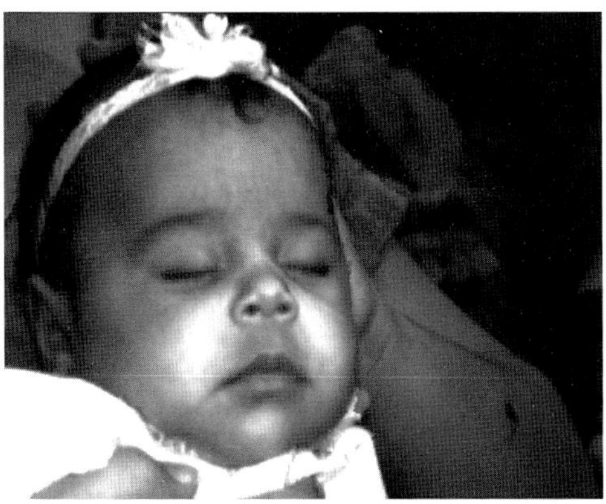

Figure 30: Neonates and young babies are obligate nasal breathers and sleep with the mouth closed while breathing through the nose.

the respiratory passage will set off a gagging, coughing, or choking reaction. The velopharyngeal isthmus can be viewed from above by introducing an endoscope through the nose after the use of appropriate topical anesthesia (Fig. 31a). Similarly, the velopharyngeal isthmus can be viewed from the lateral aspect to determine its relation to the posterior pharyngeal wall, for example by using video-fluoroscopy during speech (Fig. 31b). In addition, dynamic MRI can also be used. Essentially, viewed from above the velopharyngeal isthmus has three basic patterns of closure: antero-posterior, medio-lateral, and a constrictor pattern of closure (Witzel and Posnick, 1989). Therefore, the functional behavior of the upper airway can vary between individuals, and this variation in behavior may impact the response to various treatments.

In addition, functional spaces can affect the facial skeleton, which provides a basis for facial appearance. Here we introduce the notion that underdeveloped faces may indicate a collapse or constriction of the upper airway. For example, the functional space of the oropharynx is required for mastication, speech, and swallowing. It is thought that a minimum speaking space is required for adults (Burnett and Clifford, 1993) as speech communication is central to the human condition. This physiologic position may be encroached upon, producing clinical signs

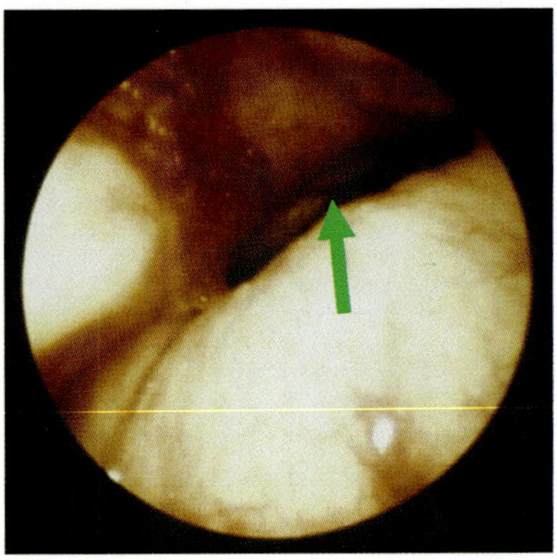

Figure 31a: The velopharyngeal isthmus (arrowed) viewed from above using nasendoscopy.

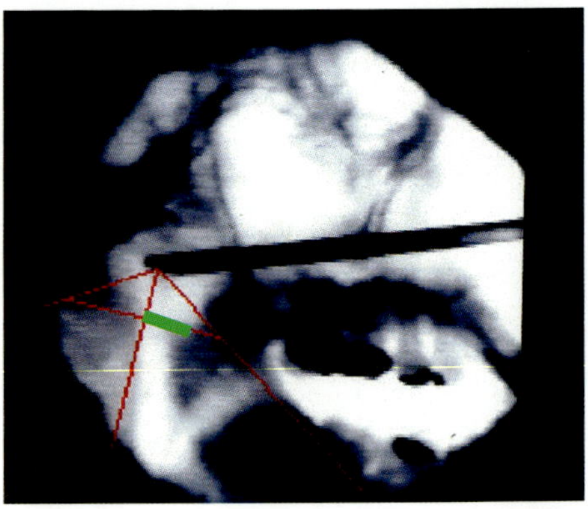

Figure 31b: The velopharyngeal isthmus (green bar) viewed from the lateral aspect using video-fluoroscopy.

such as tongue scalloping and tooth wear associated with bruxism and clenching (Weiss *et al.*, 2005). Other functional positions also exist, such as the intercuspal position, which differs from the postural or rest position by a few millimeters of the freeway space. During swallowing, the epiglottis at the back of the tongue guards the entrance to the laryngopharynx so that food and fluids are directed into the esophagus and not to the trachea. Obstruction of the oropharyngeal airway space in children can be due to enlarged palatine tonsils. In the past, tonsillectomy was carried out routinely. While it remains as an elective treatment, it is less commonly performed these days even though it may be of immense value in addressing pediatric OSA and preventing the onset of chronic mouth-breathing. Similarly, the adenoids within the posterior pharyngeal wall may cause airway obstruction in the growing child (Fig. 25b). Thus, each patient needs a thorough functional evaluation prior to the removal of any tissues such as the tonsils or teeth etc., as the upper airway space can have profound effects on facial appearance, a theme that we will return to later in this book. However, two facial features are of note even in this introductory section. First, people with a 'double-chin' appearance are likely obstructing the upper airway by the tongue base (Banabilh *et al.*, 2009), and second, people with an increased thyromandibular angle are likely to have a similar condition. For example, Lam *et al.* (2005) found that male Caucasian patients with a Class II or Class III jaw profile and Asian patients, especially those that are obese, are more likely to have snoring, sleep disordered breathing, and OSA with high apnea-hypopnea indices, which are indicative of respiratory disturbance. Males have an increased predisposition to OSA, which is likely due to temporo-spatial patterning, as males tend to deposit more fat in the submandibular space below the chin, giving a double-chin appearance with a neck girth beyond 17–18 inches. The reason for this particular storage site may be phylogenetic. For example, certain mammals, such as oxen exhibit a flap of skin, which hangs down below the lower jaw and neck. Beneath this flap of skin is the platysma muscle, enclosed in fascia. This site can act as a fat store, similar to the hump of a camel. Hanging down due to gravity, this flap of skin has little consequence to a quadruped. In the human bipedal stance, however, this very same site continues to store fat, but large accumulations will impede respiration as the tongue is displaced backward, obstructing the upper airway. The etiology, significance, and management of these features will be discussed as features of the spatial matrix hypothesis in the section below.

Periodontium: Functional space

Within the oral cavity, a series of other functional spaces exist, i.e. the periodontal 'ligament' space or periodontium. This series of functional spaces is at the heart of the development of a malocclusion, its clinical correction, and relapse, as it provides a developmental mechanism for the complex, adaptive oral system to remain in homeostasis, equilibrium, or balance. In fact, the historical nomenclature of periodontal 'ligament' is a misnomer. **The periodontium is not a ligament**. When comparing the histologic and ultrastructural components of a typical ligament and the periodontium, obvious differences become apparent (Shore *et al.*, 1984). For example, in the rat periodontium the fibril diameter is small (40μm) but in a true ligament the fiber diameter is large (Berkovitz *et al.*, 2018). In addition, in a typical ligament the fiber diameter shows a bimodal pattern of distribution, i.e. small (immature) and large (mature) fibers, while in the rat periodontium the distribution of fibers is unimodal, showing a normal distribution (Berkovitz *et al.*, 1981). These features suggest that the fibrils in the periodontium have a high rate of turnover and fail to undergo maturation, somewhat similar to fetal tissue. In addition, the extracellular matrix composition of the rat periodontium differs significantly from that of a typical ligament (Shore *et al.*, 1991). Functionally, the periodontal ligament space of the periodontium is subject to sutural homeostasis not unlike the clinical sutures of the skull (Williams *et al.*, 2011). Typically, the periodontal ligament space occupies a width of about 0.25mm (250μm). Recent research suggests that this sutural width is tightly controlled at the genetic level. For example, a sutural width

> 250μm can initiate new bone deposition until the normal sutural width has been achieved. Conversely, a sutural width < 250μm results in bone resorption until the normal width has been achieved. Thus, from this sutural homeostasis model, one can appreciate that the periodontal ligament or periodontium ought to be regarded as a modified suture or 'periodontal suture'. Sutural homeostasis explains how malocclusions are maintained and how orthodontic procedures might be deployed in their correction, including palatal expansion or induced maxillary morphogenesis. Indeed, a biomimetic oral appliance might also be utilized so that certain genes are modulated. Downstream, specific protein products are biosynthesized, which contribute to new tissue (bone) formation. At the same time, angiogenesis and the in-growth of capillaries can provide the nutrients required, such as calcium, to complete the physiologic process of sutural osteogenesis, which is monitored and subject to sutural homeostasis. In fact, it has been shown that the mammalian periodontium has a structure that is akin to fetal tissues rather than mature adult tissues (Shore *et al.*, 1984). Moreover, it is thought that the periodontium retains its fetal-like behavior into adulthood so that bony remodeling and adaptation remain viable throughout the entire life span. Using this concept, premature maturation of the periodontium would result in ankylosis of the tooth root to the alveolar bone (Fig. 32). In contrast,

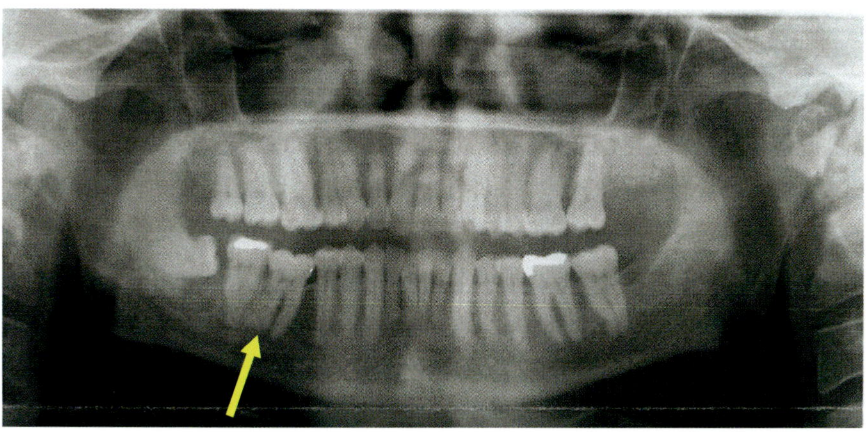

Figure 32: The lower right first molar shows ankylosis (arrowed) likely due to premature maturation of the periodontium.

ultra-light forces exerted on the periodontium are thought to provoke woven bone formation (Williams and Murphy, 2008), and woven bone is a hallmark of fetal, not adult, bone formation.

Summary of the spatial matrix hypothesis

During normal craniofacial growth and development, ossification centers arise at sites of signal transduction and lay down bone for the first time. These growing facial bones are displaced by expanding soft tissues, such as the brain and other developing functional spaces. For example, the nasal capsule proliferates, and because cartilage is pressure resistant (having very few blood vessels), the nasal cavity increases in volume, remaining encased in bone through bone deposition and remodeling. In the floor of the nose, for example, the two halves of the palatal bones (horizontal plates of the maxillae) meet in the midline midpalatal suture as they ossify. Deposition of bone (precursor) occurs at this sutural boundary and is subject to sutural homeostasis by the encoding genes that respond to environmental stimuli. The periodontal ligament space is another specialized functional space, which can affect facial appearance, according to the spatial matrix hypothesis. Thus, during normal growth and development, the spatial and functional alignment of skeletal elements (and teeth) is maintained through remodeling of bony surfaces (including the periodontium) to permit function. Environmentally induced changes in these early morphologic relationships will lead to a 'new solution' perceived as a change in facial appearance as a child grows. However, departure from the genetically encoded 'developmental program' leads to different 'new solutions' or conditions of stability even if function is somewhat compromised, such as malocclusions, TMD, OSA, etc. These variant but sometimes pathologic conditions arise due to developmental compensation, which permits compromised function rather than no function at all. **Therefore, developmental decompensation is first required before optimal function can be established clinically**, since appropriate spatial signaling can re-establish the genomic pattern formation for optimal form and function, as noted in the distraction osteogenesis example given above. Nevertheless, non-surgical, dentofacial orthopedic-orthodontic options are also available to dental professionals.

As mentioned in Chapter 2, early investigations of the effect of changing spatial relations on craniofacial growth and development were first carried out by Kingsley (1880) who introduced the concept of 'jumping the bite' for patients with a retrognathic mandible. In later studies, Breitner (1930) suggested that the forward position of the mandible might be a result of remodeling processes in the articular fossa, but later Breitner (1940) hypothesized that the tissue changes were the result of applied forces, since (retrusive) elastics applied in the opposite direction showed reciprocal changes. Perhaps the notion that bone resorption is a response to tissue pressure was not known at that time. Thus, the tissue response to mandibular repositioning was not fully understood, and it was Haupl and Psansky (1938), and Eschler (1939), who introduced the concept of a 'functional factor' as being important in 'functional' orthopedic treatment, such as Andresen monobloc or the 'functional' activator (Wahl, 2006). On the other hand, Longmire and Sanford (1949) sutured the anterior portion of the tongue to the inner surface of the lower lip to putatively stimulate the development of the mandible in cases of Pierre Robin syndrome. Not only was the obstructive apnea resolved but the subsequent growth of the lower jaw was apparently normalized even though **gentle traction with no forces were used** *per se*; in other words, the mandible was held in a forward position secondary to the tongue suture. Despite these studies supporting the effects of positional changes, Baume and Derichsweiler (1961) suggested that the mandibular response was mediated via condylar growth centers. In this way, repositioning of the mandible somehow became labeled as the work of 'functional' appliances and inadvertently created confusion and controversy in the minds of orthodontists, which has not been resolved at the time of writing. For example, experimental studies on 'functional' mandibular protrusion were done on Rhesus macaques (McNamara and Carlson, 1979) who quantified adaptations of the TMJ in mandibular protrusion. Later, McNamara and Bryan (1987) also described long-term adaptations to mandibular protrusion in Rhesus monkeys. They indicated that the mandibular length was 7mm longer in the protrusive group compared to controls after nearly 3 years and concluded that mandibular growth is not solely genetically pre-determined. But, these findings, which were made in the absence of molecular genetic techniques, support the spatial matrix hypothesis, and appear to follow the developmental mechanisms reported by Fuentes *et al.* (2003) in that **changing the position of the mandible leads to a change in the pattern of gene expression**. More recently, using digital geometric morphometric techniques, Singh and Clark (2001) localized changes in the condylar region after mandibular advancement device use in children and teenagers. In pubertal boys, we found a 28% increase in condylar length, similar to the reports of studies on Rhesus macaques. These types of findings lead me to suggest that 'functional' appliances may actually be 'formational' appliances (Singh, 2009) in the sense that bone and other tissues are being formed in response to the change in spatial relations of the jaws and teeth. Moreover, these contentions are also supported by the work of Williams and Murphy (2008) who note that Singh (2004) first captured the concept of how clinical spatial changes might invoke changes in gene expression.

According to the spatial matrix hypothesis (Singh, 2004), changing the spatial relations of the jaws changes the bite and positions of the cusp-fossa relations of the teeth, which lose their normal occlusal contacts and thus are no longer in homeostasis. These spatial changes are detected by mechanoreceptors in the periodontium (Sherrington, 1919; Suzuki, 1963) and periosteal cells. Consequently, remodeling occurs due to signal transduction, as predicted by the spatial matrix hypothesis (Singh, 2004; Singh, 2007; Singh and Krumholtz, 2009) in an effort to regain (sutural) homeostasis. Systemic examples of homeostasis include blood pressure maintenance, body temperature regulation, etc. These systems are subject to physiologic control through sophisticated feedback loops. Similarly, the craniofacial region is under spatial and functional regulation. However, the craniofacial region is also subject to developmental compensation, which differs according to genomic variation from patient to patient because of complexity. Therefore, patients may present with a range of clinical signs and symptoms, such as: malocclusions, TMD, UARS/OSA, facial asymmetry, tooth wear/bruxism, headaches, orofacial pain, etc., even though the underlying etiology may be similar in most cases, most of the time. Since craniofacial epigenetics is aimed at the overall health of the craniofacial region, appropriate treatment protocols must be provided that address the underlying etiology of the signs and symptoms of these conditions. Moreover, despite these phenotypic variations, the outcomes of these epigenetic processes require clinical decompensation prior to final correction. This decompensation is often achieved through appropriate spatial signaling, which can help re-establish (genomic) pattern formation for optimal form and function (Singh, 2004, 2007; Singh and Krumholtz, 2009). Thus, craniofacial epigenetics deploys a person's natural genes to correct and enhance the jaws, teeth, soft tissues and functional spaces, painlessly, using biomimetic oral appliances.

The spatial matrix hypothesis differs from old ideas, such as the Equilibrium theory (Proffit, 1978) which focused primarily on dental tissues, and the functional matrix hypothesis (Moss, 1997), which taught that the facial skeleton (maxilla and mandible) is formed mainly by ossification within genic membranes (such as the osteogenic periosteum and perichondrium). Moss (1997) argued that skeletal form is largely secondary and adaptive to its surrounding soft tissues and functional spaces. Here is the first point of divergence from the spatial matrix hypothesis (Singh, 2004) since the behavior of dental tissues (teeth) has been largely omitted from the old functional matrix hypothesis. I define a spatial matrix as an arena in which development events unfold as gene-environmental interactions proceed, e.g. the developmental dynamics of the orofacial complex, including tooth eruption. Next, the old functional matrix hypothesis was based on 'functional' changes to some extent. For example, if a tooth is lost (through extraction) then resorption and loss of alveolar bone ensues since bone is no longer required to accommodate that tooth in the jaw. While this example holds true in clinical practice, it does not comprehensively describe how the craniofacial region attains homeostasis after the event. Consider the loss of an upper molar tooth, say, second or third maxillary molar (Fig. 18). In these cases, it is often noted that the maxillary air sinus expands into the alveolar region post-extraction (Fig. 18a). Sometimes, an opposing tooth in the lower jaw (over)erupts into the vacated space (Fig. 18b), and the tongue learns to avoid those new occlusal contacts to avoid trauma during function. In other words, the spatial matrix hypothesis takes all four craniofacial components (hard tissues, bone; soft tissues, muscle; dental tissues, teeth; and functional spaces, sinuses/upper airway) into account with a unifying principle: craniofacial homeostasis.

On the other hand, the functional matrix hypothesis simply stated that during growth, spatial and functional alignment of the skeletal elements (such as the maxilla and mandible) is maintained through remodeling of bony surfaces (cortical bone remodeling). This statement omits the dental tissues (teeth) that are intimately and uniquely associated with the maxilla and mandible. Conversely, the spatial matrix hypothesis teaches that sutural homeostasis is a craniofacial requirement, and this may be associated with pneumatization of (new) functional spaces as noted above. The functional matrix hypothesis also taught that 'ossification centers' arise during growth but at the time of its first formulation (van der Klaauw, 1946) there was little or no information on how they arise. It is now known that these 'ossification centers' are, in fact, sites of signal transduction, based on temporo-spatial patterning. In other words, according to the genetic blueprint, certain genes will be expressed at certain sites during development. On receiving an appropriate signal these (stem) cells will undergo signal transduction and differentiate into osteoblasts that will lay down new (woven) bone. In fact, van der Klaauw (1946) correctly described how 'new' bones were displaced by soft tissues (e.g. the brain) and expanding functional spaces, e.g. the cranial cavity. In this way, cranial sutures are formed when two adjacent bones come into close proximity. In other words, two plates of bone meet at sutures as they grow by deposition of bone (precursor) at sutural boundaries. But one question remained unanswered: How do they know when to stop bone formation? The most likely answer is the mechanism of sutural homeostasis (as discussed in Chapter 2). In other words, ossification centers arise during development *de novo* and represent sites of signal transduction due to temporo-spatial patterning of genes within localized stem cell populations.

Another important difference between the FMH and the spatial matrix hypothesis is that during growth, while the spatial and functional alignment of the maxilla and mandible is maintained through remodeling of bony surfaces, this mechanism includes the periodontium, to permit function. Here, using the spatial matrix hypothesis, perhaps for the first time, dental tissues are more properly included in the equation. Teeth are important craniofacial structures in many regards. Although their spatial arrangement permits activities such as mastication, speech, and swallowing, they may have other functions, such as load distribution to protect the large and fragile human brain from (micro)trauma that might be associated with modern diseases, such as multiple sclerosis (Williams *et al.*, 2011). While the calvaria adapt to house the expanding brain, the teeth erupt through the bone and their final positions are dictated to a greater or lesser extent by sutural homeostasis in combination with tooth morphology and cusp-fossa relationships that have evolved over millennia. During their eruptive phase, the posterior maxillary teeth determine the extent of pneumatization, and this part of the upper airway provides essential components for gas exchange and oxygenation of tissues further distally. Specifically, the pneumocytes that line the paranasal air sinus produce nitric oxide (NO), and NO is a small vessel dilator *inter alia*. Following inspiration, in the proximal part of the lower airway, smooth muscle relaxation can help with vasodilation, as well as gas exchange and oxygenation in the vicinity of the pulmonary alveoli. Therefore, perturbation of normal craniofacial development can impact both the upper airway directly and the distal airway indirectly.

According to the spatial matrix hypothesis, environmentally induced changes in early morphologic relationship precipitate new clinical solutions (phenotypic variation). Using Waddington's epigenetic landscape (Waddington, 1956), which is a metaphor for how gene regulation modulates development, consider a child with a Class I genotype who becomes a habitual digit-sucker. Instead of having a normal, Class I occlusion, the overjet and/or overbite change to yield a Class II phenotype clinically. In effect, there has been a departure away from genetically encoded 'developmental program'. Because of complexity, the clinical outcome in this particular case might later present as a Class II malocclusion in a teenager; TMD as a young adult, or OSA as an older adult. In other words, developmental compensation occurs to permit compromised function. The teeth are not well-aligned but the teenager can still eat food; the young adult can chew but gets jaw pain or headaches; the older adult can breathe but has snoring or episodes of apnea at night. These three examples represent developmental compensation. Therefore, decompensation is required through treatment, and this is largely achieved through appropriate spatial signaling. Put simply, the insertion of a (biomimetic) oral device changes the position of the mandible analogous to 'jumping the bite' and initiates a change in the pattern of gene expression, which through a cascade of events, eventually leads to a new level of craniofacial homeostasis. This spatial signaling may also require remodeling (widening) of the hard palate. In so doing, the midpalatal suture would be gently stretched, activating stretch-sensitive genes in the local stem cells. In turn, these stem cells would undergo signal transduction (mechanotransduction) and differentiate into osteoblasts that would lay down new bone (Maxim *et al.*, 2015) to accommodate the tongue and alleviate any oropharyngeal airway obstruction. In addition, biomimetic devices exert ultra-light, prolonged, intermittent forces on the periodontium of the associated teeth during rest and during function (such as swallowing during sleep). These ultra-light forces are detected by mechanoreceptors on the cell surfaces of the periodontal and periosteal cells. Due to signal transduction, a cascade of events is initiated, resulting in gene transcription, mRNA biosynthesis and bone remodeling. In this way, *de novo* tissue regeneration or enhanced craniofacial structures offer a potential solution for diseases such as sleep disordered breathing.

References

ada.org/en/press-room/news-releases/2017-archives/october/ada-adopts-policy-on-dentistry-role-in-treating-obstructive-sleep-apnea.

Agrawal V. Role of salpingopharyngeal fold in lateral pharyngeal wall collapse causing obstructive sleep apnea. *Sleep Med.* 2015;16(1):S7.

Au C, Li A. Association between cephalometric measurements and severity of obstructive sleep apnoea in children and adults. *Sleep Med.* 2015;16(1):S75-S76.

Au C, Zhang J, Wing Y, Li A. Familial aggregation of obstructive sleep apnoea in children without tonsillar hypertrophy. *Sleep Med.* 2015;16(1):S209-S210.

Baik HS, Han HK, Kim DJ, Proffit WR. Cephalometric characteristics of Korean Class III surgical patients and their relationship to plans for surgical treatment. *Int J Adult Orthodon Orthognath Surg.* 2000;15(2):119–128.

Balarajan R, Soni Raleigh V, Botting B. Sudden infant death syndrome and postneonatal mortality in immigrants in England and Wales. *Brit Med J.* 1989;298(6675):716–720.

Banabilh SM, Suzina AH, Dinsuhaimi S, Samsudin AR, Singh GD. Dental arch morphology in South East Asian adults with obstructive sleep apnoea: Geometric morphometrics. *J Oral Rehab.* 2009;36:184–192.

Banabilh SM, Suzina AH, Dinsuhaimi S, Singh GD. Craniofacial obesity in patients with obstructive sleep apnea. *Sleep Breath.* 2009;13(1):19–24.

Baume LJ, Derichsweiler H. Is the condylar growth center responsive to orthodontic therapy? An experimental study in Macaca mulatta. *Oral Surg Oral Med Oral Pathol.* 1961;14:347–362.

Berkovitz B, Holland G, Moxham B. Oral Anatomy, Histology and Embryology. Elsevier. 5th Edition, 2018.

Berkovitz BK, Weaver ME, Shore RC, Moxham BJ. Fibril diameters in the extracellular matrix of the periodontal connective tissues of the rat. *Connect Tissue Res.* 1981;8(2):127–132.

Beynon AD, Wood BA. Variations in enamel thickness and structure in East African hominids. *Am J Phys Anthropol.* 1986;70(2):177–193.

Bishara SE, Treder JE, Jakobsen JR. Facial and dental changes in adulthood. *Am J Orthod Dentofacial Orthop*. 1994;106(2):175–186.

Bookstein FL. Reconsidering "The inappropriateness of conventional cephalometrics". *Am J Orthod Dentofacial Orthop*. 2016;149(6):784–797.

Braun J, Loyal L, Frentsch M, Wendisch D, Georg P, *et al.* Presence of SARS-CoV-2 reactive T cells in COVID-19 patients and healthy donors. medRxiv. doi: https://doi.org/10.1101/2020.04.17.20061440

Breitner C. Bone changes resulting from experimental orthodontic treatment. *Am J Orthodont and Oral Surg*. 1940;26:521.

Breitner C. Experimental change of the mesio-distal relations of the dental arches. *Angle Orthod*. 1930: 67–76.

Bressane LB, Guilherme J, Oltramari-Navarro PVP, Henriques JFC, Garib DG. Long-term changes of alveolar buccal bone after rapid maxillary expansion in an adolescent patient. *J World Federation Orthod*. 2016;5(2):64–69.

Broadbent BH. A new X-ray technique and its application to orthodontia. *Angle Orthod*. 1931;1(2):45–6.

Burnett CA, Clifford TJ. Closest speaking space during the production of sibilant sounds and its value in establishing the vertical dimension of occlusion. *J Dent Res*. 1993;72:964–967.

Cerajewska TL, Singh GD. Changes in soft-tissue facial profile of craniofacial microsomia patients: geometric morphometrics. *Int J Adult Orthod Orthog Surg*. 2001;16(1):61–71.

Davidson TM. The great leap forward: The anatomic basis for the acquisition of speech and obstructive sleep apnea. *Sleep Med*. 2003;4(3):185–194.

Enlow DH, Hans MG. Essentials of facial growth. Philadelphia: Saunders, 1996.

Eschler J. Inwiefern stiitzen experimentalle Studien die Formgestaltung der paradentalen Gewebe und des Kieferknochens die Grundlage der Funktions-Kieferorthopädie, Deutsch Zahn- Mund- und Kieferheilkunde. 1939;6:759.

Fuentes MA, Opperman LA, Buschang P, Bellinger LL, Carlson DS, Hinton RJ. Lateral functional shift of the mandible: Part II. Effects on gene expression in condylar cartilage. *Am J Orthod Dentofacial Orthop*. 2003;123(2):160–166.

García-García AS, Martínez-González JM, Gómez-Font R, Soto-Rivadeneira A, Oviedo-Roldán L. Current status of the torus palatinus and torus mandibularis. *Med Oral Patol Oral Cir Bucal*. 2010;15(2):e353–360.

Gonçalves RC, Raveli DB, Pinto Ados S. Effects of age and gender on upper airway, lower airway and upper lip growth. *Braz Oral Res*. 2011;25(3):241–247.

Gruetter CA, Barry BK, McNamara DB, Gruetter DY, Kadowitz PJ, Ignarro L. Relaxation of bovine coronary artery and activation of coronary arterial guanylate cyclase by nitric oxide, nitroprusside and a carcinogenic nitrosoamine. *J Cyclic Nucleotide Res.* 1979;5(3):211–224.

Guilleminault C, Abad V, Chiu H, Quo S. Obstructive-sleep-apnea and alveolo-dental synchondrosis. *Sleep Med.* 2015;16(1):S80.

Guilleminault C, Abad VC, Chiu HY, Peters B, Quo S. Missing teeth and pediatric obstructive sleep apnea. *Sleep Breath.* 2016;20(2):561–568.

Guilleminault C, Stoohs R. Obstructive sleep apnea syndrome in children. *Pediatrician.* 1990;17(1):46–51.

Häupl K, Psansky R. Histological studies on the mode of operation of the devices used in functional orthodontics. Deutsch Zahn, mund und kieferheilkunde. 1938;19;641–648.

Hay AD, Ayoub AF, Moos KF, Singh GD. Euclidean Distance Matrix Analysis of Surgical Changes in Prepubertal Craniofacial Microsomia Patients Treated with an Inverted L Osteotomy. *Cleft Palate Craniofac J.* 2000;37(5):497–502.

Hay AD, Singh GD. Mandibular Transformations in Prepubertal Patients following Treatment for Craniofacial Microsomia: Thin-plate spline analysis. *Clin Anat.* 2000;13(5):361–372.

Hosoya H, Kitaura H, Hashimoto T, Ito M, Kinbara M, Deguchi T, Irokawa T, Ohisa N, Ogawa H, Takano-Yamamoto T. Relationship between sleep bruxism and sleep respiratory events in patients with obstructive sleep apnea syndrome. *Sleep Breath.* 2014;18:837–844.

Jackson FE. Hemicrania secondary to elongated styloid process "the Eagle Syndrome". *Dis Nerv Syst.* 1974;35(11):528–531.

Johns FR, Strollo PJ Jr, Buckley M, Constantino J. The influence of craniofacial structure on obstructive sleep apnea in young adults. *J Oral Maxillofac Surg.* 1998;56(5):596–602.

Jørgensen KD. The Dryopithecus pattern in recent Danes and Dutchmen. *J Dent Res.* 1955;34(2):195–208.

Kappen C. Modeling anterior development in mice: diet as modulator of risk for neural tube defects. *Am J Med Genet C Semin Med Genet.* 2013;163C(4):333–356.

Khoury S, Rouleau GA, Rompré PH, Mayer P, Montplaisir JY, Lavigne GJ. A significant increase in breathing amplitude precedes sleep bruxism. *Chest.* 2008;134(2):332–337.

Kingsley NW. A Treatise on oral deformities as a branch of mechanical surgery. New York, 1880.

Kokich VG: The biology of sutures. In: Cohen MM (ed.): Craniosynostosis. Diagnosis, evaluation, and management. New York: Raven Press, 1986, pp. 81–103.

Korenhof CA. Evolution of upper molar morphology and remnants of the trigone in man. *Ned Tijdschr Tandheelkd*. 1978;85(11):456–459.

Korngut R. Case study: A persistent positive outcome treating OSA with a MAD following the treatment protocol. *Dialogue*. 2010;1:26–27.

Lam B, Ip MS, Tench E, Ryan CF. Craniofacial profile in Asian and white subjects with obstructive sleep apnoea. *Thorax*. 2005;60(6):504–510.

Liao F, Singh GD. Resolution of sleep bruxism using biomimetic oral appliance therapy: A case report. *J Sleep Disord Ther*. 2015;4:204–208.

Liu S, Zhou Y, Gao X. Growth and development of upper airway and surrounding tissues in non-snoring children. *Sleep Med*. 2015;16(1):S47.

Longmire WP Jr, Sanford MC. Stimulation of mandibular growth in congenital micrognathia by traction. *Am J Dis Child*. 1949;78:750–754.

Lozanoff S. Midfacial retrusion in adult brachyrrhine mice. *Acta Anat* (*Basel*). 1993;147(2):125–132.

Marks MB. Bruxism in allergic children. *Am J Orthod*. 1980;77(1):48–59.

Maxim MA, Soritau O, Baciut M, Bran S, Baciut G. The role of dental stem cells in regeneration. *Clujul Med*. 2015;88(4):479–482.

McNamara JA Jr, Bryan FA. Long-term mandibular adaptations to protrusive function: an experimental study in Macaca mulatta. Am J Orthod Dentofac Orthop. 1987;92:98–108.

McNamara JA Jr, Carlson DS. Quantitative analysis of temporomandibular joint adaptations to protrusive function. *Am J Orthod*. 1979;76:593–611.

McNamara JA Jr. Maxillary transverse deficiency. *Am J Orthod Dentofacial Orthop*. 2000;117(5):567–570.

Mithen S. The prehistory of the mind. Thames & Hudson, 1996.

Morrison MD, Tamimi F. Oral tori are associated with local mechanical and systemic factors: A case control study. *J Oral Maxillofac Surg*. 2013;71:14–2.

Moss ML. The functional matrix hypothesis revisited. 1. The role of mechanotransduction. *Am J Orthod Dentofacial Orthop*. 1997;112(1):8–1.

Moss ML. The functional matrix hypothesis revisited. 2. The role of an osseous connected cellular network. *Am J Orthod Dentofacial Orthop*. 1997;112(2):221–226.

Moss ML. The functional matrix hypothesis revisited. 3. The genomic thesis. *Am J Orthod Dentofacial Orthop*. 1997;112(3):338–342.

Moss ML. The functional matrix hypothesis revisited. 4. The epigenetic antithesis and the resolving synthesis. *Am J Orthod Dentofacial Orthop*. 1997;112(4):410–417.

Mossey P, Singh GD, Smith ME. More extensive analysis is needed when assessing facial structure in SIDS. *Brit Med J*. 1999;318:396–397.

Moyers RE, Bookstein FL. The inappropriateness of conventional cephalometrics. *Am J Orthod*. 1979;75(6):599–617.

Nada RM, Fudalej PS, Maal TJ, Bergé SJ, Mostafa YA, Kuijpers-Jagtman AM. Three-dimensional prospective evaluation of tooth-borne and bone-borne surgically assisted rapid maxillary expansion. *J Craniomaxillofac Surg*. 2012;40(8):757–762.

Nada RM, van Loon B, Schols JG, Maal TJ, de Koning MJ, Mostafa YA, Kuijpers-Jagtman AM. Volumetric changes of the nose and nasal airway 2 years after tooth-borne and bone-borne surgically assisted rapid maxillary expansion. *Eur J Oral Sci*. 2013;121(5):450–456.

Ohayon MM, Li KK, Guilleminault C. Risk factors for sleep bruxism in the general population. *Chest*. 2001;119(1):53–61.

Parsons TE, Downey CM, Jirik FR, Hallgrimsson B, Jamniczky HA. Mind the gap: genetic manipulation of basicranial growth within synchondroses modulates calvarial and facial shape in mice through epigenetic interactions. *PLoS One*. 2015;10(2):e0118355.

Proffit WR. Equilibrium theory revisited: factors influencing position of the teeth. *Angle Orthod*. 1978;48(3):175–186.

Ramoglu SI, Sari Z. Maxillary expansion in the mixed dentition: rapid or semi-rapid? *Eur J Orthod*. 2010;32(1):11–18.

Ranke J. Verst@ndigung gber ein gemainsames cranio-metrisches Verfahren (FrankfurterVerst@ndigung). *Archiver Anthropologie*. 1884;15:1–8.

Sakakibara H, Tong M, Matsushita K, Hirata M, Konishi Y, Suetsugu S. Cephalometric abnormalities in non-obese and obese patients with obstructive sleep apnoea. *Eur Respir J*. 1999;13(2):403–410.

Salama H, Salama M. The role of orthodontic extrusive remodeling in the enhancement of soft and hard tissue profiles prior to implant placement: a systematic approach to the management of extraction site defects. *Int J Periodontics Restorative Dent*. 1993;13(4):312–3.

Santiago PE, Singh GD, Yáñez MA, Dietrich RA, García P, Grayson BH, McCarthy, JG. Restitution of the temporo-mandibular joint in patients with craniofacial microsomia after multiplanar mandibular distraction: Assessment by magnetic resonance imaging. *Semin Orthod*. 2011;17(3):186–196.

Schendel SA, Jacobson R, Khalessi S. Airway growth and development: a computerized 3-dimensional analysis. *J Oral Maxillofac Surg*. 2012;70(9):2174–2183.

Schwartz AR, Smith PL, Wise RA, Gold AR, Permutt S. Induction of upper airway occlusion in sleeping individuals with subatmospheric nasal pressure. *J Appl Physiol.* 1988;64(2):535–542.

Schwarz AM, Gratzinger M. Removable orthodontic appliances. W. B. Saunders Company, Philadelphia and London (1966).

Sherwood RJ, Duren DL, Demerath EW, Czerwinski SA, Siervogel RM, Towne B. Quantitative genetics of modern human cranial variation. *J Hum Evol.* 2008;54(6): 909–914.

Shore RC, Kirkham J, Robinson C, Moxham BJ, Berkovitz BK. An assessment of the control of matrix turnover by a quantitative ultrastructural analysis of fibroblasts of the periodontal ligament in rats. *J Biol Buccale.* 1991;19(1):68–73.

Shore RC, Moxham BJ, Berkovitz BK. Changes in collagen fibril diameters in a lathyritic connective tissue. *Connect Tissue Res.* 1984;12(3–4):249–255.

Siegel MI, Mooney MP, Eichberg JW, Gest T, Lee DR. Septopremaxillary ligament resection and midfacial growth in a chimpanzee animal model. *J Craniofac Surg.* 1990;1(4):182–6.

Simmons JH, Prehn R. Airway protection: The missing link between nocturnal bruxism and obstructive sleep apnea. *Sleep.* 2009;32:A218.

Simmons JH, Prehn R. Nocturnal bruxism as a protective mechanism against obstructive breathing during sleep. *Sleep.* 2008;31:A199.

Singh GD and Chandrashekhar R. Breath of life: Complexity and heterogeneity in the integration of etiologic components associated with sleep disordered breathing. In: LeFebvre E and Moreau R (eds.) Snoring: Symptoms, Causes, Diagnosis and Treatment. New York, USA: Nova Science Publishers, 2009, pp. 109–126.

Singh GD, Clark WJ. Localization of mandibular changes in patients with Class II division 1 malocclusions treated using Twin Block appliances: Finite-element modeling. *Am J Orthod Dentofacial Orthop.* 2001;119(4):419–425.

Singh GD, Cress SE, McGuire MK, Chandrashekhar R. Case report: Effect of mandibular tori removal on obstructive sleep apnea parameters. *Dialogue.* 2012;1:22–24.

Singh GD, García AV, Hang WM. Evaluation of the posterior airway space following Biobloc therapy: Geometric morphometrics. *Cranio.* 2007;25(2):84–89.

Singh GD, Hay AD. Morphometry of the Mandible in Prepubertal Craniofacial Microsomia Patients following an Inverted L Osteotomy. *Int J Adult Orthod Orthog Surg.* 1999;14(3):229–235.

Singh GD, Heit T, Preble D, Chandrashekhar R. Changes in 3D nasal cavity volume after biomimetic oral appliance therapy in adults. *Cranio.* 2016;34(1):6–12.

Singh GD, Heit T, Preble D. Changes in 3D midfacial parameters after biomimetic oral appliance therapy in adults. *J Ind Orthod Soc.* 2014;48(2):104–108.

Singh GD, Johnston J, Ma W, Lozanoff S. Cleft palate formation in fetal Br mice with midfacial retrusion: tenascin, fibronectin, laminin, and type IV collagen immunolocalization. *Cleft Palate Craniofac.* J. 1998;35(1):219–241.

Singh GD, Kim HN. Changes in nasal airway volume after biomimetic oral appliance therapy in Korean adults. *Am J Respir Crit Care Med.* 2020;201:A2442.

Singh GD, Kim HN. Changes in pneumatization of the maxillary air sinuses in Korean adults following biomimetic oral appliance therapy. *World J Otorhinolaryngol Head Neck Surg.* 2020 https://doi.org/10.1016/j.wjorl.2020.07.007.

Singh GD, Kraver M, Chernyshev O. Restoration of sleep using a novel biomimetic protocol for adult OSA: Clinical case report. *Cranio.* 2019;37(2):136–139.

Singh GD, Krumholtz J. Epigenetic Orthodontics in Adults. *Appliance Therapy Group,* USA, 2009.

Singh GD, Krumholtz J. Epigenetic Orthodontics in Adults. *Appliance Therapy Group,* USA, 2009.

Singh GD, Liao F. Long term changes in upper airway volume and sleep architecture using biomimetic oral appliance therapy. *Am J Respir Crit Care Med.* 2019;199:A5533.

Singh GD, Maher GJ, Padilla RR. Customized mandibular orthotics in the prevention of concussion/mild traumatic brain injury in football players: a preliminary study. *Dent Traumatol.* 2009;25(5):515–521.

Singh GD, McNamara JA Jr and Lozanoff S. Thin-plate spline analysis of the cranial base in subjects with Class III malocclusion. *Euro J Orthod.* 1997;19(4): 341–353.

Singh GD, McNamara JA Jr, Lozanoff S. Allometry of the cranial base in Prepubertal Korean subjects with Class III Malocclusions. Finite-Element Morphometry. *Angle Orthod.* 1999;69(5):507–514.

Singh GD, Moxham BJ, Langley MS, Waddington RJ and Embery G. Changes in the composition of glycosaminoglycans during normal palatogenesis in the rat. Arch. *Oral Biol.* 1994;39(5):401–407.

Singh GD, Moxham BJ. Mesenchymal cell activity during 5-fluoro-2-deoxyuridine-induced cleft palate formation in the rat. *Cleft Palate Craniofac J.* 1996;33(5):395–399.

Singh GD, Olmos S. Use of a sibilant phoneme registration protocol to prevent upper airway collapse in patients with TMD. *Sleep Breath.* 2007;11(4):209–216.

Singh GD. On Growth and Treatment: The spatial matrix hypothesis. In: Ribbens KA and McNamara JA Jr (eds.) Growth and treatment: A meeting of the minds. Craniofacial Growth Series, *Ann Arbor*, USA, 2004;41:197–239.

Singh GD. On the etiology and significance of palatal and mandibular tori. Cranio. 2010;28(4):213–215.

Singh GD. Report on a Symposium "Advances in the modeling of form: Clinical and computational interfaces". *Amer J Orthod Dentofac Orthop*. 2004;125(1):124–125.

Singh GD. Response to "Oral Appliance Therapy Should be Prescribed as a First-Line Therapy for OSA during the COVID-19 Pandemic". *J Dent Sleep Med*. 2020;7(3).

Singh GD. Spatial matrix hypothesis. *Brit Dent J*. 2007;202(5):238–239.

Sjamsudin J, David DJ, Singh GD. An Indonesian child with orofacial duplication and neurocristopathy anomalies: Case Report. *J Craniomaxillofac Surg*. 2001;29(4),195–197.

Smitthimedhin A, Whitehead MT, Bigdeli M, Nino G, Perez G, Otero HJ. MRI determination of volumes for the upper airway and pharyngeal lymphoid tissue in preterm and term infants. *Clin Imaging*. 2018;50:51–56.

Spence JA, Aitchison GU, Sykes AR, Atkinson PJ. Broken mouth (premature incisor loss) in sheep: the pathogenesis of periodontal disease. *J Comp Pathol*. 1980;90(2):275–292.

Sutherland K, Cistulli P. Mandibular advancement splints for the treatment of sleep apnea syndrome. *Swiss Med Wkly*. 2011;141:w13276.

Thompson JL Jr, Kendrick GS. Changes in the vertical dimensions of the human male skull during the third and fourth decades of life. *Anat Rec*. 1964;150:209–213.

Tremble GE. Pneumatization of the temporal bone. *Arch Otolaryngol*. 1934;19(2):172–182.

Valigi MC, Logozzo S. Do exostoses correlate with contact disfunctions? A case study of a maxillary exostosis. *Lubricants*. 2019;7(2):15.

van der Klaauw CJ. Cerebral skull and facial skull. Arch Neerl Zool. 1946;7:16–37.

Wahl N. Orthodontics in 3 millennia: Functional appliances to midcentury. *Am J Orthod Dentofacial Orthop*. 2006;129(6):829–833.

Weiss TM, Atanasov S, Calhoun KH. The association of tongue scalloping with obstructive sleep apnea and related sleep pathology. *Otolaryngol Head Neck Surg*. 2005;133(6):966–971.

White JD. Expanding the jaw. *Dental Cosmos*. 1860;1(6):281–282.

Whitney MR, Sidor CA. Histological and developmental insights into the herbivorous dentition of tapinocephalid therapsids. *PLoS One*. 2019;14(10):e0223860.

Williams DE, Lynch JE, Doshi V, Singh GD, Hargens A. Bruxism and temporal bone hypermobility in patients with multiple sclerosis. *Cranio*. 2011;29(3):1–9.

Williams DE, Lynch JE, Doshi V, Singh GD, Hargens A. Bruxism and temporal bone hypermobility in patients with multiple sclerosis. *Cranio*. 2011;29(3):1–9.

Williams MO, Murphy NC. Beyond the ligament: A whole-bone periodontal view of dentofacial orthopedics and falsification of universal alveolar immutability. *Semin Orthod*. 2008;14:246–259.

Witzel MA, Posnick JC. Patterns and location of velopharyngeal valving problems: atypical findings on video-nasopharyngoscopy. *Cleft Palate J*. 1989;26(1):63–67.

Chapter 4 Biomimetic Tooth Movement: Epigenetic Orthodontics

Synopsis: In this chapter, we discuss tooth movements in their various guises. The concepts outlined here are illustrated with clinical observations in both children and adults, and the consequences of these findings are presented. Clinical identification of techniques associated with biomimetic tooth movement are noted and the novel concept of epigenetic orthodontics is re-iterated. The ideas discussed here are integrated with a new clinical 'gold standard' of 32 teeth fully erupted and in occlusion.

The entire dental specialty of orthodontics is fundamentally built around one word — 'malocclusion'. So what is a malocclusion exactly? Essentially, it is a working orthodontic diagnosis, and once any differential diagnoses have been addressed, treatment objectives can be identified, a treatment plan (including retention) can be formulated, and the likely treatment time can be estimated. The problem remains, however, that currently there is no consensus on the definition of a malocclusion. Depending on what textbook is read or organization consulted, the definition varies widely, as evidenced by the following list:

- A condition in which the upper and lower teeth do not fit together properly
- Incorrect positioning of the biting surfaces of the upper and lower teeth

- An inherited defect where the upper and lower jaws do not let teeth meet
- An abnormal or improper alignment of the teeth
- A bad bite caused by incorrect positions of the upper and/or lower teeth
- Teeth that are misaligned or fit together poorly when the jaws are closed
- Malposition and imperfect contact of the mandibular and maxillary teeth
- Abnormal contact between upper and lower teeth
- A dental disease where the teeth overgrow
- Deviation from normal occlusion, or incorrect alignment/position of the upper and lower teeth
- Disharmony in the way the upper and lower teeth come together when biting
- Abnormal relationships or malposition of the maxillary and mandibular teeth
- Abnormal occlusion of the teeth and/or jaws
- Crowded or crooked teeth with or without misaligned jaws
- A condition in which the opposing teeth do not mesh normally
- A misalignment of teeth and/or incorrect relation between the teeth of the two dental arches
- An orthodontic or orthognathic problem, including crowded/crooked, missing or extra teeth, and/or a misaligned jaw
- The World Health Organization defines malocclusion as a handicapping dentofacial anomaly, and refers to abnormal occlusion and/or disturbed craniofacial relationships, which may affect esthetic appearance, function, facial harmony, and psychosocial well-being.

Another deficiency in the modern approach to orthodontic correction of the teeth is the original classification of malocclusions (Angle, 1907). For example, Rinchuse and Rinchuse (1989) consider that classification using the maxillary first molars is inadequate and that malocclusion can be viewed not as a discrete but a continuous variable. Furthermore, conditions that are common today, such as anterior open bite, were not included in Angle's classification of malocclusions. The explanation for this omission likely includes the fact that anterior open bite was relatively rare a century ago, but it is now far more common (Lopez Del Valle *et al.*, 2006). The reasons for this change in prevalence can be accounted for if the original premises are re-assessed, and a new definition of malocclusion is applied. Singh (2007) defined a malocclusion as a solution for a complex, adaptive system to remain in equilibrium or homeostasis. The notion of 'equilibrium' as noted in the equilibrium theory (Proffit, 1978) is a prime candidate for this type of re-assessment. In traditional thinking, it seems that 'orthodontic equilibrium' is simply based on a balance of forces. This is not surprising since orthodontic theory was largely based on Newtonian physics and Darwinian genetics. Newton taught that action and reaction are equal and opposite, but that law does not apply to a biologic system, because of its innate behavior and response (in providing necessary functions). In fact, the theories of orthodontic and non-orthodontic tooth movement started with histological observations of tissue response using the light microscope. Oppenheim (1930), Gottlieb (1931), Schwarz (1932), and Reitan (1951) studied cellular changes during tooth movement and retention. Later, others such as Rygh (1972) and Davidovitch (1991) used advancements in technology, such as electron microscopy for ultrastructural observation of the sub-cellular changes during tooth movement and retention, but scant or little attention was paid to biologic behavior at the organ level even using these types of approaches. However, Meikle (2006) surmised that orthodontic tooth movement is not limited to events occurring within the periodontal ligament but also involves remodeling of alveolar bone and facial sutures, and that mandibular displacement initiates remodeling activity within the TMJ that can alter condylar growth (Meikle, 2007), in accord with the spatial matrix hypothesis.

Note that later generations of physicists talked about quantum physics, where (physical) behavior is studied on an entirely different scale. Correspondingly, the quanta of biology are genes, representing a new era of quantum biology or epigenetic orthodontics. Singh and Krumholtz (2009) were the original formulators of the term 'epigenetic orthodontics' since an epigenetic basis for the etiology of malocclusions can be advocated. This notion is probably best explained by the work of Corruccini *et al.* (1985) who described the effects of interactions between genetic and environmental variance. In their studies, it was noted that rural youths showed significantly better dental occlusion and respiratory health when compared to their urban counterparts. These changes did not support the genetic mutation basis of malocclusions since they developed rapidly in just one generation after families moved from villages to cities to find employment, indicating that epigenetic phenomena were probably induced. In probability and statistics, variance informally measures how far a set of random numbers are spread out from their average value. In the ancestral condition (say, 25,000 *Homo sapiens* genes; 50,000 years ago), every baby that was born was exclusively breast-fed or it didn't survive. There was little or no air pollution at that time, and no access to refined or processed foods. Because of these environmental conditions, the genetic variance of the human genome was suppressed by these canalizing (channeling) environmental factors. In other words, most of these children developed Class I occlusions most of the time. Over a century ago, environmental transition to the urbanized condition slowly but surely occurred worldwide. Altered environmental factors, such as a lack of breast-feeding, bottle-feeding, pacifier use, soft foods, refined foodstuffs, processed foods containing additives, such as sugar, colorants, preservatives, stabilizers, and food-like products started to produce phenotypic variation as the genetic variance of the (same) human genome increased. This means that new types of malocclusions would, at least theoretically, be produced (Fig. 33). In fact, clinical experience indicates that the range of malocclusions not classified by Angle (1907) now includes: anterior open bite, posterior open bite (unilateral or bilateral), 'gummy smile', and low clinical crown height where the anatomical crowns of the teeth have not fully erupted into occlusion. This phenotypic variation was

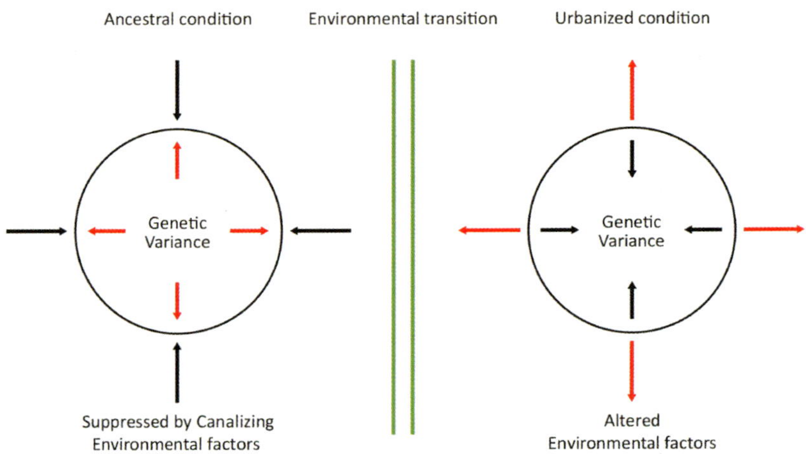

Figure 33: Interaction between genetic and environmental variance. After Corruccini *et al.*, 1983.

identified by pioneers such as Price (1897) and supported by the work of Pottenger (1983) and others such as Fonder (1984).

Weston Price traveled internationally and noted that good occlusion and robust facial architecture were features of primitive societies where modernization had not yet been implemented (Price, 1897). He surmised that the introduction of refined white sugar was somehow associated with 'physical degeneration' although he could not describe a mechanism that would explain this correlation. It is now known that one method of producing tissue degeneration is through inflammation. The endothelia that line the internal organs and systems are susceptible to inflammatory processes that disrupt their functional capabilities. Thus, endothelial dysfunction can lead to a diverse array of maladies, ranging from migraine and hypertension to inflammatory bowel disease, etc. The question remains: How can a single molecule of sugar precipitate such a spectrum of disorders? The answer may partly lie in the glycocalyx of cell membranes. The glycocalyx is a cell membrane component that consists of carbohydrate moieties of membrane glycolipids/glycoproteins. These molecules contribute to cell–cell recognition, cell communication, and cellular adhesion (McKinley and O'Loughlin, 2012). For example, Pino and Thouron (1986) identified lectin-receptor monosaccharides on the endothelium of retinal capillaries. Moreover, the binding of these receptors was inhibited by sugars that behave as haptens that elicit an immune response, such as inflammation in the conditions noted above.

In more recent years there has also been significant progress in molecular biology. New molecular phenomena such as signal transduction have been elucidated, and further advancements in molecular genetics have provided a deeper understanding of gene-environmental interactions and epigenetics. In fact, in early experiments on cats, Pottenger (1983) was able to illustrate both epigenetic effects as well as genetic potential. In a 10-year study, Pottenger investigated the impact of changing the diets in a sample of cats, who were fed on meat and milk. The control group was fed raw meat, organ meats, bone, and raw milk. The test group was fed on cooked meat and refined dairy (pasteurized milk). Overall, his results indicated that the control group stayed healthy and agile over 9 generations, while the test group suffered from numerous health issues. For example, the first generation of cats in the test group showed irregular skeletal development, and crooked teeth with swollen and inflamed gums. They also exhibited impaired coordination and were less active compared to the control group. The second generation of cats in the test group were smaller in size, showed skull degeneration and had hypoplastic teeth. The propensity for bone fractures was also increased with osteopenia and osteomalacia. These cats also exhibited impaired coordination and behavioral changes. The third generation of cats in the test group were also smaller than the control group and showed more severe skull degeneration with thin skulls/sinuses and hypoplastic teeth. There was increased prevalence of osteopenia, osteomalacia, allergies, and skin infections. These cats were the least active compared to the control group and showed pronounced exhaustion. The fourth generation cats exhibited a loss of fertility and had stillborn kittens, so that they died out without leaving any offspring. In conclusion, since the genes of the control and test cats were not changed during the study period, it can be deduced that the physical degeneration of the test cats was epigenetic in nature. **However, the genetic potential of the cats remained unchanged**. Thus, by improving the diet of the third-generation cats, it took four generations for them to be bred back to health. This classic experiment shows the labile nature of the mammalian genome being susceptible to epigenetic influences, both detrimental and beneficial. Clinical advantage can be gained from this empiric understanding.

Fonder *et al.* (1965) were some of the first to highlight that malocclusions may relate to systemic health. In a classic experiment, unilateral occlusal interference was induced in rats by placing a composite block on the molars on one side only. Radiographs after one week revealed that the spinal alignment was perturbed, mimicking the condition of clinical scoliosis. After composite placement on the balancing side, further radiographs were taken after another week, and these revealed that the spinal alignment was normalized. **This simple experiment highlights the danger of appliances that advocate the use of a unilateral bite block and validates the idea of bilateral support in oral device design**. It is thought that asymmetric occlusal interference results in mandibular misalignment and TMJ dysfunction likely through subluxation of the cervical vertebrae C1/C2 (Fonder, 1988) since these vertebrae relate to both head posture, spinal alignment and neurologic function (Fonder, 1980). Moreover, Fonder (1984) contended that there appears to be a relationship within the body whereby a dysfunctional occlusion is associated with issues in distant organs and systems of the body, which he called Dental Distress Syndrome (DDS). This rather comprehensive condition included a wide range of signs and symptoms that affect diverse systems, producing clinical outcomes such as: postural issues, auriculotemporal conditions, respiratory illnesses, ocular disturbances, skin conditions, visceral symptoms, gynecological issues, and neurologic symptoms. Fonder *et al.* (1965) implied that a balanced occlusion is essential for optimal health since he asserted that a reciprocal relationship exists between jaw posture and spinal posture. In fact, some recent studies (Kent, 2006; Chapman and Singh, 2013; Singh *et al.*, 2014) appear to support this contention. Moreover, Fonder (1973) claimed that elimination of clinical problems can be achieved in the musculature and nervous system when the dental occlusion is properly aligned and balanced (Fonder, 1985). Indeed, Fonder's claims were supported in part by Tinbergen (1973) who was awarded the Nobel prize for medicine and physiology for his work.

So how do advances in technology and our current understanding affect the notion of orthodontic 'equilibrium'? Put simply, the holy grail in orthodontics is now biologic equilibrium, otherwise known as homeostasis. In the same way that blood pressure, body temperature, etc. are subject to physiologic control, the craniofacial region, including the teeth, is no different. Thus, a malocclusion is a solution for a complex, adaptive system to remain in or maintain homeostasis or (biologic) equilibrium (Singh, 2007). In fact, it can be argued that the prime reason why malocclusions are stable conditions is partly because of sutural homeostasis. While previous generations were taught about the histologic structure of the periodontal 'ligament', more recent data (Shore *et al.*, 1984; 1991; Singh and Krumholtz, 2009) suggests that the periodontium is most likely a modified suture and, as such, is subject to sutural homeostasis (Singh and Krumholtz, 2009; Williams *et al.*, 2011), which is itself genetically encoded and epigenetically regulated. Taking the old functional matrix hypothesis as a starting point (Moss, 1997), and adding newer concepts, such as temporo-spatial patterning (Chaplin *et al.*, 1999), novel theories are generated. One such theory is my spatial matrix hypothesis (Chapter 2 and Chapter 3), which successfully predicted how we can clinically modify the conditions and still satisfy the state of biologic equilibrium. In this way, craniofacial homeostasis becomes the new norm, by addressing the hard tissues, soft tissues, dental tissues, and functional spaces, such as the upper airway. By so doing, surgical and non-surgical solutions to orthodontic dilemmas, such as relapse, start to come into focus.

Despite the above claims and expectations, most orthodontic textbooks still describe conventional phases of orthodontic tooth movement. Oppenheim (1930) was one of the first to develop a theory for the basis of orthodontic tooth movement. His pressure-tension hypothesis suggested that an alteration of blood flow was induced by (removable) orthodontic devices, which led to the release of various chemical messengers. These chemical factors produced cellular changes, involving a cascade of events, which led to orthodontic tooth movement. This empirical process, while rather unsophisticated, intuitively surmised a biologic basis for orthodontic tooth movements with osteoclastic activity accounting for bone resorption on the pressure side, osteoblastic activity accounting for bone deposition on the tension side, and odontoclastic activity accounting for root resorption. However, with new innovations such as bonded brackets, removable orthodontic appliances lost favor and fixed appliances became the preferred choice of treatment for most orthodontists. The question now became: How do teeth biologically respond to fixed orthodontic appliances? When orthodontic brackets and wires are first applied to the teeth, a pain response is initiated, and an initial phase of induced tooth movement occurs within the first 24hrs to two days (King *et al.*, 1991). During this initial phase there is rapid tooth movement within the periodontium of approx. 0.3–0.9 mm (Fig. 34). The next phase is the

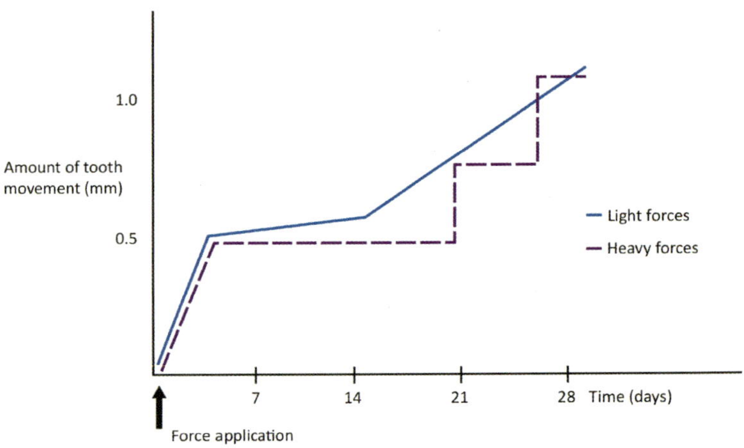

Figure 34: Idealized graph showing that less force does not produce less tooth movement since the amount of tooth movement is about the same in both cases over four weeks. After King *et al.*, 1991 and Proffit and Fields, 2000.

lag phase, which lasts about 14 days. During this phase slow or no tooth movement occurs. Histologically, a hyalinization response is often evident. Hyaline is a cement-like substance, which is deposited as a pathologic response to prevent further tooth movement; in other words, it's the body's attempt to maintain the prior level of homeostasis. However, since the orthodontic brackets and wires are still actively in situ, the ensuing inflammatory response produces an undermining resorption of the lamina dura by osteoclasts. Note that dentists monitor the health of the periodontium by looking for an intact lamina dura. Loss of an intact lamina dura suggests that the tooth has transitioned from a (pain free) physiologic state into one of (periapical) pathology. During this post-lag phase, removal of the hyalinized tissues is evident histologically, and orthodontic tooth movement occurs clinically. Thus, biologic knowledge is essential to understand the biomechanical phenomena required for successful orthodontic tooth movement.

In order for teeth to move orthodontically, the surrounding bone needs to be remodeled. Some are of the opinion that teeth can simply be moved 'through the bone'. This misconception is based on inappropriate tooth movement that leads to localized (traumatic) bone loss in the form of a dehiscence and/or fenestrations when the tooth roots are driven against the cortical plate with inappropriate forces (Bressane *et al.*, 2016). These bony defects are not easily detected by the naked eye since the alveolar bone is covered by oral mucosa; however, tell-tail signs such as a 'washboard' appearance of the mucosa can be identified in some cases as the roots of the underlying teeth begin to shine through, but dehiscence and/or fenestration are best seen after raising a flap or by using radiology. In any case, it is clear that there are different types of bone resorption during orthodontic tooth movement. According to the orthodontic literature, frontal bone resorption is the ideal mechanism for removing bone and allowing the tooth roots to take up position in the perceived vacated space. This type of bone resorption is achieved via osteoclasts lining the alveolar bone on the surface of the periodontium. In this case, lighter forces are used to move the teeth, and the movement of the tooth root is parallel with the bone surface. It is claimed that this method is less painful compared to undermining bone resorption. Using the latter technique, osteoclasts are recruited from medullary surfaces of the alveolar bone using heavy forces, which cause pain. After a period of time, sterile necrosis of the cellular elements leads to a hyalinization response. Thereafter, elimination of the hyalinized tissues takes about 2–3 weeks and the tooth moves in a stepwise manner as the undermined bone collapses under the pressures exerted. Comparing tooth movement graphically using either light forces or heavy forces (Fig. 34), it becomes apparent that more force does not produce more tooth movement or faster tooth movement. Therefore, less force does not produce less tooth movement or slower tooth movement either. In other words, force is on both sides of the equation and cancels out, meaning that **force is not, in fact, the sole arbiter of orthodontic tooth movement**. This conclusion is borne out by studies on bone biology. For example, King *et al.* (1991) demonstrated that both bone resorption and deposition can be present in any tension side, as well as in any site of compression when orthodontic forces are applied. That study indicated an early phase of bone resorption (3–5 days), reversal with bone resorption (5–7 days), followed by a late phase of further bone deposition (7–14 days). Put simply, the tooth-bone relationship (i.e. the periodontium) is doing whatever it has to do, wherever it has to do it, to maintain (sutural) homeostasis.

Looking at tooth movement from a different perspective, we note that there are many types of tooth movement, including: mesial drift, passive eruption, distal drift, orthodontic relapse, etc. The most important feature during these types of tooth movement is the absence of any directly applied forces. According to older theories, such as the functional matrix and the equilibrium hypotheses, the teeth somehow come to occupy positions where the balance of (soft tissue) forces precipitates unwanted tooth movement (relapse). On the other hand, the spatial matrix hypothesis includes the concept of the 'periodontal suture' and sutural homeostasis. It states that the spatial and functional alignment of the skeletal elements is maintained through remodeling of bony surfaces (including the periodontium) to permit function. Environmentally induced changes (e.g. digit-sucking, orthodontic tooth extraction, etc.) result in a new morphologic relationship (e.g. increased overjet, a reduced number of teeth, etc.). This phenotypic variation represents departure from the genetically encoded developmental body plan, which is influenced by temporo-spatial patterning. Subsequently, developmental compensation occurs to permit compromised function, and the subsequent attainment of sutural homeostasis can result in orthodontic relapse if teeth were orthodontically moved into cosmetically pleasing but biologically non-sustainable positions. It is also important to appreciate other types of non-orthodontic, physiologic tooth movement. For example, it is well known that tooth movements occur during mastication, and these are different from orthodontic tooth movements. These differences mean that the advice of wearing an orthodontic appliance while eating to enhance tooth movement is an incongruity. Physiologic tooth movement is called tooth support and can be investigated as an adaptation to intermittent axial forces (loading and unloading). The force, pressure, or loading of the tooth during eating results in a displacement (measured in μm) as the crown sinks into the tooth socket (Fig. 35).

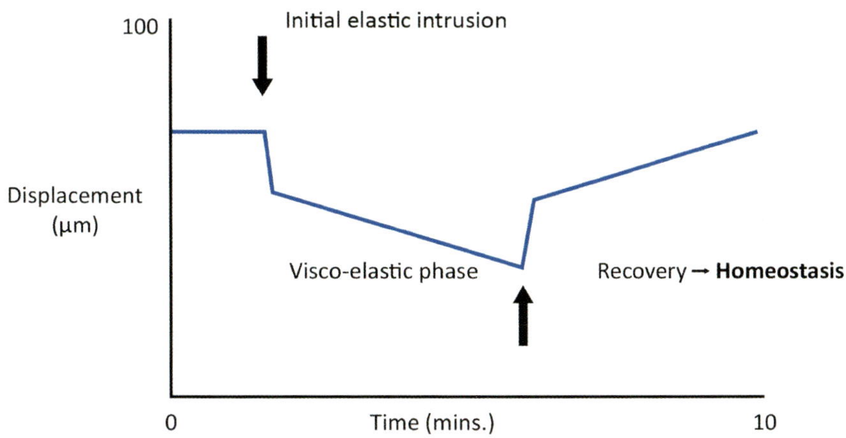

Figure 35: Graph illustrating tooth support, the adaptation of teeth to intermittent axial loading (forces).

This displacement takes time and is referred to as the initial elastic intrusion. If the force is maintained on the crown, the tooth continues to sink into the socket, so the clinical crown height becomes shorter, and this is known as the viscoelastic phase (measured in minutes). When the force is removed from the crown there is partial elastic spring back, followed by a further viscoelastic phase of recovery, so that eventually the crown reaches homeostasis when it contacts its opposing counterpart (Fig. 35). This clinical behavior is dependent on the structure of the periodontium, which does not have the components found in ligaments in other parts of the body; differences in the extracellular matrix components are evident. Originally, tooth attachment in humans was based on the idea of gomphoses (alveoli, tooth sockets) with a thecodont dentition since the early histologists identified a 'fibrous' tooth attachment, using light microscopy. We now know that the periodontium is far more sophisticated. Thus, physiologic tooth movement is a different behavior from orthodontic tooth movement. For example, during orthodontic intrusion or extrusion, the clinical crown height does not vary significantly (Salama and Salama, 1993), unlike the initial elastic intrusion during mastication, since orthodontic tooth movement is dependent on successful bone remodeling.

The early anatomists described alveolar crest fibers, horizontal fibers, oblique fibers, periapical fibers, and inter-radicular fibers within the periodontium, but this simple classification does not represent the functional response and clinical behavior of the periodontium. In fact, some studies suggest that the periodontium has 'fetal-like' behavior (Shore *et al.*, 1984). The hallmark of fetal tissues is an identifiable population(s) of stem cells that can regenerate and differentiate into new tissues and can heal without scar formation (Whitby and Ferguson, 1991; Ferguson and O'Kane, 2004). For example, in a study on fetal sheep, Stern *et al.* (1993) created lip wounds *in utero*. The fetuses were then harvested after 1–3 weeks, and when the wound sites were examined microscopically, it was found that they had healed rapidly and without any inflammation or scar formation. In fact, there was also complete regeneration of the skin, muscle, mucosa, and epidermal appendages. Surprisingly perhaps, the periodontium appears to have some of these fetal tissue-like properties to a limited extent. Newer histologic techniques have identified mesenchymal cells (adult stem cells) in the human periodontium, which can differentiate into fibroblasts, osteoblasts, and multinucleated giant cells, such as osteoclasts (Amar and Chung, 1994; Zhu and Liang, 2015). The periodontium also has a rich vascularity, and these blood vessels provide a source for both the fluid and the cells that are found in the periodontium. In addition, the capillaries within the periodontium are fenestrated or 'leaky' (Moxham *et al.*, 1985) so that fluid that is exuded can be bound by the extracellular matrix since it contains (hydrophilic) hyaluronan proteoglycan and other glycosaminoglycans. These ground substance components provide the viscoelastic cushioning mentioned above, which can resist compressive forces during mastication. In addition, collagen fibers can resist tensile stresses. Furthermore, it has been found that the fibers within the periodontium are small dimeter fibrils (≈45nm) and follow a unimodal distribution in terms of fiber size (Berkovitz *et al.*, 1981). This likely means that the fibrils in the periodontium have a high rate of turnover similar to fetal tissues that are undergoing constant remodeling. This rapid turnover rate ensures that the fibrils do not reach maturation by becoming large-diameter fibers, which are found in ligaments in other parts of the body. Berkovitz *et al.* (2018) also reported that periodontal fibroblasts are responsible for collagen fiber degradation within the periodontium. This fibroclastic activity results in the presence of intra-cellular collagen profiles, and the time taken to degrade collagen intracellularly is approx. 30mins, which is consistent with the high turnover rate characteristic of the human periodontium. This behavior, at least in part, explains the propensity for tooth movement, but a tooth needs to know where it is in space. Spatial perception is enabled by neural elements within the periodontium, including unmyelinated fibers (for pain perception) but also mechanoreceptors for proprioception. Sherrington (1917) discovered mechanoreceptors for proprioceptive capability within the periodontium. He found that the jaw opening reflex could be elicited in decerebrate cats when pressure was applied to the teeth and gingival margins. Therefore, teeth know where they are in space and changes in these spatial relations (e.g. decompensation during treatment) can provide appropriate spatial signaling to re-establish (genomic) pattern formation for optimal form and function, according to the spatial matrix hypothesis. In addition, during temporo-spatial patterning, ossification centers arise during fetal development *de novo*. These ossification centers are sites of signal transduction (temporo-spatial patterning suggests that certain genes are expressed at various places at particular times during development). The differentiation of stem cells at these ossification centers leads to the deposition of new, immature, woven bone. Woven bone differs from lamellar bone as it contains coarse (large diameter) collagen bundles, which are not well-organized, unlike lamellar bone that contains fine-fibred collagen in a well-arranged manner. Woven bone can be regarded as the body's first attempt to make new bone, for example during fracture healing in an adult, which is then remodeled and replaced by lamellar bone. This pattern of bone formation would also explain the formation of a 'periodontal suture' where intramembranous bone surrounds the tooth root. Note that tooth roots occasionally exhibit ankylosis, whereby the tooth root is attached directly to the underlying alveolar bone (Fig. 32). In these cases, it can be suggested that the stem cell population of the periodontium has been depleted due to premature synostosis or with primary failure of eruption in the absence of mechanical obstruction associated with gene mutations (Frazier-Bowers *et al.*, 2010), similar to synostoses of the craniofacial sutures due to mutations of various genes, for example FGF-2 (Moore *et al.*, 2002).

Biomimetic tooth movement

Currently, the consensus opinion is that the use of light forces is most preferable for orthodontic tooth movement. Allied with this approach is the question of whether there is a need for prolonged orthodontic forces. A force can vary in magnitude, duration, and direction, and application of these forces changes the stress-strain levels within the periodontium. Heavy forces of short duration (1-50kg, < 1sec) are exerted during mastication. These forces are addressed by the incompressible fluids within the periodontium, as alluded to above, and while no orthodontic tooth movement occurs, bending of collagen and bone results in a piezoelectric effect, which may have other (bony) effects. Similarly, light forces of short duration (< 1kg, < 1sec) during mastication are also absorbed by the periodontium, and no orthodontic tooth movement occurs (Proffit and Fields, 2000). On the other hand, considering heavy forces of long duration (1–50kg, continuous), fluid is expressed from the tooth socket and the tooth moves within the periodontium within the first 1–2 seconds. After 3–5 seconds, the periodontal tissues are compressed, and the pain response is initiated. After a few minutes, blood flow is cut off to the compressed periodontium, and after a few hours, cell death occurs in the compressed areas with subsequent sterile necrosis. After about 3–5 days, cell differentiation and undermining bone resorption is discernible and after approx. 7–14 days, osteoclasts remove the lamina dura so that tooth movement occurs in a stepwise manner following collapse of the bony architecture. Therefore, tooth movement is technique sensitive and there appears to be an environmental window that might permit optimal tooth movement. It has more recently been suggested that light forces of long duration (< 1kg, continuous/intermittent) mimic the natural environment more closely. In these conditions, after about 3–5 seconds, blood vessels are compressed on the pressure side, and dilated on the tension side. Within a few minutes, the oxygen tension begins to change; and prostaglandins and other cytokines are released. Within hours, chemical messengers are affected and enzyme levels (such as alkaline phosphatase) begin to change. After approx. four hours, increased levels of cAMP indicate cellular differentiation within the periodontium. Thus, by about two days, direct bone resorption is identifiable and progressive tooth movement occurs (Proffit and Fields, 2000). Despite these variants of clinical technique, more force does not produce more or faster tooth movement, and less force does not produce less or slower tooth movement (Fig. 34), suggesting that force is not the sole mediator of orthodontic tooth movement.

The effects of light, prolonged, intermittent forces on cytokine expression such as interleukins, for example IL-1β, and prostaglandins, such as PGE2, have been investigated, since it's known that IL-1β is a cytokine required for osteoclast activation and PGE2 is required for bone resorption. In one study, the maxillary canine on one side received a continuous force and the opposite canine received an interrupted/intermittent force. Significant increases in IL-1β and PGE2 were observed after 24 hours in both cases, but the side with intermittent signaling showed reactivation, and greater elevations of IL-1β and PGE2 were observed (Lee *et al.*, 2004). These types of studies not only provide a biochemical basis for orthodontic tooth movement but also elucidate the nature of the signal that the body responds to best. For example, in post-emergent eruption, control seems to be light forces of long duration rather than heavy forces of short duration such as those during mastication. Studies of human premolars in their passage from gingival emergence to the occlusal plane show that this phase of eruption occurs only during a few hours in the early evening. The critical hours for eruption parallel the time that growth hormone levels are highest in a growing child (Proffit and Frazier-Bowers, 2009). For maxillary molars, the maximum eruption rate is about 1mm per month (Berkovitz and Bass, 1976). Similarly, the rate of orthodontic tooth movement by conventional protocols cannot exceed about 1mm per month (Williams and Murphy, 2008). These types of studies help us to formulate clinical protocols to mimic the natural, physiologic behavior of tooth movement or **biomimetic orthodontics**. Using a biomimetic approach, it seems feasible that an oral device that targets craniofacial tissues, including the teeth and bone, should impart cyclic, intermittent forces and primarily been worn for prolonged periods of time starting in the late afternoon and early evening but not during the day or during meals while eating. However, the device should be worn all night long while sleeping to benefit from the growth hormone circadian rhythm. Hwang and Cha (2004) studied the effects of human growth hormone (rHGH) therapy on craniofacial growth and development in a child with short stature. They noted that rHGH therapy supplementation appeared to affect mandibular growth more than the maxilla, and these findings were further supported by Kjellberg and Wikland (2007). Indeed, Tsuboi *et al.* (2008) also showed that therapy with rHGH enhanced craniofacial development during orthodontic treatment of children with pituitary dwarfism. In addition, it is also thought that circadian rhythms modulate homeostatic bone metabolic pathways. Zvonic *et al.* (2007) noted that about 25% of genes associated with calvarial bone metabolism showed an oscillatory profile in mice. Ostensibly, these notions suggest that the pattern of device wear ought to focus on the evening and nighttime since appliances worn during the day may have little or no benefit in terms of craniofacial correction, especially in growing children. Furthermore, Proffit and Fields (2000) are of the opinion that during orthodontic treatments there should be brief periods of no force, and that fixed appliances need to be modified to permit this.

Despite the above guiding principles, currently there is no consensus on how much force is needed to move teeth. Newtonian mechanics teaches that:

$$F = ma$$

where 'F' is force, 'm' is mass and 'a' is acceleration. But when is a force not a force? Here, the biological phenomena need to be differentiated from the mechanical phenomena. **A force is not a force if it fails to reach a biologic threshold**. Once the detection threshold has been reached, it will be sensed, and an appropriate response will be initiated. Note also that continuous application of a signal/force will result in the system becoming refractory as the neurotransmitters are depleted. Thus, repetitive/intermittent signaling may be required to prevent force/signal decay and this behavior may lie in the properties of the materials that are being used to apply a force-signal. Another biologic question is: If a tooth moves if a force is applied, will it move even if a force is not applied? From the above discussion, it appears that force is not the sole arbitrator for tooth movement. In could be argued that teeth need three conditions to be satisfied to move orthodontically: **space, signal, and guidance**. Numerous orthodontic books teach that space is 'created' by the extraction of teeth. This erroneous assumption is disproved by quantum physics. According to the current theory of relativity, space is created at the edge of an expanding universe. Orthodontic extraction therapy simply displaces space, as taught by the Archimedes' principle. Worse still, the extraction of healthy premolar and wisdom teeth for orthodontic reasons simply decreases the associated bone volume, if the functional matrix hypothesis is to be believed. This decreased bone volume is thought to have potentially unfavorable facial effects by some (Singh *et al.*, 2005) and detrimental upper airway effects by others (Guilleminault *et al.*, 2016).

Bearing in mind the salient points of the above discussion, the design, materials, and protocols for oral appliance therapy need to be re-visited. One aspect is the nature of the signal. It appears that cyclic, intermittent signaling may be preferable over static, continuous force application. Here the biologic phenomenon of mechano-transduction may be evoked. Biomimetic oral devices are thought to exert cyclic, intermittent signals on the periodontium of the associated teeth during rest and function (such as swallowing during sleep) since one of the materials used in these particular devices is a super-elastic, nickel-free alloy. It is thought that these signals are detected by mechanoreceptors on the cell membrane surfaces of the periodontal and periosteal cells. Due to signal transduction, a cascade of events is initiated, resulting in gene transcription and mRNA biosynthesis, which can mimic natural growth and development pathways in line with the genetic potential of the individual. Moreover, biomimetic devices are worn for about 12-16 hours of the 24-hour circadian rhythm. In this way, the application of ultra-light forces has been shown to elicit cytoskeletal changes, and the ensuing cell deformation is mediated via microtubules and microfilaments, which targets bone-producing genes, such as PTH-rP (Suda *et al.*, 2001). Thus, this biomimetic protocol putatively evokes signal transduction, such as the bone morphogenetic protein (BMP) signaling pathway (Luo, 2003). Indeed, Banes *et al.* (2001) reviewed mechanical signal detection, transduction, and response pathways in connective tissue cells. Other work also suggests that biomechanical stress is linked to gene expression. For example, tensile stresses applied to mouse (calvarial) sutures induce sustained upregulation of BMP-4 gene expression, and it is possible that mechanical stimuli upregulate genes that are not typically expressed in normal suture development (Mao and Nah, 2004). The effects of biomechanical forces on sutures were studied by Kopher and Mao (2003). Using normally growing (premaxillary-maxillary and frontonasal) sutures in rabbit as controls, static and intermittent forces were applied. It was found that light static forces increased the amount of new bone matrix deposited in the suture compared to controls; while the intermittent forces increased the amount of new bone matrix deposited in the suture compared to both the control and static groups. Later, Williams and Murphy (2008) investigated the application of ultra-light forces in adults (Fig. 36). By taking tissue biopsies from volunteers, they were able to show new, immature, woven bone deposition (Fig. 37), as predicted by the spatial matrix hypothesis.

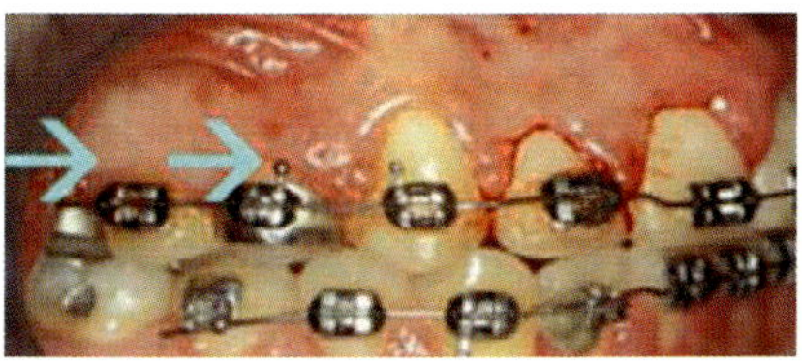

Figure 36a: Application of ultra-light forces (arrows).

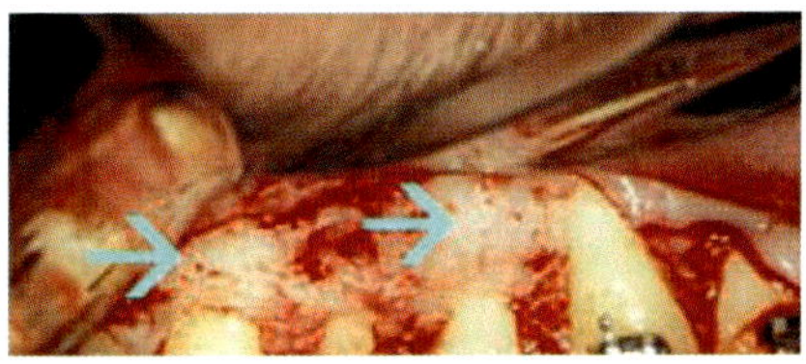

Figure 36b: Site of tissue biopsy (arrows).

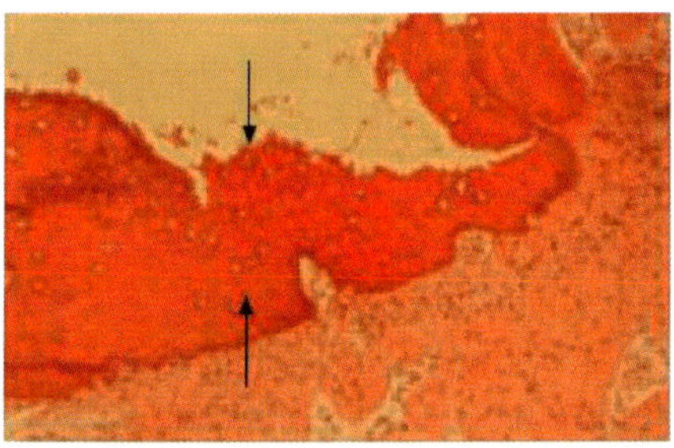

Figure 37a: New, immature, woven bone (arrows). Courtesy: Dr Neal Murphy and Dr Mike Williams

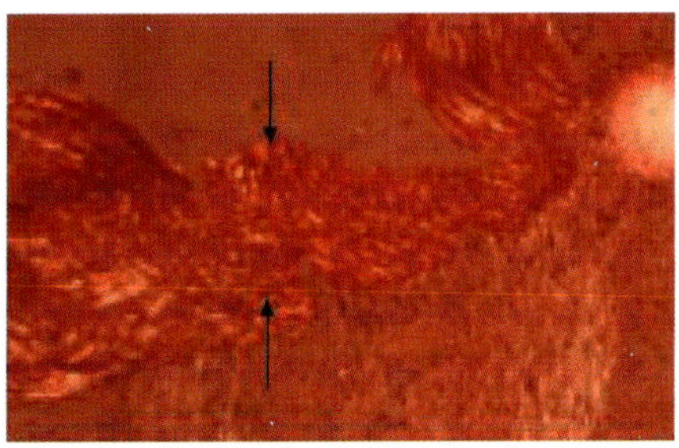

Figure 37b: New, immature, woven bone (arrows).

Cyclic intermittent signaling: vibrational response

Mao and Nah (2004) implied that biomechanical forces can modify skeletal growth and development. Unlike traditional static orthodontic forces, their work suggested that cyclic forces can induce anabolic responses in the craniofacial sutures. These intermittent forces are thought to be transmitted as tissue- and cell-borne stresses and strains that upregulate gene expression, inducing cells to proliferate, differentiate, undergo maturation, and synthesize extracellular matrix, *inter alia*. For example, in one study, Mao *et al.* (2003) compared static forces (2N) with cyclic forces (2N at 0.2Hz) during sutural osteogenesis in rabbits. It was found that cyclic forces at 0.2Hz for 10min/day over 12 days provoked significantly more craniofacial growth, sutural separation, and newly formed bone when compared to controls and static forces of the same magnitude. These data demonstrated for the first time that the application of cyclic, intermittent forces appears to induce sutural osteogenesis more effectively than static forces alone. In a similar study, Kopher and Mao (2003) applied static and cyclic forces at a magnitude of 5N to the frontonasal suture (FNS) and premaxillary-maxillary suture (PMS) in growing rabbits. Using immunocytochemistry labeling of newly formed bone tissue, they demonstrated increased osteogenesis on cyclic loading in comparison with controls and static loading. In addition, the oscillatory components of cyclic force in the stretched FNS and compressed PMS suggested that both tension and compression can produce sutural growth responses. Thus, Kopher *et al.* (2003) concluded that while the current craniofacial orthopedic therapies exclusively utilize static forces, cyclic forces are capable of inducing size- and shape-changes of craniofacial tissues via mechanically induced bone apposition and resorption. Thereafter, Peptan *et al.* (2008) investigated the effect of brief doses of tensile or compressive forces on intramembranous bones and sutures. In rabbits, cyclic tensile or compressive forces of 1N at 8Hz were applied to the maxilla for 20min/day over 12 consecutive days. Histomorphometric analyses revealed that the average sutural widths and cell densities of both the PMS and FNS loaded in either tension or compression were increased when compared to matched controls. These data further suggested that high-frequency cyclic forces in either tension or compression induce growth and remodeling in the craniofacial sutures and, due to structural craniofacial complexity, these signals are transmitted as shear stresses that upregulate genes responsible for sutural growth.

It can be ventured that this new bone formation in adults mimics the adult bone fracture repair pathway. This raises the question: Does adult fracture repair recapitulate embryonic skeletal formation? In other words, if an adult sustains a bone fracture, does it heal in the same way that a fetus produces bone *de novo*? In fact, in an earlier study, Ferguson *et al.* (1999) confirmed that the genetic mechanisms regulating fetal skeletogenesis also regulate adult skeletal regeneration. Furthermore, Singh *et al.* (2014) reported increased midfacial bone volume in adults following biomimetic oral appliance therapy, corroborating the work of Ferguson *et al.* (1998) who hypothesized that various molecular signaling pathways regulating skeletogenesis are common to both fetal bone development and adult wound healing. In fact, osteogenesis is an ongoing process that starts in fetal development and continues in adulthood in the form of bone remodeling and fracture repair. The ability of skeletal tissues to regenerate is dependent on proteins that exert their effect on pattern formation partly through regulation of BMPs and PTHrP. Thus, knowledge acquired through the study of fetal skeletogenesis can help guide the development of biologically based therapeutic interventions, such as biomimetic oral appliance therapy.

It is becoming clear that orthodontic tooth movement using traditional orthodontic forces elicits acute inflammation in the early stages of therapy. Later, bone remodeling following cell interactions permits tooth movements. Thus, during traditional orthodontic loading there is an interaction between the patient's genome and the external forces applied. This gene-environmental communication leads to the expression of specific growth factors, leading to vascular induction and invasion. Therefore, mechanically induced inflammation permits orthodontic tooth movements through changes in bone morphology via induced bone-remodeling (Roberts and Hartsfield, 2004). During the normal inflammatory process, arachidonic acid release stimulates the formation of a prostaglandin (PGE2), which in turn stimulates the formation of bone and bone remodeling. On the other hand, non-steroidal anti-inflammatory drugs (NSAIDS) have a damping effect on the inflammatory process since they block formation of PGE2, and therefore interfere with bone formation/remodeling and subsequent tooth movement. It is also known that platelet-rich plasma (PRP) has an effect on the inflammatory process. Platelets contain an interleukin (IL-1α) which stimulates PGE2 production, and since PGE2 is a potent stimulator of bone formation and remodeling, the growth factors in PRP can bypass the normal inflammatory process to induce bone formation via direct signaling of undifferentiated mesenchymal cells. Therefore, alternative biochemical pathways illustrate the degree of biologic redundancy in the human genome, but it has been suggested that novel biomimetic oral appliances evoke epigenetic signaling via these alternative pathways, which remain unelucidated at this time, providing ripe areas for future research.

In contrast to sutural bone formation, several studies investigated the notion that cyclic intermittent signaling might accelerate orthodontic movements in children. Woodhouse *et al.* (2015) investigated the effect of vibrational forces on the rate of orthodontic tooth movement with fixed appliances supplemented with 20mins of daily use of a vibrational device. However, that study did not find any evidence that a vibrational force can either increase the rate of tooth orthodontic tooth movement or reduce the amount of time required to achieve tooth alignment when used in conjunction with fixed appliances. It could be argued that the archwire ligated in the orthodontic brackets impeded the vibrational signal and/or that the application time of 20mins was too short, since Proffit (2005) contends that a device needs to be worn in the mouth for 8hrs to have a clinical effect. In addition, perhaps the vibrational signal was applied at the wrong time of day with respect to the circadian rhythm, which shows that growth hormone levels peak during sleep

(Minuto *et al.*, 1982). Despite these concerns, a similar study (Miles *et al.*, 2018) concluded that a vibrational appliance had no effect on the rate of maxillary premolar extraction space closure during orthodontic treatment with fixed appliances, while another study (Katchooi *et al.*, 2018) also found no evidence that a vibrational device enhances orthodontic tooth movement using removable clear aligners. On the other hand, it has more recently been reported (Judex and Pongkitwitoon, 2018) that mechanical vibrational devices that transfer vibrations into alveolar bone to influence bone remodeling can increased cell proliferation and gene expression in osteoblasts and fibroblasts, as well as increasing osteoclastic activity. This study suggests that specific cell types respond to different vibration characteristics involved in orthodontic tooth movements. In fact, El-Bialy *et al.* (2004) reported the effects of low-intensity pulsed ultrasound (LIPUS) on orthodontically induced root resorption in premolars. Using scanning electron-microscopy, a decrease in the areas of resorption and the number of resorption lacunae in the LIPUS-exposed tooth roots was found while histologic examination showed healing of the resorbed root surface by hypercementosis. Moreover, Singh and Krumholtz (2009) surmised that the periodontal ligament is, in fact, a modified suture. If so, periodontal stems cells (Zhu and Liang, 2015) ought to be able to respond in a similar fashion and induce the biosynthesis of skeletal tissues as determined by Mao *et al.* (2003). Thus, the design, materials, and protocol of oral devices are critical in modulating craniofacial tissue behavior. We shall return to this theme in Chapter 6.

The formation of bone (osteogenesis) is stimulated by separation (gentle stretching) of craniofacial sutures, according to the spatial matrix hypothesis. Indirect evidence for this supposition comes from clinical cases of craniosynostoses. In these rare cases, the craniofacial sutures are unable to respond to environmental stimuli because the cell membrane receptors, e.g. FGF-2, are non-functional (Moore *et al.* 2002). Depending on which sutures are affected, different clinical conditions, such as Apert syndrome, Crouzon's syndrome, Pfeiffer syndrome, etc. are precipitated, most of which are associated with midfacial hypoplasia and deficient midfacial bone volume. It can also be suggested that some malocclusions are secondary to midfacial hypoplasia, such as Class III malocclusions (Singh *et al.*, 1997; 1998; 2000), and these conditions may, in turn, be associated with systemic diseases such as sleep disordered breathing. Based on these recent findings, I developed a new definition of occlusion, as follows: **The occlusion (or bite) defines the end point of the body with respect to the plantar surfaces of the feet and, within these two biologic boundaries, all functional spaces for normal physiologic processes and functions must be accommodated**. Thus, in the same way that blood pressure, body temperature, etc. are subject to physiologic control, the craniofacial region is under spatial and functional regulation. Malocclusions that exhibit midfacial hypoplasia, mandibular retrognathia, crowding, anterior and/or posterior crossbite suggest a deficiency of functional space secondary to developmental compensation. Therefore, because of this phenotypic variation, functional spaces in the craniofacial region, such as the upper airway, need to be optimized if craniofacial homeostasis is to be enhanced and maintained.

References

Amar S, Chung KM. Clinical implications of cellular biologic advances in periodontal regeneration. *Curr Opin Periodontol.* 1994:128–140.

Angle EH. Treatment of malocclusion of the teeth: Angle's system, 7th ed. Philadelphia: SS White Dental Manufacturing Company, 1907.

Banes A, Lee G, Graff R, Otey C, Archambault J, Tsuzaki M, Elfervig M, Qi Jie. Mechanical forces and signaling in connective tissue cells: Cellular mechanisms of detection, transduction, and responses to mechanical deformation. *Current Opinion in Orthopaedics.* 2001;1:389–396.

Berkovitz B, Holland G, Moxham B. Oral Anatomy, Histology and Embryology, 5th ed. Elsevier, 2018, p. 218.

Berkovitz BK, Bass TP. Eruption rates of human upper third molars. *J Dent Res.* 1976;55(3):460–464.

Berkovitz BK, Weaver ME, Shore RC, Moxham BJ. Fibril diameters in the extracellular matrix of the periodontal connective tissues of the rat. *Connect Tissue Res.* 1981;8(2):127–132.

Bressane LB, Guilherme J, Oltramari-Navarro PVP, Henriques JFC, Garib DG. Long-term changes of alveolar buccal bone after rapid maxillary expansion in an adolescent patient. *J World Federation Orthod.* 2016;5(2),64–69.

Chaplain MAJ, Singh GD, McLachlan JC (eds.) "On Growth and Form: Spatio-Temporal Patterning in Biology". England: John Wiley and Sons Publishers, 1999. ISBN: 0-471-98451-5.

Chapman C, Singh GD. Combined effect of a biomimetic oral appliance and atlas orthogonist cervical adjustment on leg lengths in adults. *Annals Vert Sub Res.* 2013;46–50.

Corruccini RS, Flander LB, Kaul SS. Mouth breathing, occlusion, and modernization in a north Indian population. An epidemiologic study. *Angle Orthod.* 1985;55(3):190–6.

Corruccini RS, Kaul SS, Chopra SR, Karosas J, Larsen MD, Morrow C. Epidemiological survey of occlusion in North India. *Br J Orthod.* 1983;10(1):44–47.

Davidovitch Z. Tooth movement. *Critical Reviews Oral Biol Med.* 1991;2:411–450.

El-Bialy T, El-Shamy I, Graber TM. Repair of orthodontically induced root resorption by ultrasound in humans. *Am J Orthod Dentofacial Orthop.* 2004;126(2):186–193.

Ferguson C, Alpern E, Miclau T, Helms JA. Does adult fracture repair recapitulate embryonic skeletal formation? *Mech Dev.* 1999;87(1–2):57–6.

Ferguson CM, Miclau T, Hu D, Alpern E, Helms JA. Common molecular pathways in skeletal morphogenesis and repair. *Ann NY Acad Sci.* 1998;857:33–42.

Ferguson MW, O'Kane S. Scar-free healing: from embryonic mechanisms to adult therapeutic intervention. *Philos Trans R Soc Lond B Biol Sci.* 2004;359(1445):839–850.

Fonder AC, Alter JL, Allemand LE, Monks WW. Malocclusion as it relates to general health. *Ill Dent J.* 1965;34:292–302.

Fonder AC. Dental distress, respiratory and posture problems. American Dental Association Meeting, Houston, TX, 1973.

Fonder AC. The dental distress syndrome (DDS). *Basal Facts.* 1984;6(1):17–29.

Fonder AC. The Dental Distress Syndrome (Part One). *Stress.* 1980;1(1).

Fonder AC. The Dental Distress Syndrome (Part Two). J Chronic Diseases Therapeutics Res. London, England: Int Soc Prevention Stress, 1980.

Fonder AC. The Dental Distress Syndrome (Quantified). *Quantum Med.* 1988;1(1).

Fonder AC. The Dental Physician. Blacksburg, VA: Univ Publications, 1977. 2nd Rev. ed. Rock Falls, Ill: Medico-Dental Arts, 1985.

Frazier-Bowers SA, Simmons D, Wright JT, Proffit WR, Ackerman JL. Primary failure of eruption and PTH1R: the importance of a genetic diagnosis for orthodontic treatment planning. *Am J Orthod Dentofacial Orthop*. 2010;137(2):160–161.

Gottlieb B, Orban B. Die Veränderungen der Gewebe Bei Übermässiger Beanspruchung der Zähne. Leipzig Verlag von Georg Thieme, 1931.

Guilleminault C, Abad VC, Chiu HY, Peters B, Quo S. Missing teeth and pediatric obstructive sleep apnea. *Sleep Breath*. 2016;20(2):561–568.

Hwang CJ, Cha JY. Orthodontic treatment with growth hormone therapy in a girl of short stature. *Am J Orthod Dentofacial Orthop*. 2004;126(1):118–126.

Judex S, Pongkitwitoon S. Differential efficacy of 2 vibrating orthodontic devices to alter the cellular response in osteoblasts, fibroblasts, and osteoclasts. *Dose Response*. 2018;16(3).

Katchooi M, Cohanim B, Tai S, Bayirli B, Spiekerman C, Huang G. Effect of supplemental vibration on orthodontic treatment with aligners: A randomized trial. *Am J Orthod Dentofacial Orthop*. 2018;153(3):336–346.

Kent A. Catastrophic occlusion. *Br Dent J*. 2006;201(7):419.

King GJ, Keeling SD, McCoy EA, Ward TH. Measuring dental drift and orthodontic tooth movement in response to various initial forces in adult rats. *Am J Orthod Dentofacial Orthop*. 1991;99(5):456–465.

King GJ, Keeling SD, Wronski TJ. Histomorphometric study of alveolar bone turnover in orthodontic tooth movement. *Bone*. 1991;12(6):401–409.

Kjellberg H, Wikland KA. A longitudinal study of craniofacial growth in idiopathic short stature and growth hormone-deficient boys treated with growth hormone. *Eur J Orthod*. 2007;29(3):243–250.

Kopher RA, Mao JJ. Suture growth modulated by the oscillatory component of micromechanical strain. *J Bone Miner Res*. 2003;18(3):521–528.

Kopher RA, Nudera JA, Wang X, O'Grady K, Mao JJ. Expression of in vivo mechanical strain upon different wave forms of exogenous forces in rabbit craniofacial sutures. *Ann Biomed Eng*. 2003;31(9):1125–1131.

Lee KJ, Park YC, Yu HS, Choi SH, Yoo YJ. Effects of continuous and interrupted orthodontic force on interleukin-1beta and prostaglandin E2 production in gingival crevicular fluid. *Am J Orthod Dentofacial Orthop*. 2004;125(2):168–7.

Lopez Del Valle LM, Singh GD, Feliciano N, Machuca M Del C. Associations between a history of breast feeding, malocclusion and parafunctional habits in Puerto Rican children. *PR Health Sci J*. 2006;25(1):31–34.

Luo K. Negative regulation of BMP signaling by the ski oncoprotein. *J Bone Joint Surg Am*. 2003;85-A Suppl 3:39–43.

Mao JJ, Nah HD. Growth and development: hereditary and mechanical modulations. *Am J Orthod Dentofacial Orthop*. 2004;125(6):676–689.

Mao JJ, Wang X, Mooney MP, Kopher RA, Nudera JA. Strain induced osteogenesis of the craniofacial suture upon controlled delivery of low-frequency cyclic forces. *Front Biosci*. 2003;8:10–17.

McKinley M, O'Loughlin VD. Human Anatomy, 3rd ed. McGraw-Hill, 2012, pp. 30–31.

Meikle MC. Remodeling the dentofacial skeleton: the biological basis of orthodontics and dentofacial orthopedics. *J Dent Res*. 2007;86(1):12–24.

Meikle MC. The tissue, cellular, and molecular regulation of orthodontic tooth movement: 100 years after Carl Sandstedt. *Eur J Orthod*. 2006;28(3):221–240.

Miles P, Fisher E, Pandis N. Assessment of the rate of premolar extraction space closure in the maxillary arch with the AcceleDent Aura appliance vs no appliance in adolescents: A single-blind randomized clinical trial. *Am J Orthod Dentofacial Orthop*. 2018;153(1):8–14.

Minuto F, Barreca A, Ferrini S, Mazzocchi G, Del Monte P, Giordano G. Growth hormone secretion in pubertal and adult subjects. *Acta Endocrinol* (*Copenh*). 1982;99(2):161–165.

Moore R, Ferretti P, Copp A, Thorogood P. Blocking endogenous FGF-2 activity prevents cranial osteogenesis. *Dev Biol*. 2002;243(1):99–114.

Moss ML. The functional matrix hypothesis revisited. 1. The role of mechanotransduction. Am J Orthod Dentofacial Orthop. 1997;112(1):8–1.

Moss ML. The functional matrix hypothesis revisited. 2. The role of an osseous connected cellular network. *Am J Orthod Dentofacial Orthop*. 1997;112(2): 221–226.

Moss ML. The functional matrix hypothesis revisited. 3. The genomic thesis. *Am J Orthod Dentofacial Orthop*. 1997;112(3):338–342.

Moss ML. The functional matrix hypothesis revisited. 4. The epigenetic antithesis and the resolving synthesis. *Am J Orthod Dentofacial Orthop*. 1997;112(4):410–417.

Moxham BJ, Shore RC, Berkovitz BK. Fenestrated capillaries in the connective tissues of the periodontal ligament. *Microvasc Res*. 1985;30(1):116–124.

Oppenheim A. Bone changes during tooth movement. *Intl J Orthodontia, Oral Surgery and Radiog*. 1930;16:535–551.

Peptan AI, Lopez A, Kopher RA, Mao JJ. Responses of intramembranous bone and sutures upon in vivo cyclic tensile and compressive loading. *Bone*. 2008;42(2): 432–438.

Pino RM, Thouron CL. Identification of lectin-receptor monosaccharides on the endothelium of retinal capillaries. *Curr Eye Res*. 1986;5(8):625–628.

Pottenger FM. Pottenger's Cats: A Study in Nutrition. 1983.

Price WA. The Physiology of Cataphoresis. *Am J Dent Sci*. 1897;31(7):303–308.

Proffit WR, Fields HW Jr. Contemporary Orthodontics. St. Louis: Mosby, 2000, pp. 296–310.

Proffit WR, Frazier-Bowers SA. Mechanism and control of tooth eruption. *Orthod Craniofac Res*. 2009;12(2):59–6.

Proffit WR. Contemporary Orthodontics, 3rd edition. Elsevier, 2005.

Proffit WR. Equilibrium theory revisited: factors influencing position of the teeth. *Angle Orthod*. 1978;48(3):175–186.

Reitan K. The initial tissue reaction incident to orthodontic tooth movement as related to the influence of function. An experimental histological study on animal and human material. *Acta Odont Scand*. 1951;9(6).

Rinchuse DJ, Rinchuse DJ. Ambiguities of Angle's classification. *Angle Orthod*. 1989;59(4):295–298.

Roberts WE, Hartsfield JK Jr. Bone development and function: genetic and environmental mechanisms. *Semin Orthod*. 2004;10(2):100–122.

Rygh P. Ultrastructural cellular reactions in pressure zones of rat molar periodontium incident to orthodontic tooth movement. *Acta Odont Scand*. 1972;30:575–593.

Salama H, Salama M. The role of orthodontic extrusive remodeling in the enhancement of soft and hard tissue profiles prior to implant placement: a systematic approach to the management of extraction site defects. *Int J Periodontics Restorative Dent*. 1993;13(4):312–3.

Schwarz AM. Tissue changes incidental to orthodontic tooth movement. *Intl J Orthodontia, Oral Surgery and Radiog*. 1932;18:331–352.

Sherrington CS. Reflexes elicitable in the cat from pinna vibrissae and jaws. *J Phys*. 1917;51:404–431.

Shore RC, Kirkham J, Robinson C, Moxham BJ, Berkovitz BK. An assessment of the control of matrix turnover by a quantitative ultrastructural analysis of fibroblasts of the periodontal ligament in rats. *J Biol Buccale*. 1991;19(1):68–73.

Shore RC, Moxham BJ, Berkovitz BK. Changes in collagen fibril diameters in a lathyritic connective tissue. *Connect Tissue Res*. 1984;12(3–4):249–255.

Singh GD, Chapman C, Preble M. Craniofacial changes after combined atlas-orthogonal and biomimetic oral appliance therapy. *Annals Vert Sub Res*. 2014;4:112–118.

Singh GD, Heit T, Preble D. Changes in 3D midfacial parameters after biomimetic oral appliance therapy in adults. *J Ind Orthod Soc.* 2014;48(2):104–108.

Singh GD, Krumholtz J. Epigenetic Orthodontics in Adults. *Appliance Therapy Group*, USA, 2009.

Singh GD, Maldonado L, Thind BS. Changes in the soft tissue facial profile following orthodontic extractions: a geometric morphometric study. *Funct Orthod.* 2005;22(1):34–40.

Singh GD, McNamara JA Jr, Lozanoff S. Finite Element Morphometry of the Midfacial Complex in Subjects with Angle's Class III Malocclusions. *J Craniofac Genet Devel Biol.* 1997;17(3):112–120.

Singh GD, McNamara JA Jr, Lozanoff S. Localization of Deformations of the Midfacial Complex in Subjects with Class III Malocclusions Employing Thin-plate Spline Analysis. *J Anat.* 1997;191:595–602.

Singh GD, McNamara JA Jr, Lozanoff S. Midfacial morphology of Koreans with Class III malocclusions investigated with finite-element scaling analysis. *J. Craniofac Genet Devel Biol.* 2000;20(1):10–18.

Singh GD, McNamara JA Jr, Lozanoff S. Morphometry of the Midfacial Complex in Subjects with Class III Malocclusions: Procrustes, Euclidean and Cephalometric Analyses. *Clin Anat.* 1998;11(3):162–170.

Singh GD. Outdated definition. *Brit Dent J.* 2007;203(4):174.

Stern M, Dodson TB, Longaker MT, Lorenz HP, Harrison MR, Kaban LB. Fetal cleft lip repair in lambs: histologic characteristics of the healing wound. *Int J Oral Maxillofac Surg.* 1993;22(6):371–374.

Suda N, Baba O, Udagawa N, Terashima T, Kitahara Y, Takano Y, Kuroda T, Senior PV, Beck F, Hammond VE. Parathyroid hormone-related protein is required for normal intramembranous bone development. *J Bone Miner Res.* 2001;16(12):2182–2191.

Suzuki H. Responses of the mechanoreceptors in the periodontal membrane to vibratory stimulus on the canine of the cat. *Nihon Seirigaku Zasshi.* 1963;25:415–441.

Tinbergen N. Nobel prize for medicine and physiology, 1973. https://www.nobelprize.org/prizes/medicine/1973/summary/

Tsuboi Y, Yamashiro T, Ando R, Takano-Yamamoto T. Evaluation of catch-up growth from orthodontic treatment and supplemental growth hormone therapy by using Z-scores. *Am J Orthod Dentofacial Orthop.* 2008;133(3):450–458.

Whitby DJ, Ferguson MW. The extracellular matrix of lip wounds in fetal, neonatal and adult mice. *Development.* 1991;112(2):651–668.

Williams DE, Lynch JE, Doshi V, Singh GD, Hargens A. Bruxism and temporal bone hypermobility in patients with multiple sclerosis. *Cranio.* 2011;29(3):1–9.

Williams MO, Murphy NC. Beyond the Ligament: A Whole-Bone Periodontal View of Dentofacial Orthopedics and Falsification of Universal Alveolar Immutability. *Semin Orthod*. 2008;14(4):246–259.

Woodhouse NR, DiBiase AT, Johnson N, Slipper C, Grant J, Alsaleh M, Donaldson AN, Cobourne MT. Supplemental vibrational force during orthodontic alignment: a randomized trial. *J Dent Res*. 2015;94(5):682–689.

Zhu W, Liang M. Periodontal Ligament Stem Cells: Current Status, Concerns, and Future Prospects. *Stem Cells Int*. 2015;2015:11.

Zvonic S, Ptitsyn AA, Kilroy G, Wu X, Conrad SA, Scott LK, Guilak F, Pelled G, Gazit D, Gimble JM. Circadian oscillation of gene expression in murine calvarial bone. *J Bone Miner Res*. 2007;22(3):357–365.

Chapter 5 Craniofacial Diagnostics and Treatment Planning

Synopsis: The hallmark of successful treatment is comprehensive diagnosis. The findings of this multi-part procedure are converted into treatment objectives, and a treatment plan can then be formulated, which includes appliance design and an estimate of the treatment time. Nevertheless, for any treatment plan to be successful, patient compliance must be of the highest order, and it is imperative to ascertain the chief concerns of the patient and to determine the severity of the case at the outset. This chapter lays out a methodology that has been successfully used for several years in the pneumopedics and craniofacial epigenetics (PACE) protocol delivered clinically as biomimetic oral appliance therapy.

Introduction

Prior to accepting a new patient for treatment, it's important to screen and educate the individual and share these findings with family members in pediatric cases. The dental profession is widely experienced in screening for dental diseases, ranging from caries to oral cancer, but conditions such as sleep disordered breathing (SDB) affecting the upper airway are less likely to be on the general dentist's radar. Screening can also be carried out by other dental personnel, especially dental hygienists, etc. since patients often report regularly to the dental office for check-ups and other routine hygiene procedures. These appointments can be also be used for preventive advice, including patient education and information on airway, breathing, and sleep issues; alternatively, special patient education events can be scheduled by a patient coordinator perhaps targeting particular groups, for example women of child-bearing age or parents with young children, etc. These screening sessions can be used to identify individuals who are suspected of either having an undiagnosed sleep disorder, which encapsulates a wide range of clinical entities, including upper airway resistance syndrome (UARS), primary snoring and obstructive sleep apnea (OSA) in its various degrees of severity, or at risk of developing it in later life. Once identified, these individuals need to be professionally diagnosed, following screening.

Adequate records need to be taken to reach a working diagnosis prior to any intervention. This step may entail collaboration with a medical colleague, for example a sleep physician, radiologist, etc. to determine the extent of the conditions suspected since co-morbidity of temporomandibular dysfunction (TMD) and SDB is not uncommon. For example, Sanders *et al.* (2013) reported that it is highly likely that symptoms of OSA are associated with chronic TMD. In fact, Heit *et al.* (2016) identified a patient with severe OSA who initially reported to a dental office with TMJ pain symptoms. Once a definitive diagnosis has been reached, a treatment plan needs to be formulated, based on specified treatment objectives, including a finishing phase, if appropriate, as outlined below. Prior to initiating treatment, however, two other factors need to be addressed. One issue is the financial arrangement since these types of treatments may or may not be fully covered by various insurance healthcare plans but, perhaps more importantly, one has to gauge patient compliance. Although diagnosis is the key to successful treatment outcomes, a lack of patient compliance is an absolute contra-indication and an exclusion criterion that must be rigorously applied to biomimetic oral appliance therapy. In effect, the patient's body is doing the work of healing and/or enhancement and, if the protocol is not adhered to, the chances of success are jeopardized. Patient compliance is essentially behavior modification, which is outside the scope of this chapter *per se*. Nevertheless, an oral device needs to be worn in the mouth for at least 8hrs per day to have any clinical effect (Proffit and Fields, 2000). In the pneumopedics and craniofacial epigenetics (PACE) protocol, the device is worn in line with the circadian rhythm, which necessitates 12-16hrs of wear, including all-night long. Patients with less than excellent compliance will either have an inferior result or prolong the treatment plan unnecessarily. On the other hand, patients need to take ownership and responsibility for their improvements. The professional team can help to encourage the patient, and enhance compliance using various techniques, including teamwork, reward systems and even gamification, especially in pediatric cases. Once a patient takes pride in ownership, the hurdle of compliance can be surmounted, and the chances of a good outcome are increased. Thus, a three-part process emerges involving a thorough working diagnosis, excellent patient compliance, and comprehensive clinical adjustments of the devices at each appointment till treatment is completed.

Dental disease patterns in modern adults

In modernized societies there has been an increased awareness in dental and oral health. More adults have larger numbers of healthy teeth with less caries-experience and less gingival disease. The consequences of this improved oral health are that there is a decreased demand for 'drilling and filling' accompanied by an increased demand for more advanced procedures, such as: CAD/CAM restorations; lasers for soft tissue management; dental implants; veneers and other cosmetic procedures including whitening, and limited orthodontics using clear tray systems. Orthodontic treatments, however, are still primarily aimed at children, and adult orthodontic treatment needs may be unmet. In one study, it was estimated that nearly 70% of European adults have malocclusions (Willems *et al.*, 2001). Another study found an additional 50% of residual need and demand for orthodontic treatment not related to measurable malocclusions in adults (Lilja-Kurlander *et al.*, 2003). In other words, although modern adults tend to have healthier teeth, these may present in the context of underdeveloped faces/smaller jaws, etc., accompanied by systemic sequelae that may remain untreated. The recognition, consequences, and correction of these conditions form the basis of this book.

Consequences of underdeveloped faces and jaws in adults

In the past, in nearly all cultures of the world, underdeveloped faces were found to be less attractive than faces that were more fully developed. Generally speaking, movie stars, singers/models, and athletes still tend to have better developed facial features. In addition, less developed faces may have a more asymmetric facial appearance (Fig. 38). It is also thought that features of malocclusion are more likely to be visible in the underdeveloped pediatric or adult face, and the smile esthetics may be less attractive. Sometimes the patient presents with a 'gummy' smile (Fig. 21a) or with dark buccal 'corridors' (Fig. 39a), which likely emanate from a narrow or constricted upper arch (Fig. 39b).

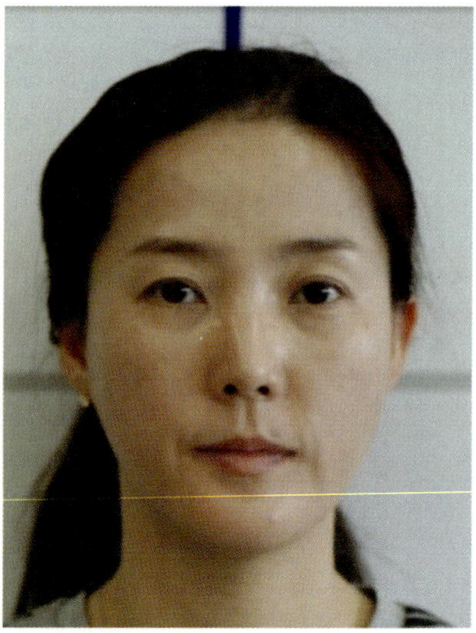

Figure 38a: Pre-treatment frontal photograph with minor facial asymmetry. Courtesy: Dr Hee Nam Kim

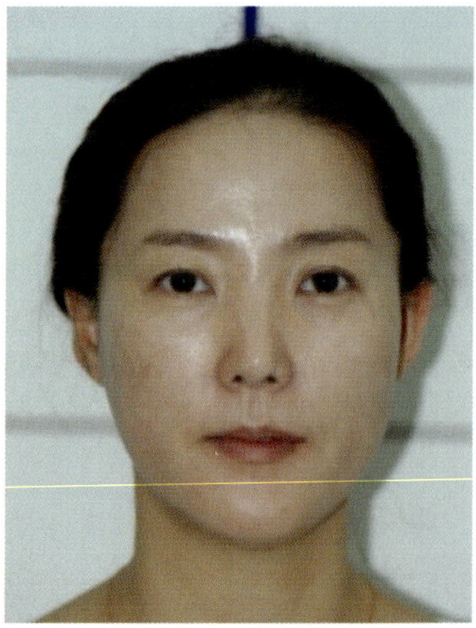

Figure 38b: Post-treatment frontal photograph with improved facial symmetry.

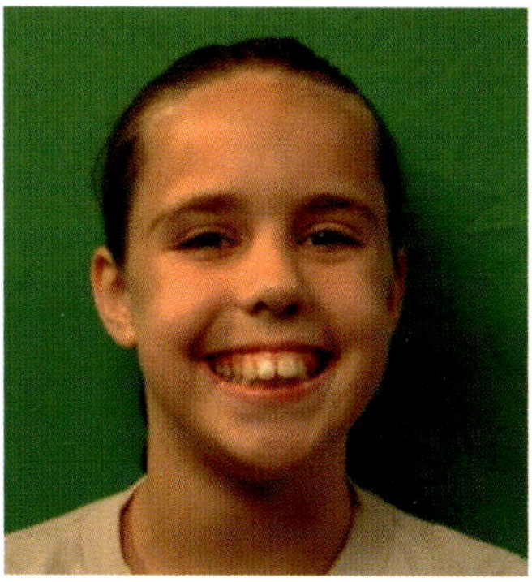

Figure 39a: Pediatric case with 'gummy smile' and dark buccal 'corridors'.

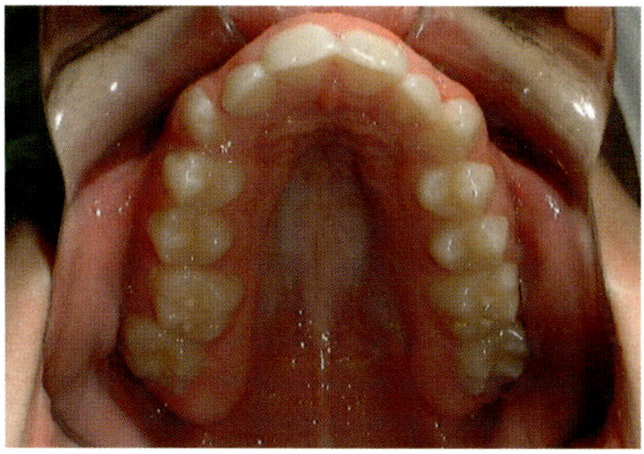

Figure 39b: A narrow or constricted upper arch associated with 'gummy smile' and dark buccal 'corridors' of Fig. 39a.

But, aside from the cosmetic detractions, other conditions of craniofacial co-morbidity may exist in these cases, such as temporo-mandibular dysfunction, headaches, bruxism, snoring, sleep disordered breathing, and obstructive sleep apnea. In addition, systemic conditions such as hypertension, cardiovascular disease, diabetes, cerebro-vascular incidents (strokes), etc., particularly in obese patients with OSA, may be present, which are associated with a decrease in longevity (Fletcher, 1996). These serious life-threatening consequences make the diagnosis of craniofacial underdevelopment mandatory for the modern dental professional. The dental clinician should recognize the significance of craniofacial underdevelopment in the same way that evidence supports the notion that periodontal disease is an indicator of heart disease. Thus, as snoring, SDB and OSA are often associated with malocclusions, they should also be viewed as indicators of decreased longevity, and efforts should be made to address their causative agents.

Assessment of craniofacial features

Prior to any assessments, a thorough medical history needs to be taken. In addition, the chief concerns of the patient have to be noted and addressed. Diagnostic craniofacial features can be quantified using the science of faciometrics, which makes craniofacial measurements, such as those used in anthropometry and forensic reconstruction. More rigorously, geometric morphometrics goes beyond simple measurement, and can be employed to quantify and localize the amounts of craniofacial size- and shape-change in both 2D and 3D data. We will return to this theme when we analyze the outcomes of the clinical PACE protocol outlined in the final chapter of this book. At this point in time, the predominant concept is that the basis for facial appearance is largely the craniofacial skeleton, which encloses functional spaces (Watanabe *et al.*, 2002). For example, the form of the head is determined by the cranial cavity, which consists of the cranial base and calvaria. The cranial cavity is a functional space in the sense that it houses the brain and upper portions of the central nervous system. The function of the brain is to process neural signals, but in order for this function to be accomplished, a functional space is needed. In this case, the functional spaces known as synapses are at the dendritic endings of individual neurons. Taken together, the microscopic functional spaces of the brain add up to a cranial volume. This volume of brain tissue has a specific morphology and is supported by the bony cranial base. The synaptic distance between two neurons is 9nm and neurotransmitters traverse these spaces to excite the cell membrane of the post-synaptic cell. Without this small but crucial functional space, brain function would be severely impeded. For example, in cases of hydrocephalus (blockage of cerebro-spinal fluid flow) and intra-cranial hemorrhage, cerebral function is critically compromised, as the space available for neural function is decreased (while intra-cranial pressure is increased). In these cases, the pressure must be relieved so that the volume of the cranial cavity available for neuronal function is restored. In addition, mild traumatic brain injuries, such as concussions that occur during contact sports or military action, are also thought to disrupt these synaptic spaces; sometimes with long-term sequelae, such as post-traumatic stress disorder, especially if the traumatic events occurred repeatedly. Therefore, assessment of functional spaces is an integral part of craniofacial diagnosis.

Comprehensive working diagnosis

Current imaging techniques such as 3D stereo-photogrammetry, cone-beam CT scans, laser scans, digital study models, etc., can be used to capture 3D data, and 3D analysis of these data can transform these techniques into powerful diagnostic tools. In addition, new, analytical software can be used for diagnostics, treatment planning, and outcome analysis, which specifies, quantifies, characterizes, localizes, models, and animates differences in size, shape, and directionality of 3D objectives or patient data using geometric morphometrics (Singh, 2008). Three-dimensional modeling of digital data may therefore have added value for clinical diagnosis, treatment planning, and post-operative assessments, including audit, but these resources may not be readily available in a dental practice. In the previous chapter, we noted that a malocclusion is a working diagnosis. However, it's likely that malocclusions don't exist in isolation and may represent a clinical sign with other craniofacial and systemic symptoms. Therefore, for clinical treatment planning utilizing the PACE protocol, a three-part diagnosis is formulated. Classification of a presenting malocclusion is only the first part of reaching a comprehensive working diagnosis, noting that malocclusions not included in Angle's classification, such as anterior open bite might need to be specified. The second part is to identify any other differential craniofacial diagnoses, e.g. temporo-mandibular joint dysfunction, bruxism, craniofacial obesity, etc. The third part is to identify any upper airway co-morbidities, such as airway, breathing, and sleep issues. In the past, orthodontic cephalometry was the hallmark of orthodontic diagnosis and treatment planning. However, recent developments in 3D imaging techniques (Singh, 2008) and mathematical modeling algorithms (Chaplain *et al.*, 1999) have highlighted the deficiencies of 2D cephalometry and the plethora of 2D cephalometric analyses that were used in the past (Moyers and Bookstein, 1979; Bookstein, 2016). For example, some still favor the outdated Sassouni analysis even though the three planes used to define the center of the facial arc that is relied upon for assessment in this particular method sometimes fail to intersect. This means that these methods of analysis may amount to simple guesswork, since a 3D object compressed into a

2D plane cannot give consistent information. For example, in these types of 2D analyses, it is assumed that the landmark called gonion is reliable; however, this landmark does not lie in the mid-sagittal plane, either the right or left gonion has to be chosen arbitrarily. For these reasons, Moyers and Bookstein (1979) and Bookstein (2016) are of the opinion that 2D cephalometric analyses are wholly inappropriate for (orthodontic) diagnosis and treatment planning. Furthermore, over-reliance upon cephalometric radiography diverts attention away from a patient's face, and important screening facial features for SDB can sometimes be overlooked.

Frontal photography

Faciometric findings can be used to help formulate a comprehensive diagnosis. In the PACE protocol, a frontal photograph of the head and neck, including the shoulders, is taken with the patient standing at rest and looking straight ahead (horizontal gaze) in the natural head position (Fig. 40a). Looking at this standardized photograph from the front, any clockwise or

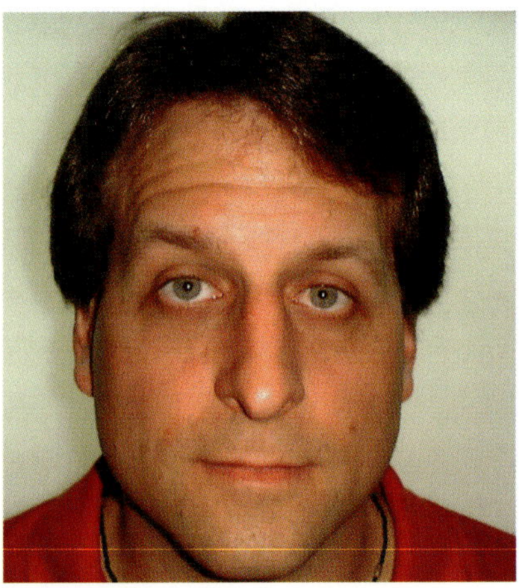

Figure 40a: Standardized photograph from the front, showing mild counterclockwise rotation of head and mild temporal bone asymmetry. The sclera is seen on both sides along with venous pooling.

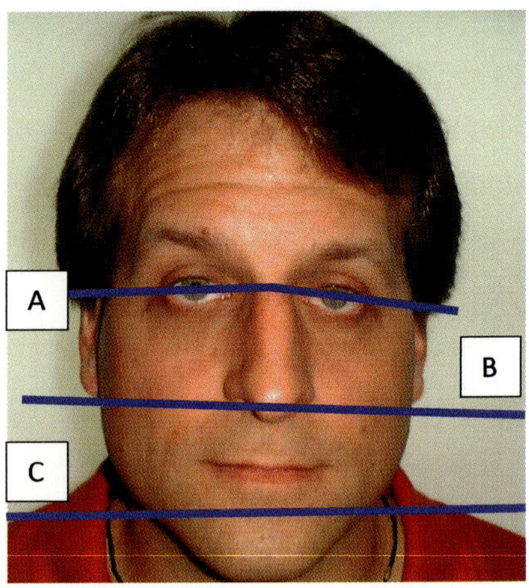

Figure 40b: Plane A is the intercanthal angle: Plane B is the inter-ear angle, and Plane C shows the left shoulder is at a lower level than the right, associated with developmental/postural compensation.

counterclockwise rotation of the head can be assessed. And, if one shoulder is found to be at a lower level than the other, we can suspect cervical subluxation as a consequence of postural compensation. This finding would warrant further investigation of the cervical region, as noted below. In addition, a brief survey of the cranium may show evidence of temporal bone asymmetry and subsequently, as discussed previously, the ears may appear to be asymmetric. For example, the left ear may be rotated anteriorly or posteriorly in comparison to the right, and vice versa. The ears may also be at different horizontal levels with either the right or left ear appearing to be higher/lower. This rotational angle can be measured by drawing a plane through the point of intersection of the pinna of the ear lobe and the ramus of the mandible on both sides (Fig. 40b). Using a simple convention, e.g. a positive or negative sign, a clockwise rotation of the inter-ear angle can be ascribed a positive value whereas a counterclockwise rotation of the inter-ear angle can be assigned a negative value. Ear displacements, as discussed in the case of deformational plagiocephaly, represent directional asymmetry. This deformation is sometimes erroneously described as 'internal or external rotation' of the temporal bones. This example highlights the need for 3D imaging so that the pitch, roll and yaw of the head can be more easily mapped in 3D space using x, y, z Cartesian coordinates, and the sites of deformation can be localized. Digital techniques, such as stereophotogrammetry, are now readily available, and these fast, non-invasive techniques are far superior since the digital data can be subjected to geometric morphometric analysis in 3D space (Singh, 2008).

Another feature that is measured on the frontal photograph is the intercanthal angle. This is the angle formed by the intersection of two lines that pass through the lateral and medial canthi (corners of the eyes on both sides; Fig. 40b). A positive intercanthal angle suggests that there is sufficient midfacial support for the orbit since the floor of the orbit is the roof of the maxilla. Conversely, a negative intercanthal angle suggests that there is a degree of midfacial hypoplasia, which needs additional investigation. This further assessment includes looking at the patient's eyeballs. The sclera may or may not be visible below the iris on one or both sides (Fig. 40a). If sclera is visible, it suggests that there is insufficient support for the lower eyelid, likely secondary to midfacial hypoplasia. In fact, drooping of the lower eyelids may be apparent as eversion or partial lower eyelid eversion, with the palpebral conjunctiva visible when looking at the face from the front. Note that the lacrimal caruncle is the structure found at the medial aspect of the eye and collects tears, which are produced by the lacrimal glands, and drain into the nasolacrimal duct. Notice also that in individuals of Asian origin, an epicanthal fold may cover the caruncle, which is a normal finding. In some other cases, the sclera may be visible above the iris. This rare finding may suggest an underlying endocrine disturbance, such as exophthalmos or goiter, which would require referral to a physician or endocrinologist. It is also thought that lax eyelids found in floppy eyelid syndrome may be related to adenoidal hypertrophy and obstructive sleep apnea (Gao *et al.*, 2018).

In other cases, venous pooling may be present below the lower eyelids (Fig. 40a). These dark circles are associated with a range of anatomical features of the skin, subcutaneous tissues, orbicularis oculi muscle, ligamentous architecture, and venous vasculature of the lower eyelid (Vrcek *et al.*, 2016). Sometimes referred to as 'allergic shiners', venous pooling may also be present in patients with nasal obstruction perhaps associated with allergic rhinitis. The pattern of venous blood drainage of the face is from superficial to deep. Classically, the nasal veins empty into the pterygoid venous plexus, which is found in the infra-temporal fossa, surrounding the lateral pterygoid muscle. From there, the venous blood enters the retromandibular vein and then drains into the internal jugular vein. In cases of mandibular retrognathia, however, it's likely that congestion occurs in the pterygoid venous plexus and retrograde flow means that venous blood pools under the lower eyelids, via the inferior ophthalmic and infra-orbital veins, producing a bluish tinge or dark circles. In this case, drainage is achieved via the angular facial vein, which drains into the external jugular vein and then on to the internal jugular vein. In addition, the thin lower eyelid skin with minimal underlying subcutaneous tissue, allied with ageing of the midfacial bone volume that can result in orbital rim recession, may lead to worsening of the shadowing (Vrcek *et al.*, 2016).

Assessment of craniofacial features also includes nasal morphology and function. From the frontal aspect, nasal asymmetry can be gleaned with narrowing of the nares on one or both sides. Nasal asymmetry may be indicative of alar cartilage collapse with or without nasal obstruction. Symmetric narrowing of the nares may also increase the risk of upper airway resistance syndrome. In the absence of 3D facial imaging, nasal asymmetry may be gauged in the 'submento-vertex' view photograph (Fig. 41a). For this image, the patient is lying in the dental chair and the camera is aimed through the chin toward the forehead at about 45°. It is sometimes surprising to see that a smaller left naris in the frontal view might contrast with a narrower right naris in the 'submento-vertex' view. In this view a submandibular pannus (double chin) might also be discernible (Fig. 41b), emphasizing the need for 3D craniofacial imaging. Nevertheless, frank nasal asymmetry is often seen in babies born with unilateral cleft lip and/or palate. In these cases, the degree of alar collapse is evident but can be non-surgically corrected (Singh *et al.*, 2005; 2007). On the other hand, to test for nasal valve collapse in non-cleft patients, the Cottle maneuver can be carried out. In this test, the individual breathes slowly through the nose, and then the nostrils are gently widened by stretching the nose using the index fingers. If an enhancement in nasal breathing is detected, then alar cartilage collapse might be the source of nasal airflow resistance. In fact, in

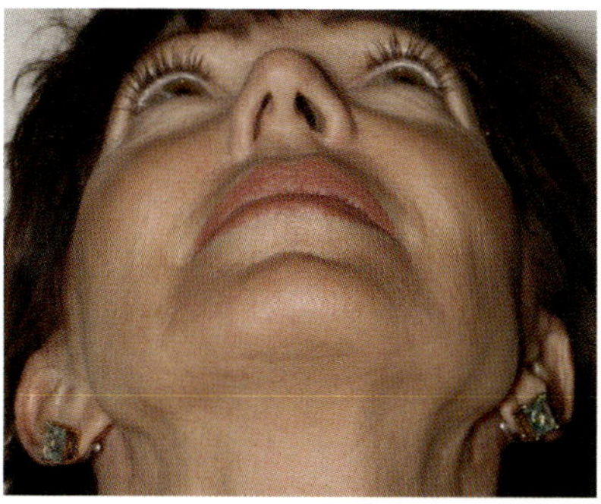

Figure 41a: Nasal asymmetry may be gauged in a 'submento-vertex' view photograph. Courtesy: Dr Myles Preble

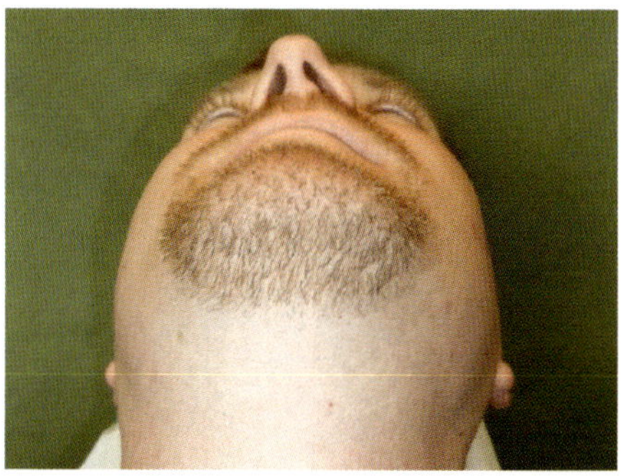

Figure 41b: A submandibular pannus (double chin) may also be discernible in a 'submento-vertex' view. Courtesy: Dr TerryLynn Tennant

some patients, a wide smile can indicate the clinical potential for increased nasal width and/or symmetry (Fig. 42), and clinical experience indicates that soft tissue nasal asymmetry and narrow nares may be amenable to correction using biomimetic oral appliance therapy (Fig. 43). Note that some are of the opinion that widening of the nares may improve arterial oxygenation (Herulf *et al.*, 1999).

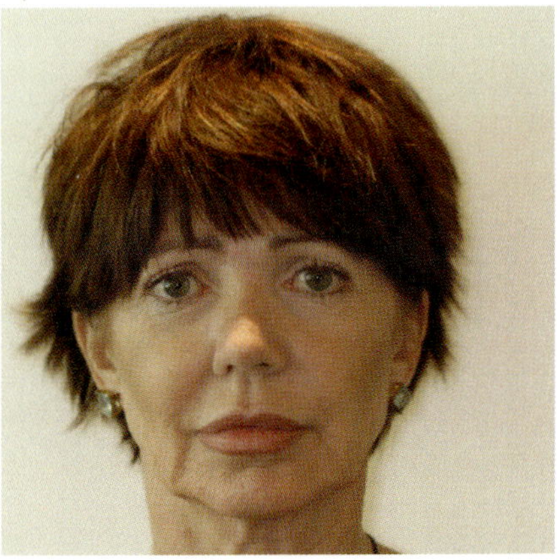

Figure 42a: Nasal asymmetry may be evident in a standardized photograph from the front.

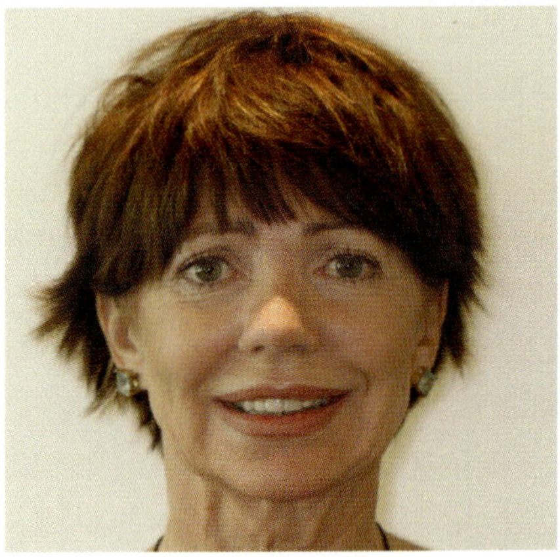

Figure 42b: Wide smile indicating the clinical potential for increased nasal width and/or symmetry. Courtesy: Dr Myles Preble

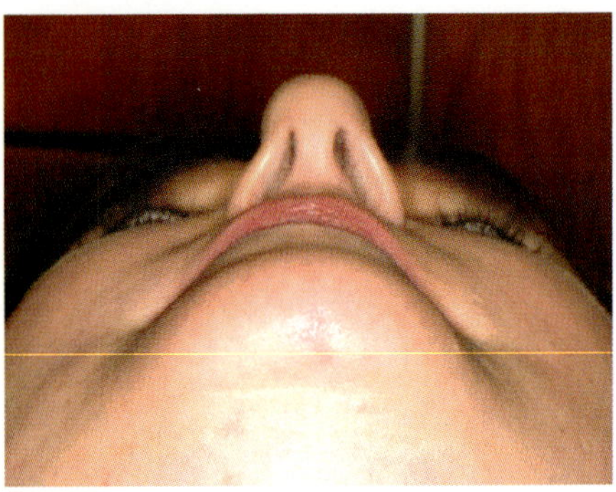

Figure 43a: Pre-treatment, alar cartilage collapse may be evident in a 'submento-vertex' photograph. Courtesy: Dr Bradley Sievert

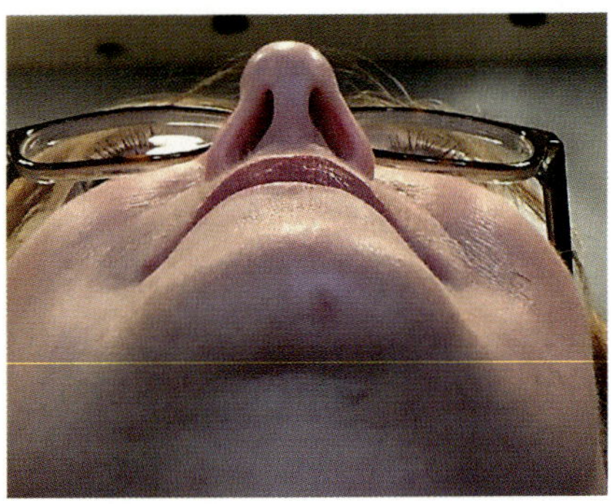

Figure 43b: Post-treatment, increased nasal width/symmetry after oral biomimetic appliance therapy.

Similarly, a slightly asymmetric upper lip with extended oral commissures can sometimes reveal reduced smile esthetics, such as a 'gummy smile'. Therefore, even simple, non-invasive techniques, such as 2D photography, can disclose useful diagnostic features.

Lateral profile (right)

In conjunction with the frontal views noted above, standardized lateral profile photographs have routinely been used in orthodontic treatment planning. Note that North Americans prefer to image the right side of the face, leading to the classification of dolicocephalic or brachycephalic facial types, while Europeans prefer to image the left side of the face. Viewing from the right side, a counterclockwise rotation of head is often associated with a forward head posture (Fig. 44a), which may in turn be a sign of a compromised upper airway. In these cases, the mandible is being protruded to maintain the patency of the upper airway, but a posterior sloping of the forehead may be more easily detected (Fig. 44a) since mandibular morphology can vary quite widely. The forehead (frontal bone) articulates

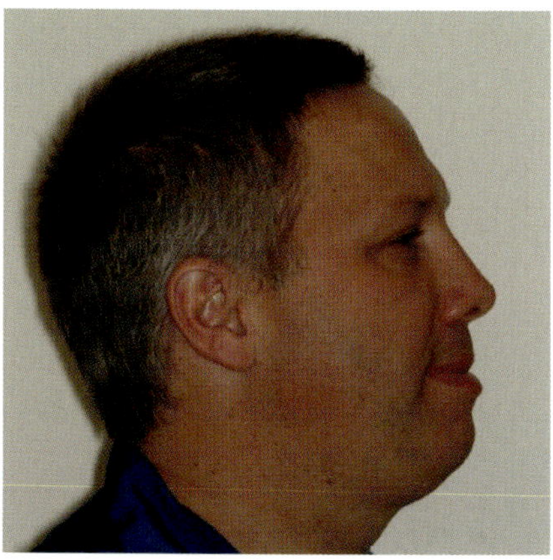

Figure 44a: Standardized lateral photograph, showing counter-clockwise rotation of head. Notice the forehead is sloping posteriorly in attempt to maintain the airway. Courtesy: Dr William Payne

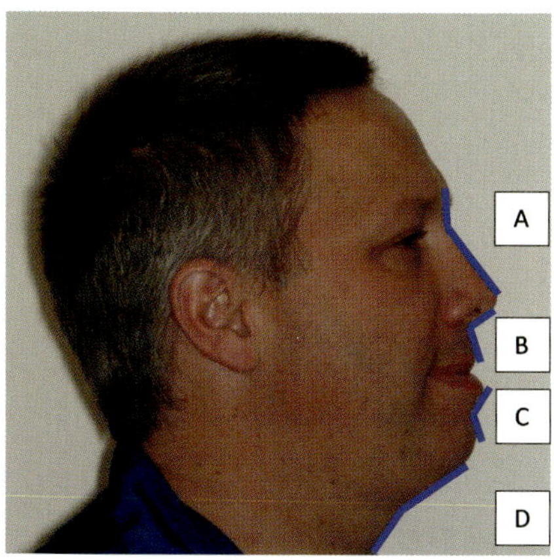

Figure 44b: Angle A shows the frontonasal angle: angle B shows the nasolabial angle, angle C shows the labiomental angle, and angle D shows the thyromental angle.

with the bridge of the nose (the nasal bone) at the frontonasal suture, which can clearly be seen on a lateral radiograph. In a lateral photograph, however, the frontonasal angle can be measured on the surface of the skin. It is formed by three homologous landmarks: soft tissue glabella (the most prominent point of the frontal bone), soft tissue nasion (the most anterior point of the frontonasal suture on the skin), and pronasale (the most anterior point on the tip of the nose; Fig. 44b). However, nasal morphology shows both heterogeneity and complexity. Humans have a 3 x 3 nasal matrix, comprising: Soft tissue nose, cartilaginous nose, bony nose; nose at the front, nose in the middle, nose at the back. In fact, most people don't realize that the nasal septum is not the nose at all; it is the non-ossified cartilage continuation of the anterior cranial base.

As mentioned previously, the cranial base develops as a series of cranial base cartilages. The nasal septum is a component of the nasal capsule that persists as cartilage even in adulthood. The significance of this finding is that modern humans have two cranial base phenotypes: A long cranial base or a short cranial base phenotype. Peoples of Asian and African descent tend to have a short cranial base phenotype (Fig. 45a), while Caucasian peoples from Europe, the Middle East, and South Asia may have a long cranial base phenotype (Fig. 45b). This dichotomy explains the craniofacial heterogeneity that is encountered in clinical practice. Typically, the frontonasal angle varies between approx. 130° and 150°. As the frontonasal angle gets larger (becomes obtuse; Fig. 45a) there is a greater likelihood of a short anterior cranial base tendency. Conversely, as the frontonasal angle gets smaller (becomes relatively acute; Fig. 45b) there is a greater likelihood of a long cranial base tendency. As a clinical indicator, the distance between the eyeball and the dorsum of the nose gets longer (Fig. 45b). These measurements can be obtained from either 2D cephalographs or 3D CBCT scans, but these simple measurements from a single photograph (Fig. 45) can help classify the morphology of the cranial base, since 'the cranial base sets the pace for the rest of the face'.

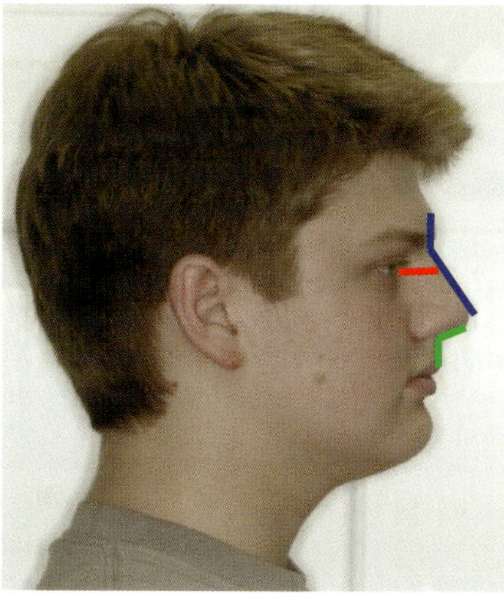

Figure 45a: Long cranial base phenotype. Notice the frontonasal angle is relatively acute (blue lines) and the distance between the eyeball and dorsum of nose is long (red line). The columella is directed upward (green lines). Courtesy: Dr Alex Pavlenko

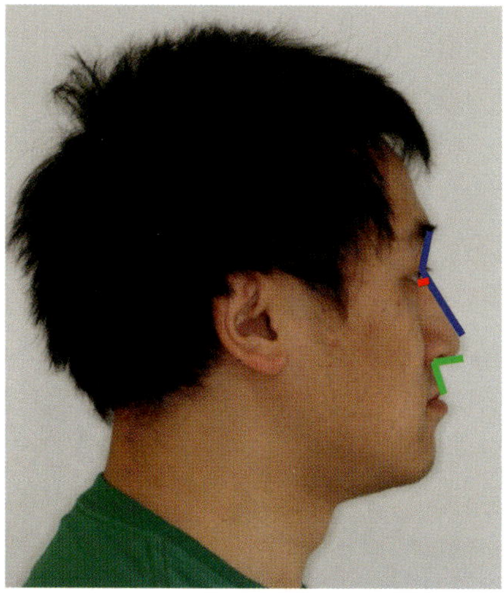

Figure 45b: Short cranial base phenotype. Notice the frontonasal angle is obtuse (blue lines) while the distance between the eyeball and dorsum of nose is very short and almost absent. The columella is horizontal (green lines). Courtesy: Dr Lihua Zhang

Further down, the nasolabial angle can also be measured. Figure 44b shows that this angle is formed between pronasale, the base of the columella (the deepest point of the concavity below the nose and above the upper lip), and prolabiale (the most anterior point of the upper lip). A value of approx. 105° is typically deemed to be within normal limits (WNL) (Armijo *et al.*, 2012). Note that the columella itself may be directed upward (Fig. 45a), downward, or horizontally (Fig. 45b). Its orientation may itself be secondary to the morphology of the nasal septum, which articulates with the nasal bones. Thus, in some cases a 'dorsal hump' or bump can be seen on the nose (Fig. 46a). This hump or bump is a consequence of the fact that the nasal septum also articulates with the maxilla via the septo- and vomero-maxillary sutures in the midline. This means that maxillary retrusion and/or midfacial hypoplasia can precipitate a 'dorsal hump' since the nasal bones are attached to the cranial base and are relatively immobile while the more flexible nasal septum is deformed or bent as it complies

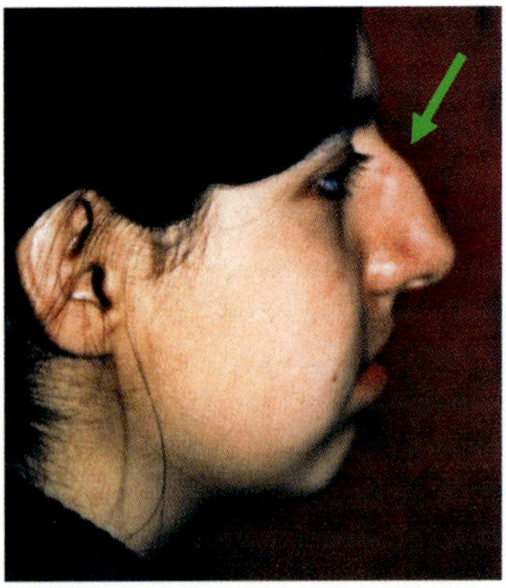

Figure 46a: Maxillary retrognathia. Notice the 'hump' or 'bump' in dorsum of nose (green arrow).

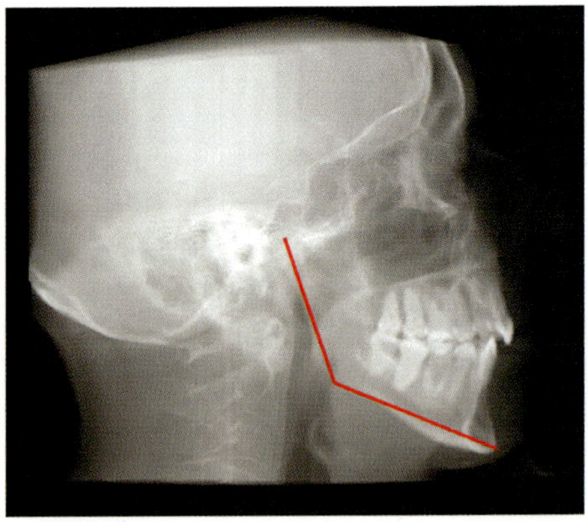

Figure 46b: High gonial angle case where the angle formed by condylion, gonion, and pogonion is > 125°.

with the (retruded) position of the bony maxilla. Therefore, this diagnostic feature is seen either superficially in photographs and/or radiographically.

Note that some people advocate measuring the distance between the tip of the nose and the incisal edge of an upper incisor as some form of 'indicator' line. This approach appears to be flawed since the tip of the nose is determined, at least in part, by cranial base morphology — not to mention differences in incisor angulation. Thus, the nasolabial angle is preferred in the medical, dental, and orthodontic literature. Specifically, as the nasolabial angle becomes more acute, the antero-posterior projection of the midface is more anteriorly positioned in the sagittal plane. A more acute nasolabial angle appears to be beneficial for nasal airway flow (Armijo *et al.*, 2012). Conversely, as the nasolabial angle becomes more obtuse, it represents midfacial retrusion and/or hypoplasia. In this case, the mandible might also be retrognathic, leading to a diagnosis of bimaxillary retrognathia. Note that in the orthodontic literature, there is much debate about bimaxillary protrusion or bialveolar protrusion. In fact, in most cases there is little or no protrusion. The angle of the upper incisors with respect to the cranial base may be slightly proclined (> 90°) but this is likely a developmental compensation for midfacial hypoplasia in the context of a short anterior cranial base morphology. In these cases, it is not unusual for the mandibular incisors to follow suite and be proclined (> 90°) with respect to the mandibular (gonion-pogonion) plane. Note also that the mandibular plane angle (condylion-gonion-pogonion) can also vary; a high gonial angle phenotype (Fig. 46b) predisposes to the risk of developing an anterior open bite tendency.

The craniofacial soft-tissue morphology also differs in people of diverse ethnic origins. For example, in Caucasian-American children, soft tissue dynamics in the prepubertal postnatal phase may contribute to the development of Class III malocclusions (Singh *et al.*, 1999). In these cases, an area of negative allometry (relative size-reduction) can be localized near soft subspinale with an increase in size in the mental region. When these children were compared with their Korean-Asian counterparts (Singh *et al.*, 1999) it was found that the Asian mental regions were generally smaller, allied with a local increase in size for the lower lip. This feature appears to be associated with an underlying skeletal Class III phenotype. In this way, further information on the mandible's morphologic behavior can be gleaned from measuring the labiomental angle. This angle is formed between the landmarks; inferior prolabiale (the most anterior point of the lower lip), soft tissue point B (the deepest point of the concavity below the lower lip and above the chin), and soft pogonion (the most anterior point of the chin). A normal value is expected of around 130° in Class I cases. On the other hand, a relatively acute labiomental angle (< 130°) indicates an increased overbite or a deep bite tendency. Conversely, an obtuse labiomental angle (> 130°) indicates a decreased overbite, a Class III phenotype or an anterior open bite tendency. In fact, Singh and Kim (2016) found that the labiomental angle improved to 118.5° from 126.5° in adults treated using biomimetic oral appliance therapy, and this feature is sometimes associated with a prominent lower lip. In addition, when examining the labiomental angle, other features are often discernible, such as a labiomarginal groove, which may merge or blend with a nasolabial groove, extending below the side of the nose. In these cases, it's worth assessing the lower border of the

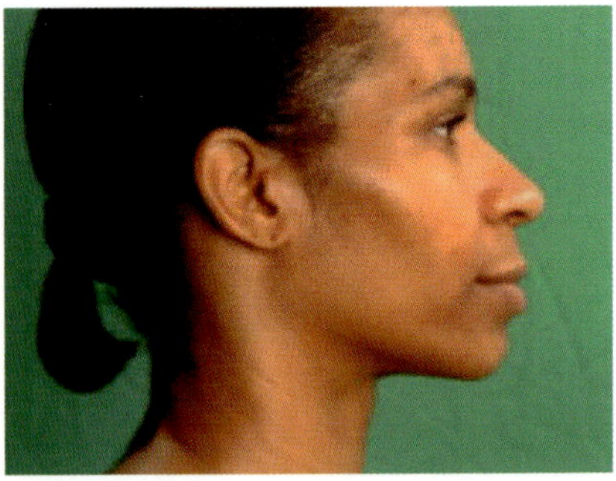

Figure 47a: A well-defined lower jaw is associated with good facial development and upper airway health.

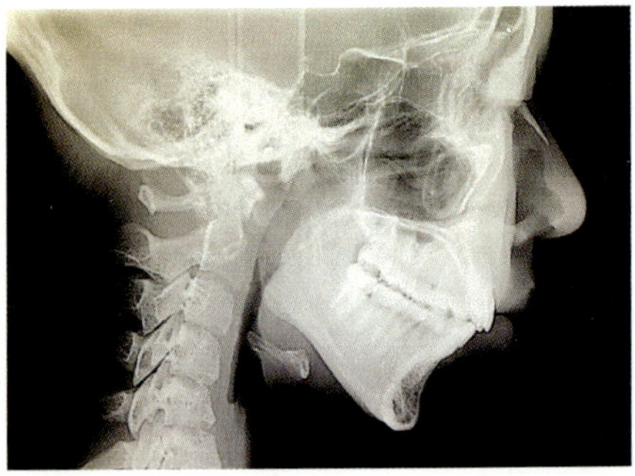

Figure 47b: Mandibular retrognathia with a diminutive mental process associated with the appearance of a receding chin.
Courtesy: Dr Lihua Zhang

mandible, which may or may not be clearly visible. A well-defined lower jaw (Fig. 47a) is often associated with good facial development and may include the mental region. Thus, the chin button or mental process needs to be assessed also. In some cases, the chin button is in itself well-developed and may give a balanced facial appearance. In other cases, the mental process may diminutive and, especially if the mandible is also retrognathic, will give the appearance of a receding chin (Fig. 47b). On the other hand, some cases may have perturbed chin features associated with genioglossal advancement surgery or chin implants for cosmetic camouflage. Thus, both the morphology and position of the mandibular structures need to be thoroughly surveyed, since the shape, size, and position of various craniofacial components contribute to craniofacial architecture, and variations can have functional consequences. For example, below the chin, the angle formed by the following three landmarks: pogonion; the deepest point of the concavity below the chin and above the neck; and the laryngeal prominence (the most anterior point of the thyroid cartilage) is known as the thyromental angle (Fig. 44b). The value of this angle varies between, say, < 100° and > 180°. In one study (Lam *et al.*, 2005), it was found that a small thyromental angle was associated with mild OSA or a low risk of SDB. As the angle got larger, the risk and severity of OSA was increased. In separate study (Banabilh *et al.*, 2009), it was found that the mechanism by which the thyromental angle increased was twofold: first, the presence of a submandibular pannus (double chin), which represents fat deposition associated with craniofacial obesity; and second, inferior displacement of the hyoid bone, which is associated with an increased risk of SDB. In non-obese Asian adults, Singh and Kim (2016) found that the thyromental angle improved from 126.5° to 118.5° following biomimetic oral appliance therapy. Thus, a simple lateral photograph can be used to screen individuals for a potentially life-threatening condition. However, corroboration of these external diagnostic craniofacial features and correlation with intra-oral signs and symptoms is warranted.

Intra-oral photographic findings

Standardized upper occlusal photographic views of the maxillary arch have long been used in orthodontic diagnosis. Although this 2D media loses some 3D information, it can provide some useful diagnostic data. When observing these images, it's important to think about size, shape and positional information since the essence of craniofacial architecture is spatial patterning and not tooth morphology or positioning. Thus, the shape of an archform may appear to be deformed or asymmetric with a tapered or square shape (Fig. 39b). The shape may also be distorted in 3D with a high palatal vault with or without a torus palatinus or other features, such as bulbous, postero-lateral aspects of the tuberosity regions. In terms of size, the arch may be narrower transversely than required or shorter antero-posteriorly than anticipated. A narrow arch refers to the width of the bone, not the teeth, which can be measured in the molar, premolar, or canine regions. Specifically, the transpalatal bone width ought to be approx. 38mm in most adult cases, measured at the mesio-palatal cusp of the first permanent maxillary molar at the cervical margin/cemento-enamel junction (McNamara, 2000). If the bone width is too narrow, anterior or posterior crowding may be observable since the midfacial bone volume is inadequate. On the other hand, if the archform is too short, there may be partial-eruption, impaction or absence of the maxillary third molars.

Note that the crowns of the third molars calcify at the age of about 8–9yrs. Thus, the need for midfacial development can often be estimated with a panoramic radiograph well before the teenage years. The biomimetic approach aims to accommodate 32 teeth, symmetrically arranged within the craniofacial architecture. Not working in isolation, apart from dentoskeletal requirements, the soft tissues and functional spaces also need to be addressed. Thus, the transpalatal bone width needs to be able to easily accommodate the tongue both at rest and during swallowing. As the previous studies have indicated, midfacial development is associated with an enhanced upper airway, and the concept of waiting for 'growth to cease' prior to instituting corrective measures appears to be an outdated concept.

One feature that helps to determine the extent of development required is the position of the permanent second maxillary molars. The hard palate is composed of two bones: the palatine process of the maxilla and the horizontal plate of the palatine bone. This design suggests that there may be two diverse functions for this one, two-part structure. It can be posited that the function of the maxilla, specifically the alveolar process, is to accommodate the teeth, while the function of the palatine bone, specifically its horizontal plate, is to maintain the patency of the upper airway at the posterior nasal apertures. The junction between the palatal processes of the maxilla anteriorly and the horizontal plates of the palatine bone posteriorly is the transverse palatine suture and, lying almost directly in line with this suture, are the crowns of the second molars (Fig. 25a). It can be ventured that maxillary hypoplasia would likely have a more direct effect on teeth anterior to the transverse palatine suture, and since the second molars erupt later, they may be guided by the palatine bone to some extent; thus maintaining their positions better than the first permanent molars (Fig. 48a). In this case, the buccally positioned second molars may give an indication of the extent of development needed, and the discrepancy between the first and second molar may reflect the degree of midfacial hypoplasia (Fig. 48b). Notwithstanding the above, it is known that midfacial development permits inferior remodeling of the posterior nasal spine (of the palatine bone), which enhances the upper (nasopharyngeal)

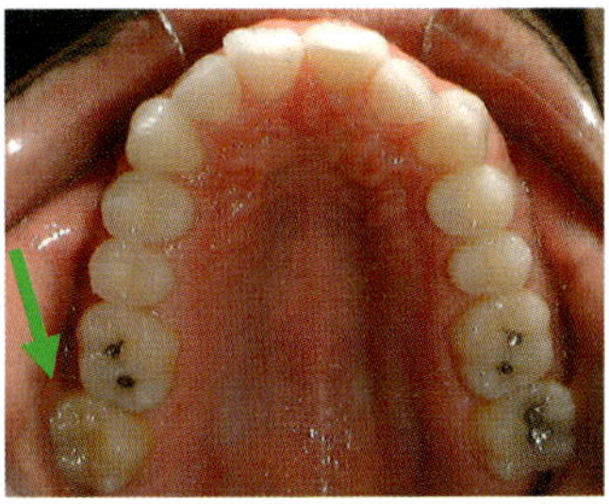

Figure 48a: Occlusal view. Notice the second molar orientation compared with the first molar orientation.

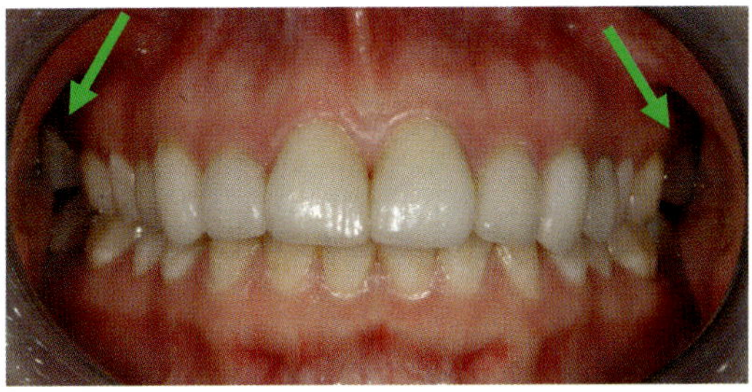

Figure 48b: Anterior view. Notice the upper second molar position compared with position of the upper first molars. Courtesy: Dr Dennis Klemp

airway as evidenced by studies in both children and adults (Singh *et al.*, 2007; Singh and Krumholtz, 2009). Thus, it is imperative to view midfacial development as a 3D phenomenon and avoid the old concept of 'palatal expansion'. In fact, unpublished data using 3D modeling suggests that when the dental arch becomes wider, the zygomas are displaced upward and outward, while the posterior nasal spine remodels inferiorly. Taken as a whole, the phenomenon increases the midfacial bone volume (Singh *et al.*, 2014), increases the upper (nasal) airway volume (Singh *et al.*, 2016; Singh *et al.*, 2020), increases the volume of the maxillary sinuses (Singh and Kim, 2020) while increasing the space necessary to accommodate 16 teeth (Fig. 49), and putatively providing sufficient space to accommodate the tongue.

Following the cranio-caudal gradient of development, the lower arch is downstream from the upper arch, and it sometimes magnifies the degree of developmental compensation. In other words, the lower arch can sometimes be more crowded than the upper arch, and the lower occlusal photograph can provide this invaluable information (Fig. 50b). The same principles apply in terms of shape, size, and position of the lower archform since it can be tapered, square, or asymmetric. However, while the position of the maxilla is largely influenced by anterior cranial base allometry, the mandible is influenced by both the posterior cranial base as well as the maxilla. For example, a relatively acute cranial base angle would predispose to the formation of a Class III phenotype, and the mandible may escape some of the developmental compensations imposed by the maxilla.

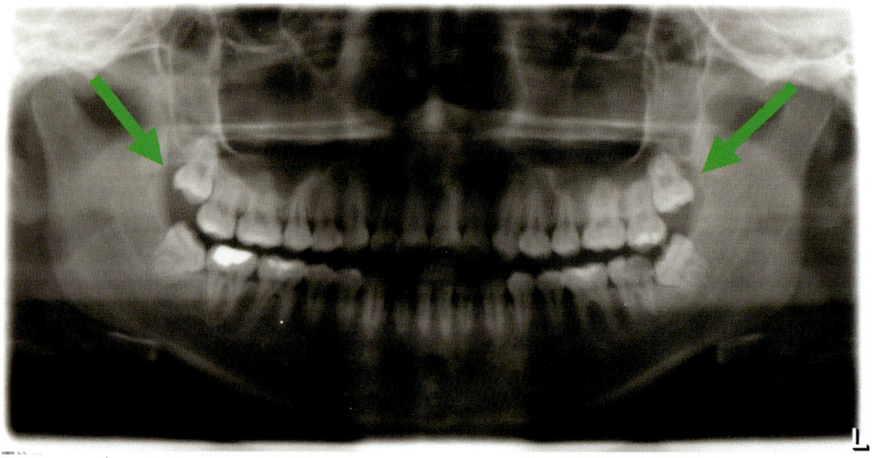

Figure 49a: Panoramic radiographic view. Notice the unerupted third molars (green arrows) at age 19yrs old. Courtesy: Dr Sang Min Lee

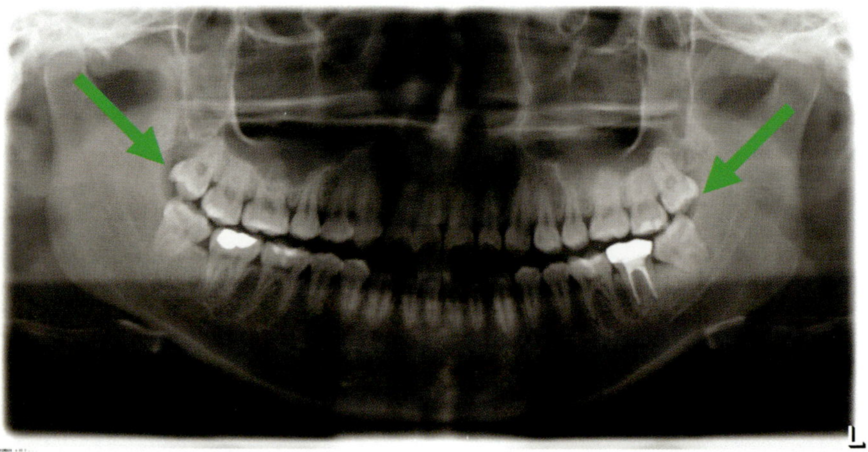

Figure 49b: Panoramic radiographic view. Notice the biomimetic eruption of the third molars by age 21yrs old.

In this case, an anterior crossbite could be precipitated even with normal maxillary morphology. More commonly, however, the lower arch may be tapered or narrowed, reflecting the deficient functional space afforded by the hypoplastic/compensated upper arch, which encroaches on the functional space of the mandible. For example, as well as showing more severe anterior crowding than the upper arch (Fig. 50), in the lower arch

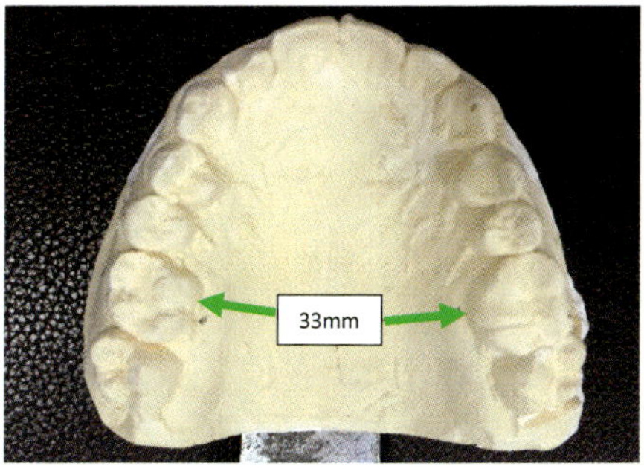

Figure 50a: Upper study model showing minor crowding. Notice the transpalatal bone width is < 38mm (≈33mm). Courtesy: Dr Hwasub Hwang

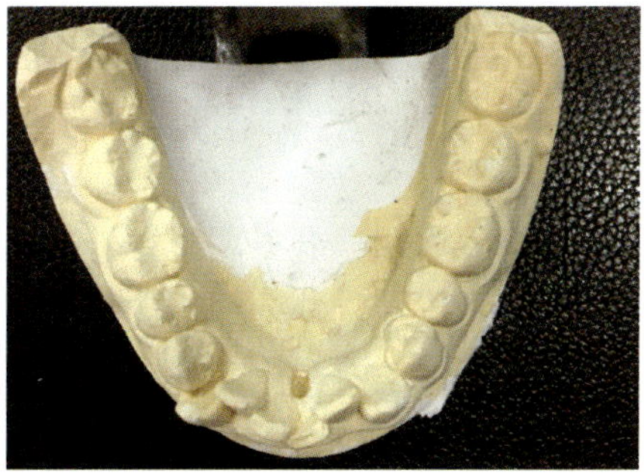

Figure 50b: Corresponding lower study model showing severe lower anterior crowding/lack of functional space. Courtesy: Dr Charin Hwang

there may be partially erupted, impacted, or missing lower third molars. Alternatively, there may be unilateral or bilateral posterior crossbite if the mandible is influenced by the cranial base morphology. In any case, apart from the alveolar region, it's also important to survey the medial aspect of the mandible. Here, mandibular torus formation may be identified, which may be unilateral or bilateral, typically in the first premolar region. The presence of tori is contentious. While some believe they are of no consequence, others associate torus formation with sleep bruxism and SDB, including OSA. Tori will be discussed in later chapters that deal with sleep bruxism but at this juncture, it is at least safe to say that large mandibular (and palatal) tori take up valuable functional space intended for the tongue. Therefore, it is necessary to assess tongue features as part of the oral examination.

It is worth noting the size, shape, and position of the tongue as part of the intra-oral examination. If the tongue appears to be large, it's possible to suspect craniofacial obesity (Banabilh *et al.*, 2009) and (rare) conditions, such as macroglossia. However, most tongues are not enlarged, rather the tongue space has been reduced. A classic example of this reduction in functional space for the tongue is Down syndrome. While syndromic contributions directly affecting the tongue can't be ruled out, one underlying anomaly in Down syndrome is cranial base dysmorphology. This genetic mutation (Trisomy 21) has epigenetic consequences. Parsons *et al.* (2015) showed that genetic mutations of the cranial base are associated

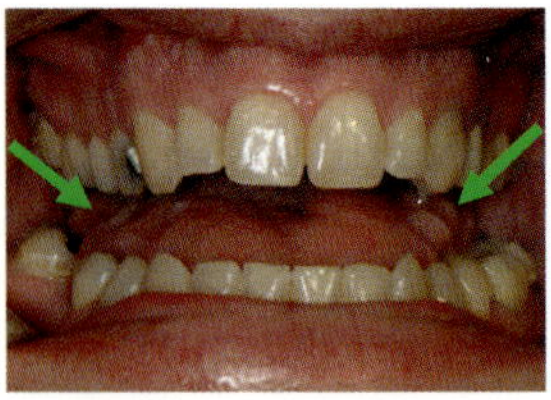

Figure 51a: Intra-oral view showing lateral tongue crenation/scalloping (green arrows).

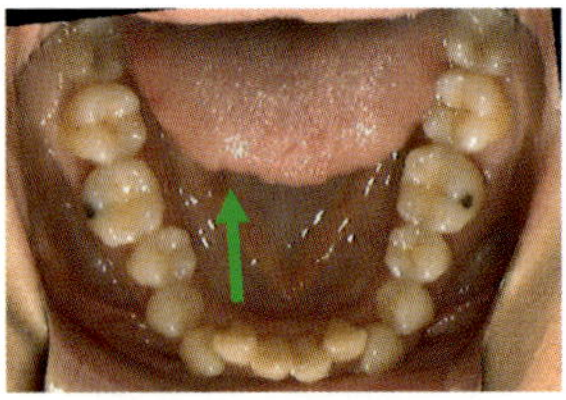

Figure 51b: Intra-oral view showing anterior tongue scalloping (green arrow).

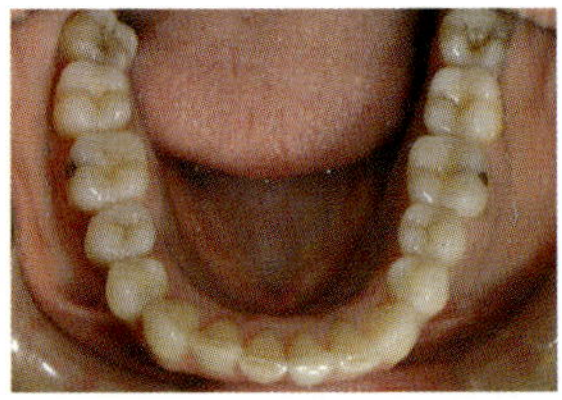

Figure 51c: Post-treatment intra-oral view with smooth contour of tongue.

with epigenetic facial shape changes (in mice). Thus, it's also likely that the typical facies identified as Down syndrome are epigenetic facial changes secondary to genetic mutation affecting the cranial base. Suppose the cranial base is shorter in patients diagnosed with Down syndrome, that would mean that the maxilla is positioned further posteriorly in the craniofacial architecture, and, if the mandible is largely unaffected, the tongue would appear to be more anteriorly placed, giving the clinical impression of macroglossia. But another feature to look for is the shape of the tongue. A deficiency of space to house the tongue would mean that the tongue would take the path of least resistance and occupy whatever space is left available. Classically, a crenated or scalloped tongue is produced (Fig. 51a and 51b). The scalloping represents the interproximal/interdental regions where the tongue comes to rest, since the intrinsic muscles of the tongue can change the shape of the tongue. In fact, tongue crenation/scalloping is a positive sign of OSA (Weiss *et al.*, 2005).

Another feature to assess is the position of the tongue. Is the tongue lying in the back of the mouth below the occlusal plane? Ideally, the tongue should be in light contact with the hard palate at rest and while asleep. If the tongue is habitually lying in the back/floor of the mouth, there may be an increased risk of nocturnal upper airway obstruction. The Mallampati score is used to classify tongue posture but I introduced functional assessment of the upper airway aperture, simply asking the patient to say "Aaaaahhhh" and observing if, say a Class 3 Mallampati score (Fig. 52a) changed to, say a Mallampati Class 2. In these cases, the use of a pharyngeal stent may be

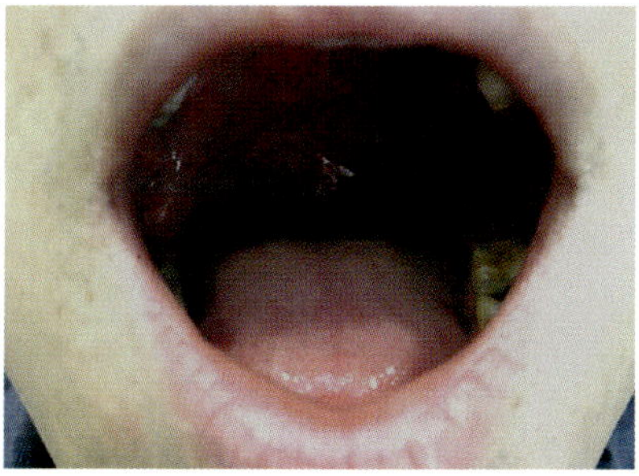

Figure 52a: Intra-oral view showing Mallampati Class 3 oropharyngeal airway aperture. Courtesy: Dr Sang Min Lee

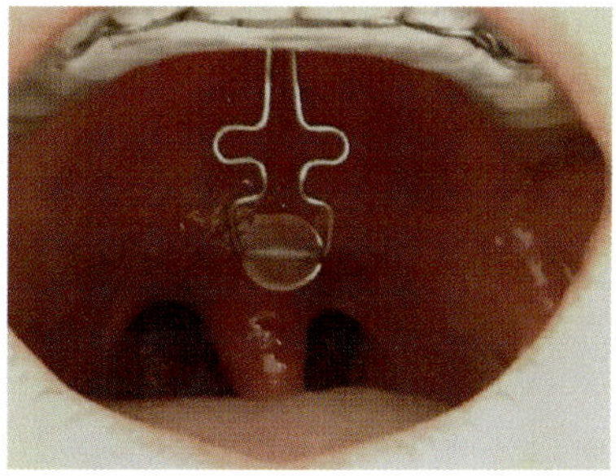

Figure 52b: Intra-oral view showing a pharyngeal stent that has improved the airway to Mallampati Class 2.

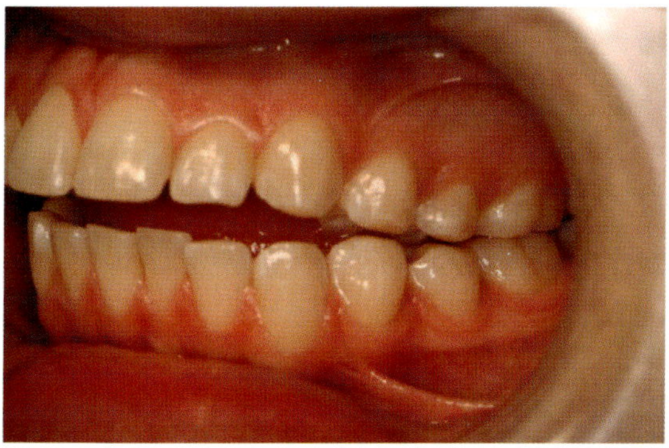

Figure 53: Intra-oral view showing anterior open bite secondary to tongue protrusion/thrust. Courtesy: Dr Felix Liao

considered (Fig. 52b). In other cases, the tongue comes to lie in a forward position instead. In these cases, the tongue posture can precipitate an anterior open bite (Fig. 53) with or without an increased risk of SDB. Tongue posture may also be influenced by the lingual frenum. In an intra-oral exam, it is necessary to decide if the lingual frenum is restrictive. In this case, a specific photograph of the ventral surface of the tongue is taken (Fig. 23a). The frenum can then be classified as being long or short, thick or thin but if it appears to be blanched when the tongue is raised to sit on the palate with the mouth wide open then it's likely that a degree of restriction is present (Fig. 23b). Note that surgical release of the frenum may not be the first stage of correction. After thorough myofunctional assessment by a qualified oral myofunctional therapist, the first phase may be 4 weeks of myofunctional exercises prior to any excision, followed by a further 8 weeks of exercises. In the absence of a planned protocol, the frenum may heal back in its original position.

Another integral part of the structural intra-oral examination is an assessment of the dental occlusion. Here, standard orthodontic photographs are taken of the occlusion (Fig. 54). The features to be assessed in the anterior view of the occlusion include the degree of overbite and overjet, including any anterior crossbites. The lower dental midline may be shifted to one side or the other, usually by a few millimeters (Fig. 54b). Assuming there are no teeth missing that contribute to the asymmetry, then one has to postulate whether the upper jaw is too narrow. If so, has the lower jaw simply changed its position in an attempt to maintain compromised function, as predicted by the spatial matrix hypothesis? If the upper jaw is narrow, the lower jaw will show developmental compensation, following the cranio-caudal gradient of development. However, because of complexity the upper and lower midlines might be well aligned even if the maxilla is not fully developed. In these cases, both the upper and lower posterior segments may be lingually inclined in response to bimaxillary hypoplasia. In yet another example of phenotypic variation, a patient with midfacial hypoplasia may exhibit either unilateral or bilateral posterior crossbites, perhaps indicating a Class III tendency. Therefore, the posterior dental occlusion on the right and left sides needs to be examined as part of the craniofacial analysis. Specifically, as well as the first molar relationship, the position of the second molars needs to be assessed. As noted above, buccally positioned second molars (Fig. 54a and

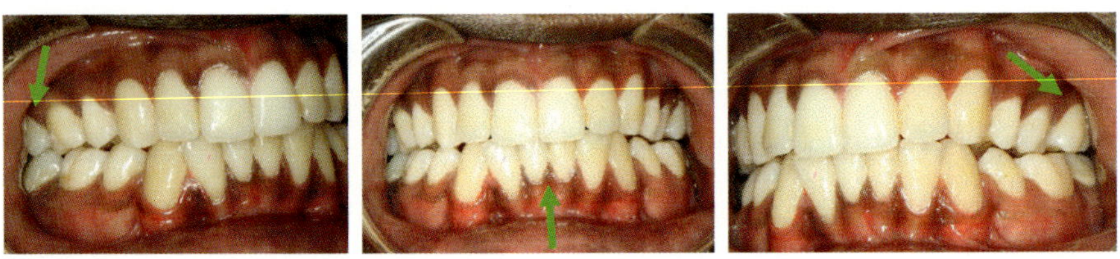

Figure 54a: Intra-oral view showing right side buccally displaced second molar.

Figure 54b: Intra-oral view showing anterior occlusion and midline shift (arrowed).

Figure 54c: Intra-oral view showing left side with buccally displaced second molar (arrowed).

Fig. 54c) may indicate the degree of midfacial hypoplasia, especially if the third molars are unerupted, partially erupted, or impacted. Therefore, the overall aim of these photographic surveys is to identify diagnostic features of the skeletal tissues, the functional spaces, the soft tissues as well as the dental tissues. But, reliance on 2D photographs only provides qualitative assessments that need to be confirmed with 3D data.

In the past, 2D cephalometrics was the mainstay of orthodontic diagnosis and treatment planning. This technique has been largely superseded by 3D cone-beam CT scans, which show that if the proper CBCT machine settings are used, the effective radiation dose is about one-tenth of the radiation of a medical CT scan for the same area (Ludlow *et al.*, 2003). Generally speaking, it is claimed that US residents receive about 3 millisieverts (3000μSv) of radiation exposure per year from natural sources, such as the ground and the sun. During a 7hr flight from New York to London, travelers receive about the same dose of radiation as a chest radiograph, which is generally up to 0.06 millisievert (60μSv), while a typical CBCT scan dose is around 100μSv (Ludlow, 2011). One further advantage of CBCT scans is based on the idea that 2D cephalometric findings cannot be relied upon. For example, Gribel *et al.* (2011) compared the accuracy of measurements made on 2D lateral cephalograms and on 3D CBCT images. Cephalometric measurements were found to be significantly different from direct measurements; some were smaller, but mid-sagittal measurements were consistently enlarged. Thus, 2D cephalometric norms cannot be readily used for 3D data, and therefore 3D CBCT scans are preferred for craniofacial diagnostics and treatment planning. But, while CBCT scans are accurate, the imaging technique is sensitive and more demanding on orientation accuracy. Because of this shortcoming, some are of the opinion that CBCT data is not reliable (Obelenis *et al.*, 2019).

Despite the above contentions, one measurement that has routinely been taken is the cranial base length, which is measured as the linear distance from basion to nasion. For most modern humans this length is typically 100mm approx. although slightly longer or shorter measurements are not uncommon. Even after correcting for size, there are various ways that the cranial base length can vary since it has three components: the anterior cranial base; the posterior cranial base, and the cranial base angle. The anterior cranial base length varies according to ethnicity, but on average it is about 65mm. Its variation has been well established in the medical and orthodontic literature. For example, in ethnic groups of northern and eastern Asia, a shorter than average anterior cranial base length has been demonstrated. For example, when compared to Caucasian-Americans, Asian-Korean children appear to develop Class III malocclusions because of shorter anterior cranial base and midfacial dimensions (Singh *et al.*, 1998), in conjunction with a larger and less favorable mandibular morphology. Presumably, heterochrony during development may contribute to ethnic craniofacial heterogeneity. This notion was investigated by Singh *et al.* (1999) who studied cranial base morphology in Korean and Caucasian children. We surmised that spheno-ethmoidal allometry could be associated with ethnic heterogeneity of the midfacial profile. Pseudo-color-coded finite element (FEM) analysis revealed that in the anterior cranial base, the Korean spheno-ethmoidal and sella turcica regions were smaller but local increases in size were found in the posterior region of the Korean cranial base. Therefore, a spheno-ethmoidal mechanism of midfacial retrognathia appears to be implicated in the development of a skeletal Class III morphology but posterior cranial base morphology must also be taken into account. The posterior cranial base length on a CBCT scan is measured from basion to sella on the mid-sagittal slice. The average value is around 45mm; however, it can be shorter in some cases. Banabilh *et al.* (2007) compared cranial base and upper airway morphology in adult Malays with and without OSA. Using pseudo-colored FEM analysis, we found an approx. 60% decrease in nasopharyngeal airway area above and behind the soft palate. As well, an approx. 30% decrease in oropharyngeal airway area was located behind the base of the tongue, with an approx. 20% decrease in hypopharyngeal area near the level of the hyoid bone. In contrast, an increase in area associated with a downward displacement of the hyoid bone was also detected. We therefore concluded that functional airway impairments are associated with OSA in Malays and are predominantly associated with the posterior region of the cranial base. In addition, inter-landmark analysis revealed that the cranial base saddle angle was more acute in the OSA group compared to the control group. Therefore, the cranial base angle, which is typically approx. 130°, needs to be assessed since it can impact both the mandible and the nasomaxillary architecture.

One way to investigate nasal airway morphology is to use acoustic rhinometry. In a study in Asians with and without OSA, adults underwent clinical examination and polysomnography (Banabilh *et al.*, 2010). Using acoustic rhinometry, we found the mean minimal cross section area to be significantly smaller in the OSA group compared to the control group. Specifically, we found decreases in size of approx. 10-20% in the nasal valve/head of inferior turbinate regions but these could not be localized precisely since acoustic rhinometry does not provide specific shape information. On the other hand, CBCT scans can be used to measure the minimum inferior nasal concha distance from the nasal septum on both the right and left sides of the nasal cavity (Singh and Liao, 2019), as well as surface area measurements of posterior nasal apertures at level of posterior nasal spine in the coronal plane in both the axial and coronal planes (Singh and Kim, 2019). In addition, much qualitative information on the nasal architecture can be obtained. Historically, clinicians have observed septal deviation and correlated this with impairment of nasal function. While septal deviation is undoubtedly important to note, further diagnostic information can be gained from the amount of available functional space. In other words, even in the presence of septal deviation, if there is sufficient space between the nasal concha and the nasal septum, nasal function may not be affected significantly. Conversely, if a deviated septum causes an obstruction of the nasal airway, then this deformity needs to be addressed to permit laminar airflow through the nose for breathing, as well as turbulent airflow upward toward the cribriform plate of the ethmoid bone in the roof of the nose for olfaction. Other qualitative factors may also perturbate nasal airflow. Singh and Chandrasekhar (2009) discuss the physics of laminar flow whereby Poiseuille's equation determines that the resistance to flow is inversely

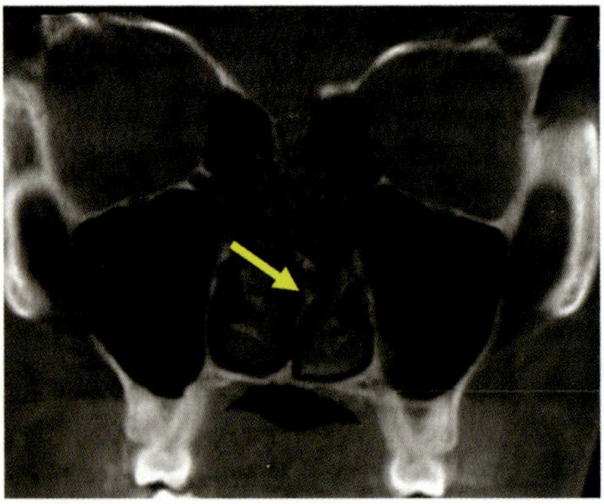

Figure 55a: Coronal slice from a CBCT scan showing septal spur formation, which can impede nasal airflow.

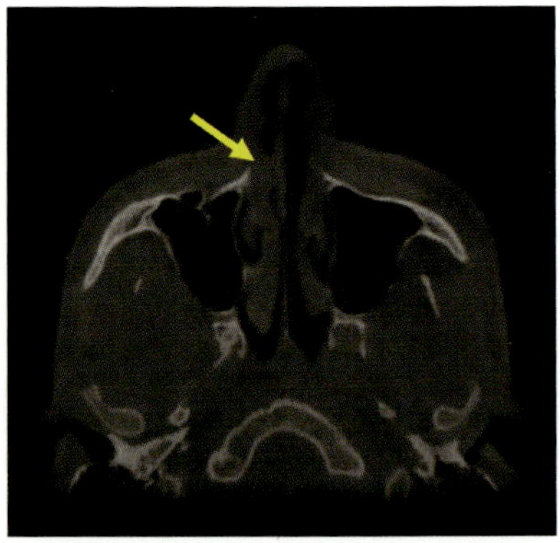

Figure 55b: Axial view from a CBCT scan showing a septal spur that is in continuity with the inferior nasal concha.

proportional to the radius of the tube to the fourth power (see Chapter 3). This means that even a small decrease (or increase) in the distance from the nasal septum to the (inferior) nasal concha can dramatically affect the quality of breathing. Indeed, the presence of a septal spur (Fig. 55a) where a nasal concha is in direct continuity with the nasal septum (Fig. 55b) ought to be surgically addressed. Recalling that the structure of the human nose can be understood as a 3 x 3 matrix, the soft tissues nose, which is mostly the nares and nasal valves; the cartilaginous nose, which is formed from the alar and septal cartilages; and the bony nose, which consists of the nasal bones and conchae/turbinates, all need to be assessed in the anterior, middle, and posterior regions of the nose. Perhaps the most important aspect is to ask the question: Is there sufficient functional space?

Starting at the front of the nose, alar cartilage collapse can impede nasal breathing. In the middle of the nose, hypertrophy of the nasal mucosa, which is the soft erectile tissue covering the conchae/turbinates can cause nasal obstruction and precipitate mouth-breathing. Similarly, insufficient space at the bony posterior nasal apertures (choanae) can impede nasal airflow at the back of the nose. In rare cases, a congenital condition, called choanal atresia, can cause a narrowing of the back of the nasal cavity that makes nasal breathing difficult. Far more commonly, adenoidal hypertrophy in children (Fig. 25b) impedes airflow at the posterior nasal apertures and needs to be addressed either directly through adenoidectomy (with or without tonsillectomy) or indirectly through biomimetic oral appliance therapy. Singh *et al.* (2016) used a biomimetic oral device that had not previously been deployed as an adjunctive treatment and reported some success in a chronic case of pediatric rhinosinusitis using this novel approach. In this non-surgical approach, it is speculated that nitric oxide (NO) somehow induces atrophy of the hypertrophied adenoids.

It well known that the paranasal air sinuses communicate with the nasal cavity through various ostia. Recently, it has been reported that the sinuses are lined by epithelial pneumocytes, and their function is to produce nitric oxide (NO) since paranasal sinus pneumocytes express NO synthase that generates NO (Lundberg, 2008). Nitric oxide has many beneficial properties, producing vasodilation through its action of smooth muscle relaxation. In addition, NO is known to be anti-bacterial, anti-fungal, and anti-viral, and it also stimulates mucociliary activity within the paranasal sinuses. Thus, the maxillary sinus produces and stores high concentrations of NO, while being protected from contamination by inspired environmental air since the structure of the nasomaxillary complex, specifically the uncinate process/infundibulum, effectively isolates the maxillary sinus from inspired contaminants during nasal airflow. In fact, Saunders *et al.* (1998) reported that patients with rhinosinusitis are more likely to develop it on the side with a more laterally positioned uncinate process. It is also thought that NO is inhaled during inspiration and on reaching the pulmonary alveoli in a more diluted form, it enhances oxygen uptake via local vasodilation. But, the developmental process of pneumatization and midfacial development remain incompletely understood.

Singh *et al.* (2000) proposed a spheno-ethmoidal model of midfacial retrognathia. We suggested that deficient cartilaginous proliferation in the anterior cranial base may be associated with inadequate anterior translation of the midfacial complex, resulting in Class III malocclusions. In that study, we compared Asian-Korean and Caucasian-American children using graphical analysis. Pseudo-color-coded finite-element scaling analysis (FESA) indicated that increases in size were present in the posterior palatal regions in the Caucasians, while the Korean anterior nasal spine regions were generally smaller. This change in morphology could affect the upper airway, which is partially located posterior to the nasopalatal complex. Therefore, various nasopalatal airway parameters need to be assessed, including: the retropalatal antero-posterior airway distance; the length of the soft palate; the medio-lateral retropalatal width; and the retropalatal airway area in the axial plane at the same level. Indeed, some are of the opinion that an anatomically narrow upper airway, which is highly likely to collapse, is one of the main causes of OSA (Carberry *et al.*, 2016). Despite this assertion, the normal limits of these parameters are still to be decided upon, but for practical purposes a minimal retropalatal A-P distance of < 10mm in the sagittal plane is regarded as being decreased. On the other hand, a soft palate length when measured from the posterior nasal spine to the tip of the uvula ought not exceed 30-35mm to be within normal limits (WNL); thus, a measurement of > 35mm represents an elongated soft palate. A minimum medio-lateral retropalatal width of < 25mm is considered to be decreased and ought to be > 25mm to be WNL. This width measurement is typically associated with a minimum retropalatal area of > 120mm^2, which is WNL whereas a retropalatal area of < 120mm^2 is less than expected and may contribute to either increased upper airway resistance or airway obstruction if the critical collapsing pressure (Pcrit) is achieved during sleep. Interestingly, biomimetic oral appliance therapy appears to target these areas non-surgically during treatment and provides a promising approach to upper airway issues, such as OSA (Singh and Liao, 2019; Singh and Kim, 2019).

In adults that have been diagnosed with OSA but are refractory to CPAP (continuous positive air pressure) or surgery, mandibular advancement devices (MADs) are currently preferred. There is a plethora of MADs that are currently used for the management of mild to moderate obstructive sleep

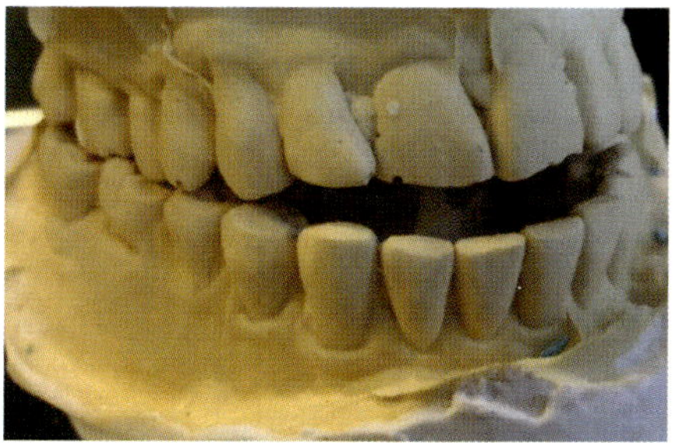

Figure 56a: Study models of a patient after long-term MAD use showing anterior open bite formation.

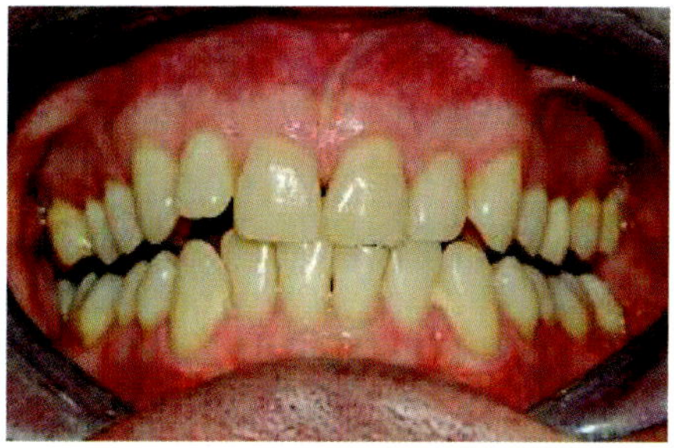

Figure 56b: Intra-oral photograph of a patient after long-term MAD use showing bilateral posterior open bite.

apnea in adults. Virtually all of these MADs have the sole purpose of holding the mandible forward during sleep to prevent upper airway collapse. However, numerous side effects (Fig. 56) have been reported with MADs, but the major issues are that these devices represent a lifetime of wear and the underlying condition can worsen with long-term use (Marklund, 2016). In addition, some patients of Asian/African ethnicities with a short cranial base/prognathic mandibular phenotype are at risk of developing an unfavorable facial profile and worsening malocclusion if treated for OSA with MADs. In view of these deficiencies, biomimetic oral appliance therapy might be considered since it differs from MADs as it aims to mimic natural craniofacial growth and development, and targets the site and severity of the obstruction. In view of this requirement, it's important to assess the following parameters on a pre-treatment CBCT scan of a potential patient: the minimum A-P retroglossal airway distance; the minimum medio-lateral retroglossal airway width; the minimum retroglossal airway area in the axial plane at the same level, and the gonial angle. In our experience over several years, a minimum A-P retroglossal distance of 11mm is required in females, and a minimum of 13mm is required in males. Classically, obstruction in this region is caused by the tongue during sleep, and an indication of this may be gleaned from the position of the hyoid bone. In these types of cases, the requirement of stabilizing the mandibular position during sleep must be addressed, if obstruction by the tongue is to be avoided.

Note that in patients that respond well, mandibular advancement is thought to increase the minimum medio-lateral retroglossal width (Sutherland and Cistulli, 2011). Thus, a medio-lateral retroglossal width of > 25mm is considered to be WNL. This width measurement likely produces a minimum retroglossal area (in the axial plane at the same level as above) of > 180mm^2, which is considered as WNL. Note that simply protruding the mandible anteriorly can prove to be ineffectual (Sutherland and Cistulli, 2011) since the muscle fibers of the pharyngeal constrictors vary in their behavior (Witzel and Posnick, 1989). Therefore, each case needs to be individually assessed, including the gonial angle. This angle is formed by three landmarks on the mandibular profile (condylion-gonion-pogonion) and it indicates the morphology of the mandible. In cases where the gonial angle is high (> 124°), the likelihood of precipitating an anterior open bite with long-term MAD use is increased significantly (Fig. 56a). Thus, in addition to assessing the mandibular phenotype prior to treatment, it is wise to survey tomographs of the temporo-mandibular joints (TMJs). In this survey the position and condition of the condyles with respect to the glenoid fossae are assessed. For example, the condyles might be postero-superiorly positioned in the glenoid fossae, which is often diagnostic of mandibular retrognathism. However, in addition to positional information, the condylar heads may show pathologic changes, such as flattening, bending, or 'beaking' with epiphyte formation on one or both sides. These features represent undiagnosed temporo-mandibular dysfunction (TMD), which may be exacerbated during mandibular advancement therapy; thus, patients need to be informed of these types of findings prior to proceeding with any appliance therapy. Once the TMJ assessment has been completed, it's important to ask the question: Which is the next bone below the mandible?

Despite flaws, 2D cephalographs do have some clinical utility since they are a form of lateral radiography. For example, the gonial angle is measured from a lateral radiograph even though the landmarks condylion and gonion do not lie in the mid-sagittal plane, unlike pogonion. Chiropractors, physical therapists, and osteopaths, etc. have also used these plane films to assess the positioning of the cervical vertebrae. This assessment is vital in craniofacial diagnosis and treatment planning since the cervical vertebrae define the posterior boundary of the upper airway (posterior pharyngeal wall; Fig. 57).

In Fig. 57, the ideal cervical spine posture and angulation are illustrated. However, more often than not, craniocervical relationships are compromised (Fig. 58) through compensatory mechanisms. So, where does (descending)

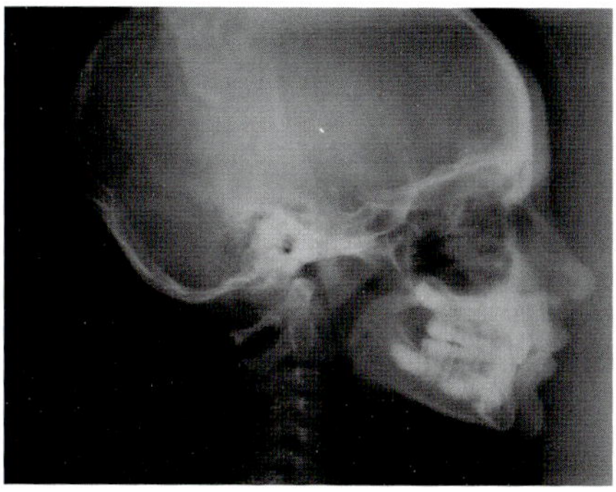

Figure 57a: Lateral cephalography of a pediatric patient showing the posterior boundary of the upper airway.

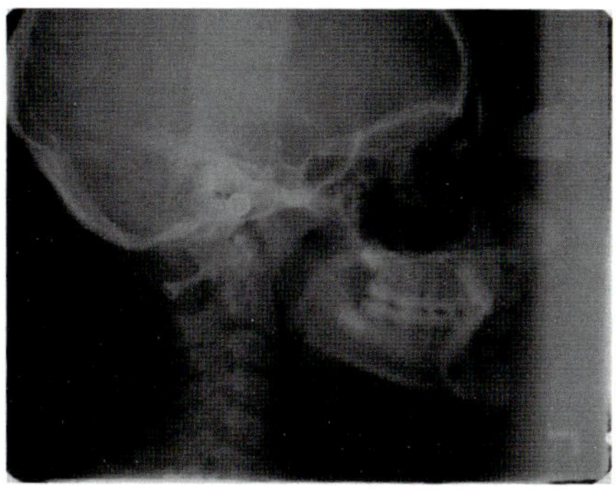

Figure 57b: Lateral cephalography of an adult patient showing the position of C1 relative to the condyle. Courtesy: Dr David Arnold

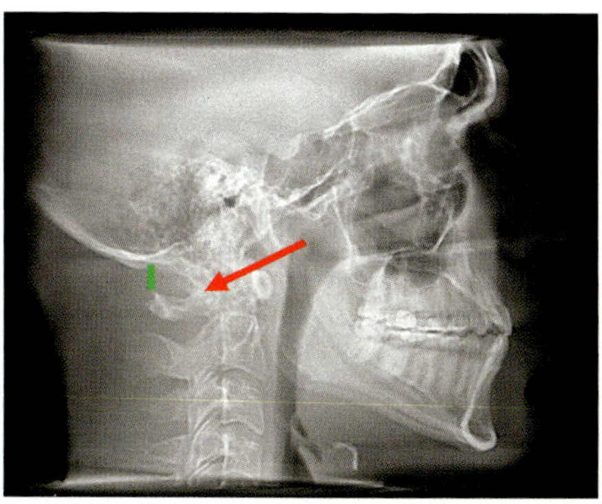

Figure 58a: Lateral cephalography of an adult patient showing double posterior boundary of C1 (red arrow).

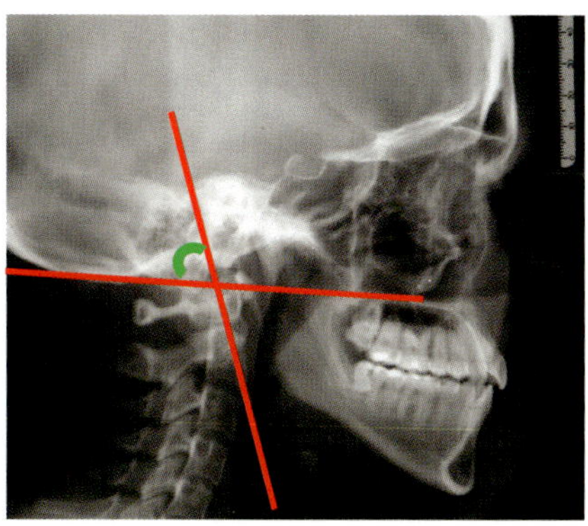

Figure 58b: Lateral cephalography of an adult patient showing the measurement of the cranio-vertebral angle.

developmental compensation meet (ascending) postural compensation? On the lateral radiograph, the next bone below the condyle of the mandible is C1 (the first cervical vertebrae, not the hyoid bone). A diagnostic feature that is often observed is a double posterior arch of the atlas (Fig. 58a). This feature usually suggests cervical subluxation, which means that the cervical vertebrae are not well-aligned. Following a biomimetic approach to enhance functional spaces, such as the upper airway, it's important to address causes from a general to specific perspective. In other words, in terms of the PACE treatment protocol, **it's best to first align the body (including the cervical vertebrae), then align the jaws, and finally align the teeth in that sequence to enhance the functional space of the upper airway**. Thus, in our preferred diagnostic protocol, the lateral cephalometric view is used to measure the occipito-atlas distance. This linear distance between the lowest point of the occipital bone (opisthion) and the highest point on the posterior arch of C1 gives an indication of head posture. As the occipito-atlas distance (green line in Fig 58a) becomes smaller, the head is rotated more posteriorly, likely in an attempt to maintain upper airway patency. In fact, in some chronic cases, occipital 'lipping' can be detected as the insertion of trapezius in the occipital bone hypertrophies with persistent overuse.

But, head rotation for upper airway patency competes with another biologic phenomenon, horizontal gaze. Human cephalization appears to follow the predator blueprint. Predators need to be able to catch prey and need to be able to estimate distances precisely. For this purpose, the eyes are located at the front of the face, so they have binocular/stereoscopic vision to judge their attack accurately. Binocular vision produces visual perceptual skills, such that two separate images from two eyes are successfully combined into one image in the brain using binocular depth perception and stereopsis (stereoscopic vision). However, in the case of head rotation for upper airway patency, horizontal gaze would be lost, and postural compensation ensues, which is known as 'forward head posture'. Therefore, individuals with a forward head posture (Fig. 44) are likely to have a compromise of their upper airway, and on the lateral radiograph a double posterior arch of the atlas is often discernible (Fig. 58a) with a reduced craniovertebral angle (Fig. 58b). The craniovertebral angle is measured by: a plane passing through the posterior nasal spine (PNS) and opisthion (the midpoint of the posterior margin of the foramen magnum); and the odontoid plane, passing through the superior-most point of the dens and the antero-inferior point of the body of the axis (C2) vertebra (Fig. 58b). In addition, while a forward head posture opens the upper airway it also increases the spinal 'moment arm', which is the perpendicular distance from a pivot to a point undergoing torque. Therefore, the head becomes relatively heavier, increasing in weight from about 5kg (approx. 12lbs) in the erect posture to some 19kg (approx. 42lbs) in a chronic forward head posture. Therefore, this forward head posture, while opening the upper airway, increases the loading on the anterior segments of the spine and intervertebral disks. It also compresses the thoracic cavity and causes the spine to deviate from the optimal sagittal posture, which subsequently undergoes pathological, epigenetic remodeling (neuro-escalator model; Burwell *et al.*, 2008). Thus, patients can present to a physician with back pain, shoulder pain, neck pain, wrist pain, etc., while being unaware that upper airway compromise may be exacerbating a bulging or slipped disk, which is compressing a nerve or nerve root to cause referred pain. Therefore, an initial assessment of cervical alignment on a lateral radiographic view is mandatory.

Moya *et al.* (1994) measured various cervical parameters and studied vertebral alignment to determine the effect of an occlusal splint on craniocervical relationships. The occipito-atlas distance is measured from the base of the occipital bone (opisthion) to the postero-superior point of C1 (Fig. 58a; green line) and a value of around approx. 10mm is considered to be within normal limits. Distances < 4mm represent posterior rotation of the head, while distances > 10mm represent anterior rotation of the head. To assess head rotation, the cranio-cervical angle is measured, using a plane formed by opisthion and the posterior nasal spine, and the odontoid plane, which starts at the apex of the odontoid process of C2 to the antero-inferior point of the body of C2 (Fig. 58b). The cranio-cervical angle is thus used to assess the antero-posterior position of the cranium relative to the cervical spine. Generally speaking, its value varies between approx. 96° and 106°. Angles $< 96°$ represent posterior extension of the head, while angles $> 106°$ represent anterior flexion of the head. Qualitative assessment of cervical posture can also be made by classifying deviations from the normal lordotic posture. In this way, some cervical vertebrae appear to be hypolordotic (reduced lordosis). If this feature is intensified, the cervical vertebrae appear to be straight and sometimes so straight that they are referred to as a 'military neck'. As the cervical vertebrae lose their normal posture even further, they appear to be kyphotic, so that the normal lordotic posture is reversed. Apart from sagittal deviations, transverse changes in the normal lordotic posture of the spine are referred to as scoliosis. It is also important to avoid asymmetric spinal alignment through asymmetric occlusal loading (Fonder, 1980; 1988), such as that associated with appliances that incorporate an asymmetric, unilateral bite block.

In children, in the lateral cephalometric view, cervical maturation is also assessed in an effort to predict the mandibular growth spurt. According to the cranio-caudal gradient of growth and development, the cranial base undergoes rapid growth first (at about 3–5yrs), followed by the midface (at about 8–10yrs), followed by the mandible (at about 11–13yrs). More detailed information about the developmental status of the mandible can be gleaned from the cervical vertebrae in terms of their morphology. Specifically, Bench (1963) was the first to note the relationship between cervical vertebrae growth and craniofacial growth, while Lamparski (1972) classified cervical vertebrae morphology and mandibular maturation. Later, Román *et al.* (2002) determined that the concavity of the lower border of the cervical vertebra body is best able to estimate the stage of maturation of the individual. These findings were repeated by Baccetti *et al.* (2005) who assessed cervical vertebrae maturation by looking at the lower borders of C2-C3 on cephalographs and deciding if they are flat or concave. A concave appearance of the lower borders of C2 and C3 suggests that peak mandibular growth is likely occurring. On the other hand, by deciding if the vertebral body is trapezoidal or rectangular in shape, it can be surmised that mandibular growth has likely ceased if at least one of the bodies of C3 and C4 is square/vertical-rectangular in shape. But, in addition to mandibular maturation, it is also important to note that the cervical vertebrae lie directly behind the posterior pharyngeal wall and, as such, they define the posterior boundary of the upper airway (Fig. 57 and Fig. 58), which is best assessed from 3D CBCT scans. Since there is no current consensus, in our preferred PACE protocol, the 3D upper airway volume is calculated from the posterior nasal spine to the inferior border of C3/hyoid bone in the vertical axis. The volumetric value varies depending on several factors, such as patient positioning during imaging and the location of certain structures, such as the mandible and tongue. In any case, an upper airway volumetric reconstruction of approx. 15-25cm^3 is considered to be WNL for most adults. The algorithms used in commercial software for 3D airway rendering are proprietary in some cases. However, we were one of the first groups to publish an edge detection algorithm to calculate the volume of the upper airway from 3D CBCT scans (Celenk *et al.*, 2010). These data can be used in the clinical evaluation of a patient who has a concern with sleep disordered breathing, in conjunction with a functional, overnight sleep study to evaluate the site(s) and severity of the obstruction(s). If it's found that a subject is suitable for oral appliance therapy, then customization of the design of these devices will be largely determined on the study models.

Study models

Once the facial photographs, intra-oral photographs and 3D CBCT scans have been assessed, a final few structural items need to be evaluated prior to appliance design on the study models. One of these items is the panoramic/panoral radiograph, which can be obtained from the 3D CBCT scan data. This view is a useful survey of the upper and lower dentitions, and it can help identify features that are not readily viewed in the other media, such as unerupted, missing, or partially erupted teeth and maxillary sinus health, etc. The results of orthopantomography can be augmented by carefully inspecting the upper study model for further diagnostic features. One of the first things to look at is the archform, and simply classify it. It can be described as being tapered, square or 'reduced', which means that (unhealthy or healthy) permanent teeth, such as premolars or third molars, were removed, likely for caries or orthodontic reasons (Fig. 59a). In addition, other diagnostic features that might be seen on the upper study model are torus palatinus and/or buccal exostoses. It is commonly presumed that a palatal torus is of little consequence, but we will return to this topic in further detail later in this book. Meantime, other dental features can be identified such as anterior crowding. 'Crowding' is a historical orthodontic term used to describe the crowns of teeth that are misaligned. In fact, crowding is one sign of overall craniofacial disharmony associated with developmental compensation.

Due to an incomplete appreciation perhaps, healthy teeth are often extracted in cases showing crowding to 'create space' for the remaining ones. This is a fallacy since it is now known that space cannot be created, except at the edge of an expanding universe, according to current thought in astrophysics. Instead, space can simply be displaced, as described by

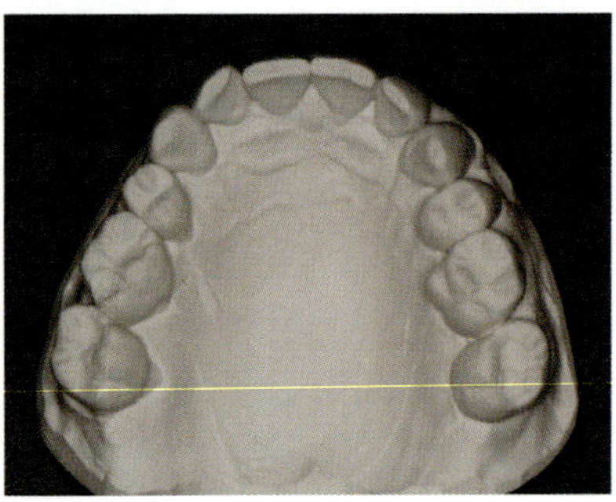

Figure 59a: Upper study model of an adult showing 'reduced' archform with anterior crowding/wear facets and missing first premolars and third molars. Courtesy: Dr Shamshudin Kherani

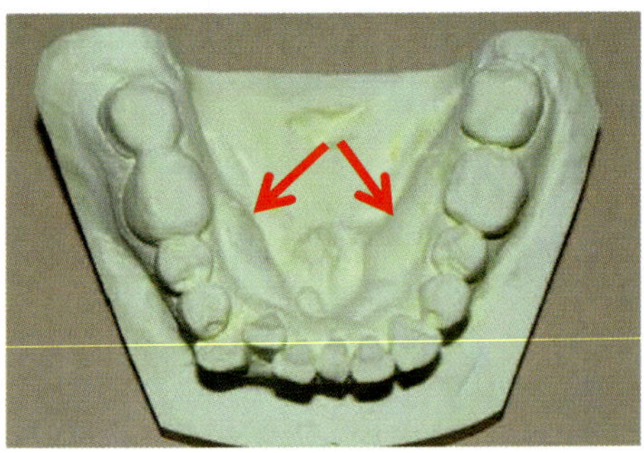

Figure 59b: Lower study model of an adult patient showing 'square' archform with extensive mandibular tori (red arrows) and severe anterior crowding. Courtesy: Dr Han

the Archimedes principle. More specifically, in a crowded arch there is a lack of functional space. This concept is encapsulated by the spatial matrix hypothesis (Singh, 2004; 2007; Singh and Krumholtz, 2009). During craniofacial growth, the spatial and functional alignment of skeletal elements is maintained through remodeling of bony surfaces (including the periodontium) to permit function. In other words, the maxilla and mandible are growing/developing and the 32 genetically determined crowns of the teeth will erupt into symmetric occlusion in an orderly fashion if gene-environmental interactions permit. This temporo-spatial pattern represents the genetic blueprint that has evolved over millennia to promote human survivability, by facilitating chewing, swallowing, speech, breathing, sleeping, etc. However, this temporo-spatial patterning is now often disrupted by environmentally induced changes, e.g. lack of breast-feeding, bottle-feeding, pacifier use, digit-sucking, soft/processed foods, nasal allergies, tooth extraction, etc. These environmental factors in turn produce epigenetic changes in the early morphologic relationship, e.g. crowding, increased overbite, increased overjet, etc., and these new solutions (malocclusions) represent phenotypic variation. In other words, a child may have inherited a (skeletal) Class I phenotype but developmental compensation means that the child reports to the dental clinic with, say, a Class II malocclusion, a 'gummy smile', or an anterior open bite, etc. Note that the child still has the genetic potential of achieving a Class I occlusion with 32 teeth fully erupted and in occlusion if the correct growth guidance is initiated early enough and complied with. Thus, crowding is a new, clinical solution, representing a departure from the genetically encoded developmental body plan, which is achieved through temporo-spatial patterning. Essentially, temporo-spatial patterning means that certain genes are expressed at specific locations at various times. For example, the genes needed to make enamel (matrix) for a permanent maxillary central incisor crown are expressed close to the midline of the maxilla at around 3 months postnatally. On the other hand, the enamel for the crowns of the third molars calcifies at about 8 years of age. Thus, if the third molars are to be accommodated, sufficient bone development needs to be attained by the age of, say, 9 years if the crowns of these (important) teeth are not to be displaced and impacted due to a lack of space, which is in fact, bone volume. More often than not, in modern societies, developmental compensations occur to permit compromised function. In other words, a baby may have deformational plagiocephaly but the bald patch on the occiput goes unnoticed or is ignored; the child is able to chew but has a malocclusion and is advised to wait for orthodontic treatment till 'growth has ceased'; the young adult has impacted wisdom teeth and may develop TMD as she gets older; the older adult develops OSA and the mandibular tori (Fig. 59b) remain undiagnosed. These are examples of developmental compensation — so what can be done at these various stages of life? Since the genes we inherited and are born with are kept for life, decompensation is required through treatment with appropriate spatial signaling using the PACE protocol since we retain our genetic potential to a large extent (but not completely) throughout life. In other words, as long as there is a viable population of stem cells, it's possible to re-establish the genomic pattern formation, at least in part, for enhanced or optimal form and function even in adult life, to an extent to be therapeutically worthwhile. Spatial signaling is a fundamental feature of human existence. In a unique study, Garrett-Bakelman et al. (2019) reported that an astronaut who came back to earth after a year on the International Space Station experienced physical changes such as changes in BMI, carotid artery and ocular structure, as well as genetic alterations, including telomere elongation, genomic instability and DNA methylation changes, compared to his identical twin brother who remained on earth during that time. In fact, it is thought that cells in the human body know where they are located in space (directly or indirectly) through proprioceptive capability, and cell-cell communications lead to various developmental consequences based on spatial signaling. For example, in one study (Singh *et al.*, 1998), the hypothesis that altered expression of extracellular matrix molecules (such as tenascin-C, TN) is associated with altered craniofacial morphology (such as cleft palate) was tested in mice. It was found that in normal mice, TN dissipated beneath the oral membrane but, in mice with a genetic mutation for cleft palate, TN remained beneath the oral membrane. It was concluded that differences in TN expression are associated with cleft palate formation in mice. In the simplified clinical analogy of malocclusion, the positions of the teeth change (for example, the angle of upper central incisor to the cranial base plane becomes retroclined), and we recognize this as crowding on the upper study model, which is one sign of a malocclusion.

The changes in tooth alignment in the upper arch do not occur in isolation. First, there is the cranio-caudal gradient of development that dictates that the maxilla will develop/mature ahead of the mandible. In addition, the body essentially consists of a series of functional spaces, and if these are deficient, there will be consequences. For example, blood pressure is to a large extent determined by the caliber of blood vessels. A control system of vasoconstriction and vasodilation exists to keep blood pressure in homeostasis. Similarly, neurologic control is through a system of nerve endings or synapses. These small gaps of 9nm permit neurotransmitters to traverse the space and cause post-synaptic excitation to enable nerve pulses to pass along the nerve fiber. Now, if the upper incisors are retroclined, the lower incisors will likely follow suite, since the envelope of mandibular motion is, at least in part, determined by the position of the maxilla in space. This encroachment of mandibular functional space may result in the posterior displacement of the mandible, including the condyles. In addition, if the mandible is retrognathic in order to articulate with the maxillary dentition, then the tongue will likely follow the retrusive direction and will precipitate upper airway obstruction, especially if the upper incisors are limiting its functional space. In fact, the lower arch can sometimes 'magnify' or exaggerate the changes in the upper arch. Thus, the lower arch may be tapered but it may show more severe anterior crowding than the upper arch (Fig. 50a and Fig. 50b). In this case, when the upper and lower arches are in articulation, there will likely be an increased overbite and decreased overjet (Class II malocclusion). In addition, it's likely that the lower midline will be displaced to either the right or left side by a few millimeters. Thus, the simple act of retroclining the upper central incisors, for example by bottle-feeding or pacifier use, can set off a domino effect of unwanted changes. If the tongue is also displaced by bottle-feeding or pacifier use into the floor of the mouth, then the vault of the palate will be unsupported and, given the downward and forward developmental gradient of facial development, a high-arched, narrow palate may be observable. In this case, it's likely that even if the first molars are in a Class I relationship, the second molars might be more buccally-positioned (Fig. 54), since the second maxillary molars are, to some extent, guided by the palatine bone during eruption. Therefore, in terms of treatment planning, addressing the underlying etiology of the condition diagnosed becomes key in craniofacial correction.

Diagnostic impression

After reviewing the data collected, a comprehensive working diagnosis is required. In order to achieve this, three areas of concern need to be borne in mind to thoroughly appreciate the sorts of corrections needed, and how to communicate these to fellow professionals. One component when formulating a comprehensive working diagnosis is to classify the malocclusion. Here, we realize that the historic norms, such as Angle's classification, appear to be deficient. For example, in Angle's classification there is no mention of anterior or posterior crossbite, which is more commonly seen these days compared to, say, 100 years ago when Angle's classification was published (Angle, 1907). According to Corruccini *et al.* (1985), the interaction between genetic and environmental factors leads to a greater degree of genetic variance following our environmental transition from an ancestral to an urban lifestyle. This essentially means that if canalizing environmental factors are not sufficiently suppressed, the interaction with altered environmental factors results in a greater amount of phenotypic variation. For example, in one study, Lopez del Valle *et al.* (2006) found that about 6% of 5yr-old Puerto Rican children exhibited anterior open bite. Thus, the developmental compensations that result in a particular malocclusion need to be identified and addressed. In addition, however, malocclusions don't exist in isolation and there may be other differential diagnoses, e.g. craniofacial obesity, TMD, mandibular tori, etc. Therefore, in the second component of the diagnosis it is important to suspect any other co-morbidity, e.g. bruxism, TMJ issues, etc. when formulating a comprehensive working diagnosis. Furthermore, TMJ dysfunction shows an overlap with airway, breathing, and sleep issues. Shapira (2013) considers that TMJ issues are often accompanied by poor sleep quality, while Talley (2019) suggests that TMJ and OSA are co-morbidities. Earlier, Singh and Olmos (2007) investigated upper airway behavior in patients with TMD. When the residual volume of the upper airway after forcible expiration was compared to the residual volume with a phonetic bite registration, a 15% increase was found. These findings suggested that patients diagnosed with TMD show upper airway collapse, and that the use of an oral device constructed to a phonetic bite registration may be useful in preventing it. Therefore, in the third component of the diagnosis it's important to suspect any upper airway co-morbidities. In summary, when formulating a working diagnosis, each of the four tissue components of the craniofacial system needs to be addressed, by simply asking the questions: What are the dental tissues (teeth) doing? What are the (bony) hard tissues doing? What are the soft tissues doing? And, what is the upper airway doing? By systematically visiting each of these areas of concern, a 3–4-part working diagnosis can often be reached, such as "Class II malocclusion with sleep bruxism. Suspect undiagnosed TMD/SDB". This broad statement provides insight into possible treatment objectives for optimal patient management.

Treatment objectives

Desired treatment objectives often follow a comprehensive working diagnosis. These objectives together address craniofacial correction with it four groups of target tissues. In other words:

- Correct the skeletal tissues, e.g. reposition the mandible, widen the maxilla, and realign the cervical vertebrae
- Correct the craniofacial soft tissues (e.g. tongue, frenae, lips, soft palate, nasal symmetry, etc.)

- Correct the functional spaces (e.g. upper airway, TMJ spaces, etc.)
- Correct the dental tissues, e.g. an increased overbite (malocclusion)

Note that the above summary is not a linear sequence of events. There is both overlap and simultaneous correction. For example, in a case with an increased overjet, repositioning the mandible anteriorly to normalize the incisor relationship will likely address nocturnal upper airway obstruction simultaneously. Generally speaking, the dental tissues/teeth are the last tissues to be corrected, using limited orthodontic treatments if indicated. As an analogy, when building a house, the foundations are laid first and then the walls/roof are constructed prior to the interior design. In this analogy, the teeth represent the interior design, so orthodontic finishing (Fig. 97) is reserved as the last option, if needed. Thus, for a specific case, the treatment objectives may include improving the overjet and overbite to WNL and/or correcting an anterior/posterior crossbite. There may be a need to resolve upper anterior crowding and increasing the transpalatal bone width to accommodate the tongue within the palate. In other cases, there may be a requirement to re-position the mandible antero-inferiorly in the midline to address sleep disordered breathing, perhaps secondary to mandibular retrognathia. If the mandible is either retrognathic and/or micrognathic, there is likely to be anterior crowding which will need to be resolved, along with the need to correct a midline discrepancy most likely. In so doing, another objective of improving the upper airway parameters might be achieved, especially if OSA was diagnosed because the tongue was positioned low in the floor of the mouth, occupying the oropharynx instead of being in contact with palate. These issues can be addressed by formulating a multi-disciplinary treatment plan.

Treatment plan

Once a list of treatment objectives has been compiled, a suggested (multi-disciplinary/inter-disciplinary) treatment plan can be formulated. Since a 3D CBCT scan has likely been taken, it's good clinical practice to have this read by a radiologist for a report. This report differs from the structural assessment detailed above. The radiologist's report is necessary to exclude any pathologic incidental findings, including any features that might interfere with efficient breathing. For example, septal deviation or, perhaps more importantly, septal spur formation (Fig. 55a) is sometimes discernible. This feature might impede nasal airflow and midfacial development since the midline structures of the nose are directly attached to the middle and/or inferior conchae (Fig. 55b). In these cases, an ENT consultation with an otolaryngologist or rhinologist might be recommended. Similarly, nasal and/or maxillary air sinus congestion, if identified, often calls for an ENT consult. In rare cases, pineal gland calcification is sometimes encountered on CBCT scans in adults. More commonly, the status of the TMJs can be readily reviewed on a CBCT scan. From a structural point of view, one is concerned with the positioning of the condylar head within the glenoid fossae. In the radiologic assessment, the health of the TMJs in terms of resorption, flattening, bending, 'beaking'/epiphyte formation needs to be assessed to exclude a pre-existing TMJ condition, such as anterior disk displacement with or without reduction prior to initiating any oral appliance therapy.

The 3D CBCT scan might also indicate regions where the upper airway is constricted. These areas may be located near the middle of the nasal cavity or the posterior nasal apertures. Other areas that might be affected include the retropalatal and retroglossal areas in both the sagittal and transverse axes, or a combination of any of these regions. If upper airway collapse is suspected or found, an overnight sleep study may be indicated. In these cases, a sleep questionnaire ought to be first completed, and the opinion of a sleep physician should be sought. In terms of diagnosing a sleep breathing disorder, overnight polysomnography (PSG) in a sleep laboratory can be prescribed by a physician or a home sleep apnea test (HSAT) can be suggested if OSA is suspected. There is much debate on the pros and cons of HSATs versus PSGs. In 2015, the International Classification of Sleep Disorders, Second Edition (ICSD-2) classified 96 sleep disorders. Currently, there are about 67 known sleep disorders (ICD-10).

Of these, only sleep disordered breathing (SDB) lies within the remit of a dental professional. In 2017, the American Dental Association (ADA, 2017) adopted a policy on the role of general dentists in the treatment of sleep-breathing disorders. It emphasized that general dentists should screen for sleep disordered breathing and that dentists should be able to provide oral appliance therapy only after diagnosis by a physician. In turn, the range of sleep-related breathing disorders varies from upper airway resistance syndrome (UARS) and primary snoring to mild-, moderate- and severe-obstructive sleep apnea (OSA). Current practice parameters suggest that oral appliance therapy can be considered as the first line of treatment for mild-moderate OSA (ADA, 2017). Given the prevalence of this specific condition, widespread screening/testing with HSATs by dentists appears to be a feasible approach. Regardless, the HSAT needs to be interpreted by a sleep physician prior to initiating any therapy. However, one of the issues with HSATs is that the algorithms deployed can under-estimate the severity of the condition, so the results from HSATs need to be viewed with some caution. Specifically, a negative result for pediatric OSA with an HSAT cannot be relied upon, and the sleep study may need to be repeated as an in-lab PSG to exclude pediatric OSA in the presence of clinical symptoms. Note that attention deficit hyperactivity disorder (ADHD) may masquerade as pediatric OSA and vice versa; a theme we will return to later in this book. In general terms, therefore, close collaboration with a sleep physician should be an integral part of treatment planning in patients that have airway, breathing or sleep issues.

Prior to any oral appliance therapy, in the PACE protocol, it is suggested that the opinion of a chiropractor (such as an atlas-orthogonist), an osteopath, or a physical therapist should be sought, especially if cervical subluxation is suspected. Recall that rotation of the head allied with asymmetry of the shoulders might be detected in the frontal photograph (Fig. 40). Furthermore, inspection of the cervical vertebrae on the lateral radiograph might demonstrate misalignment, especially of the first cervical vertebrae (Fig. 58). In these cases, collaboration with a chiropractor or similar professional can help to improve alignment of the patient's body, representing postural decompensation. Next, a dentist can align the jaws, using an appropriate bite registration, such as the phonetic bite (Singh and Olmos, 2007) or a neuromuscular bite registration (Singh *et al.*, 2014; Singh *et al.*, 2016). Finally, the dentist/orthodontist can align the teeth, using conventional fixed appliances or clear tray systems. Following this 'general to specific' sequence appears to enhance the functional space available for the upper airway. The reason for this sequence is based on the cranio-caudal gradient. Going from top down, the next bone below the mandible (condyle) is C1, not the hyoid bone (Fig. 57). It is known that the horizontal axis of growth rotation of the condyles is associated with C1 (Huggare, 1989). Thus, if the upper cervical vertebrae are misaligned/subluxated, it is impossible for the mandible to rotate freely and function optimally. Neuromuscular techniques, such as transcutaneous electrical nerve stimulation (TENS) involves the use of low-voltage electric currents to relax the muscles of mastication in order to achieve the physiologic rest position of the mandible (Cooper *et al.*, 1991). However, unless C1-C2 are well-aligned, the mandible will not be able to achieve its optimal position. In one study (Singh *et al.*, 2014), craniofacial improvements were enhanced using a combination of chiropractic adjustment and biomimetic oral appliance therapy. In fact, given the kinetic chain and the concept that the occlusion represents an end-point of the body with respect to the plantar surfaces of the feet (Chapter 4), equalization of leg length discrepancy was achieved using a combination of chiropractic adjustment and biomimetic oral appliance therapy (Chapman and Singh, 2013). Therefore, a biomimetic bite registration can be achieved using a chiropractic or physical adjustment prior to an appropriate bite registration and biomimetic oral appliance therapy in an effort to optimize the upper airway, since the posterior boundary of the upper airway is largely determined by cervical posture (Fig. 57).

Apart from structural alignment issues, soft tissue pressure can also cause upper airway collapse. In fact, in some mammals, such as the New Zealand Obese (NZO) mouse, the size of the airway is smaller because the pharyngeal fat pads, tongue volume, and soft palate volume are greater compared to lean control mice. Interestingly, these NZO mice appear to sleep in an upright posture, presumably to protect their upper airway from collapse during sleep (Brennick *et al.*, 2009). Earlier, Watanabe *et al.* (2002) had suggested that both craniofacial size and obesity can alter upper airway size. In the control subject, the craniofacial skeletal and soft tissues produce a proportionate upper airway size. However, in the non-obese case, bimaxillary underdevelopment can cause a relative increase in tissue pressure, leading to upper airway collapse. Similarly, craniofacial obesity can precipitate upper airway collapse and the risk of OSA by increasing soft tissue pressure (Banabilh *et al.*, 2009). In fact, in obese patients, fat is deposited within the tongue, which can exacerbate upper airway obstruction (Nashi *et al.*, 2007). Thus, as an integral part of patient care, nutritional counseling/dietary review is often suggested, and this includes screening for possible food allergies that may lead to nasal obstruction. Various professionals can provide dietary advice, and these individuals range from registered dietitians to naturopaths. Thus, an interdisciplinary approach is inclusive in its nature and may rely on behavior modification for a successful clinical outcome. Indeed, another significant component of the craniofacial soft tissues that may rely on behavior modification is the tongue. It is well-known that tongue position during sleep can be obstructive and precipitate apneas. Thus, in the multi-disciplinary approach to craniofacial correction, a review of the tongue for restriction/frenectomy is mandatory often in conjunction with oral myofunctional therapy.

During the screening process, tell-tale signs of tongue position can usually be readily observed. For example, simply asking the patient to open the mouth often leads to a habitual tongue posture. In this position, it is not uncommon for scalloping or indentations to be observed (Fig. 51a and Fig. 51b), leading to a crenated appearance of the tongue. Tomooka *et al.* (2017) showed that tongue-scalloping is associated with nocturnal intermittent hypoxia but not pathognomonic for SDB. Alternatively, the tongue may be fissured in appearance or asymmetric as the intrinsic muscles change the shape of the tongue to fit the available space, following the path of least resistance. In some cases, the anterior-most tip of the tongue can show mild inflammation in response to chronic friction against the (lower) anterior teeth. In these cases, it's imperative to increase the functional space required to accommodate the tongue in 3D space (Fig. 51c). Prior to any orthopedic/orthodontic therapy, however, the tongue needs to be further assessed by asking the question: Is the tongue restricted? To address this issue, the ventral surface of the tongue needs to be inspected. By asking the patient to raise the tongue to the roof of the mouth with the mouth wide open, a clear image of the ventral surface of the tongue can be gained (Fig. 23). Classic anatomy textbooks described the ventral surface of the tongue centuries ago. The lateral-most features are the bilateral fimbriated folds. These are also called the plica fimbriata, which represent a slight fold of the mucous membrane on the underside of the tongue. The free edge of the fimbriated fold typically exhibits a fringe-like appearance, which likely represents the apoptosis which occurred to free the ventral surface of the tongue from the floor of the mouth during development. Medial to the lingual veins is the midline lingual frenum, which can be long or short, thick, or thin, and blanched or not blanched when viewed with the mouth wide open (Fig. 23). Thus, a short, thick frenum, which is blanched, is likely characteristic of an increased risk of tongue-tie or ankyloglossia. In these cases, frenotomy or frenectomy might be indicated but before so doing, it is wise to implement oral myofunctional therapy for, say, 4 weeks prior to any surgery to prevent the frenum healing back in its original position. Post-tongue release, whether it was achieved by scalpel or laser, it's suggested that a further 8 weeks of oral myofunctional therapy be provided to ensure the tongue maintains its new position in light contact with the palate at rest, and not in the floor of the mouth. Note that the transpalatal bone width has to be sufficient to accommodate the tongue easily. Therefore, during treatment planning the need to realign/procline the anterior segment of the upper arch, allied with an increase in the upper intermolar bone width, needs to be considered to accommodate the tongue easily. By so doing, maintenance/stability is being in-built into the correction rather than delegated as an after-thought post-treatment. In fact, the notion of relapse is typically addressed by 'retention for life' using orthodontic retainers. This notion contrasts with the biomimetic approach adopted here. Orthodontic relapse likely represents a failure to address craniofacial homeostasis. The teeth might show an improved alignment but sometimes this is achieved at the cost of reduced functional spaces of the TMJs and/or upper airway. This scenario may result in disparate symptoms, such as tooth wear, OSA, headaches, etc. as the patient gets older. Since the ageing process is a natural component of the human lifespan, the alternative approach is to utilize the tongue as the 'pink retainer'. In other words, while it's known that a vertical drift of the face occurs with age, leading to lower incisor crowding, an active regimen of oral myofunctional therapy may permit retardation of the ageing process, at least to some extent. **This maintenance routine can be augmented by wearing a biomimetic device 'passively', say, 2–3 nights per week to retard or arrest the craniofacial ageing process**, which includes bone loss through osteoporosis and decreased facial muscle tone and volume. In that respect, the craniofacial region is no different from other musculo-skeletal systems in the rest of the body. For example, in the same way that regular exercise in a gym, perhaps with weights, is recommended to prevent premature ageing, **oral myofunctional therapy with occasional biomimetic oral appliance use may be beneficial to maintain enhanced craniofacial homeostasis in the longer term**.

Although emphasis has rightly been placed on the midfacial structures, such as the nasomaxillary complex, there needs to be re-coordination of the upper and lower arches. Part of this re-integration is, of course, the tongue since it is attached to the mandible while being in contact with the palate at rest. In contrast to the biomimetic approach adopted here, the sole premise of conventional oral appliance therapy in dental sleep medicine is anterior re-positioning of the mandible. That this is not attempted in isolation is warranted by the side-effects associated with this limited type of approach. There are numerous cases in the literature that witness the precipitation of anterior crossbite/Class III facial profile (Korngut, 2010), anterior open bite (Fig. 56a), or posterior open bite (Fig. 56b), sometimes with TMJ issues after long-term mandibular advancement device (MAD) use. Worse still, some data suggest that long-term MAD use is associated with worsening of the underlying condition. Marklund (2016) performed overnight sleep studies with and without a MAD in the mouth at the start of treatment and some 15 years later. For those cases that had been continuously treated with MADs, the severity of OSA increased from moderate (15 > AHI < 29) to severe (AHI > 30) after long-term use with or without the MAD in situ. It was concluded that worsening of the underlying condition and deterioration in treatment efficacy is associated with long-term MAD use.

In addition, for a case with a Class III phenotype that is diagnosed with OSA, one has to ponder: Where is the best position to place the already prognathic mandible? Note that mandibular prognathism can be produced by non-mandibular factors. For example, the brachyrrhine gene is associated with the short-face phenotype in both mice (Lozanoff *et al.*, 1994) and bulldogs (Fig. 60). Historically, dogs were artificially bred for facial and other characteristics. Thus, although the mandible might appear to be prognathic in English bulldogs, they have the short-face phenotype that resides in a genetic mutation of the cranial base and midface. Unfortunately, these short-face breeds, including the French bulldog, pugs, etc., exhibit

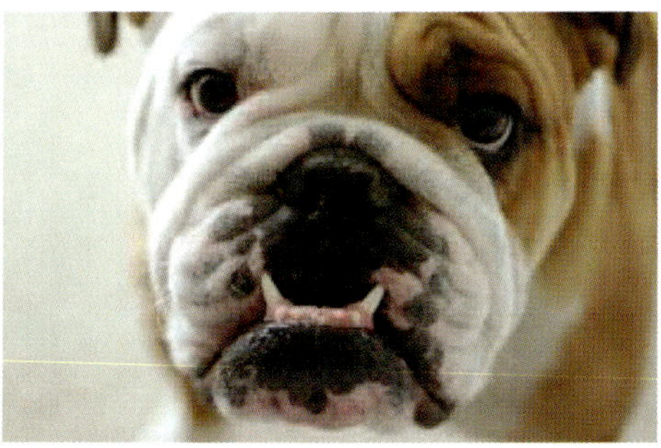

Figure 60a: Frontal photograph of an English bulldog showing an anterior crossbite.

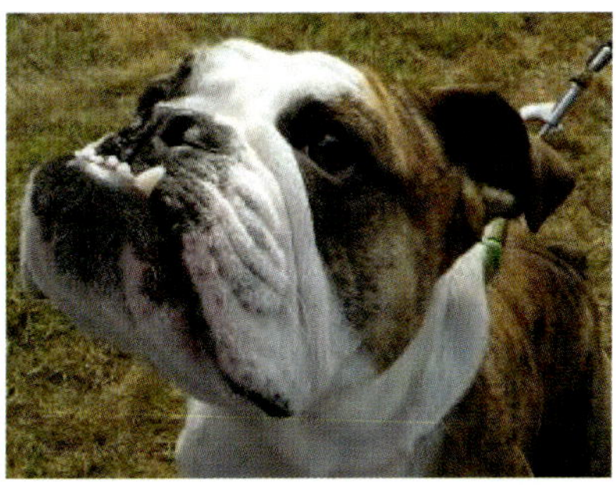

Figure 60b: Lateral aspect of an English bulldog showing features of mandibular prognathism and a severe anterior crossbite.

respiratory distress and decreased longevity (Sabino *et al.*, 2013; Lilja-Maula *et al.*, 2017). Therefore, while the mandible often needs to be manipulated clinically for the resolution of OSA, it needs to be done in coordination with midfacial development both in children and adults.

Controversy exists as to whether the mandible can be developed in both children and adults, and maintained in a new spatial matrix. In fact, there are those who propose morning positioners for the prevention of mandibular prognathism associated with long-term MAD use. In this counter-intuitive method (Singh, 2015), the mandible is protruded during sleep to prevent nocturnal airway collapse; but in the morning the mandible is retruded again using morning positioners, presumably to prevent the mandible from attaining its desirable nocturnal position during the daytime. Alternatively, it can be ventured that instead of simply maintaining the malocclusion with the mandible in a retruded position, would it not make more sense to redevelop the midface and re-coordinate the mandible in the midline anteriorly? This protocol would putatively provide more functional space to realign the lower segment (Fig. 61) and correct any midline discrepancy. In fact, a successful case following the biomimetic PACE protocol is illustrated in Figure 62. On the other hand, Table 4 shows the clinical stages for arch re-coordination. Typically, the

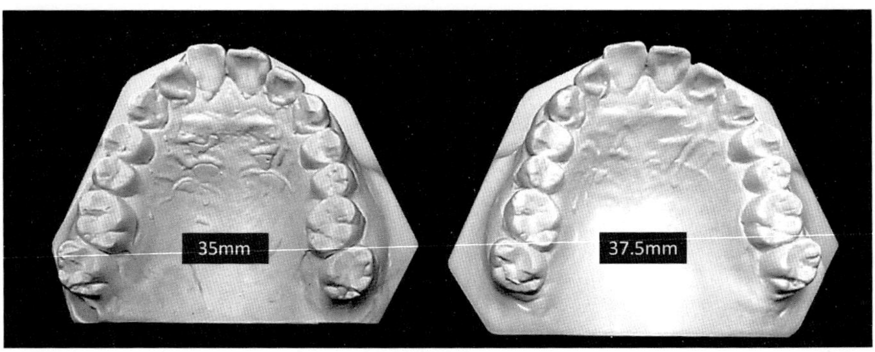

Figure 61a: Pre-treatment (left) and post-treatment (right) upper study models. Note the increased transpalatal bone width after biomimetic oral appliance therapy.

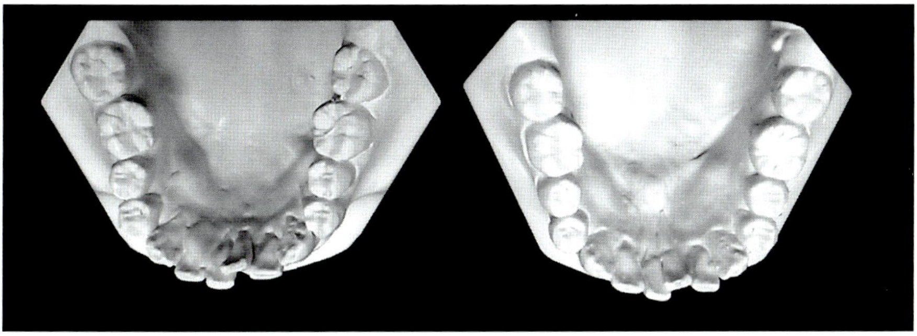

Figure 61b: Pre-treatment (left) and post-treatment (right) lower study models. Note the reduced anterior crowding after biomimetic oral appliance therapy.

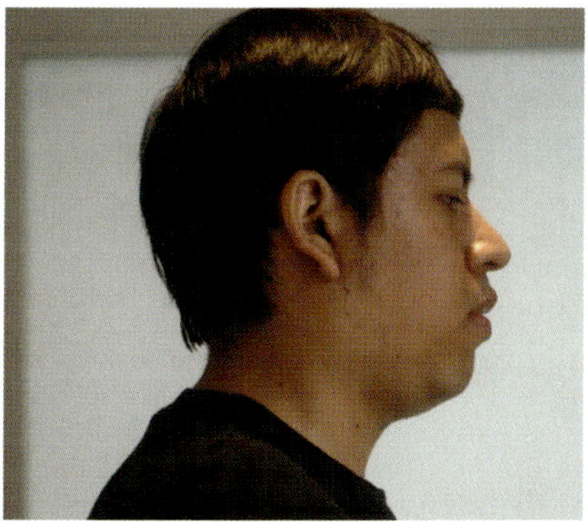

Figure 62a: Lateral photograph of an adult showing mandibular retrusion prior to treatment. Courtesy: Dr Martha Cortes

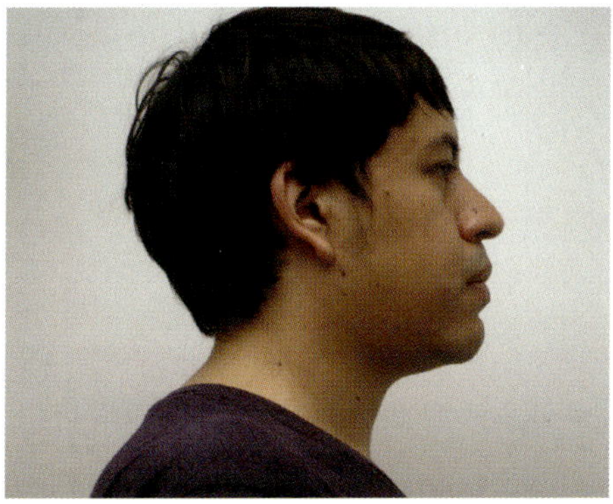

Figure 62b: Lateral photograph of same adult showing improved mandibular positioning and facial balance after biomimetic treatment.

upper device is worn for approx. 1–3 months and the lower arch is carefully observed during that time. After approx. 1–3 months a lower device is then provided if indicated. At this time arch re-coordination commences, so that changes in the upper arch are coordinated using the lower device so that only minor changes in the occlusion are produced between each appointment of treatment. This procedure follows the cranio-caudal gradient of development with the lower arch catching up with changes in the upper arch at a slightly later date (Table 4).

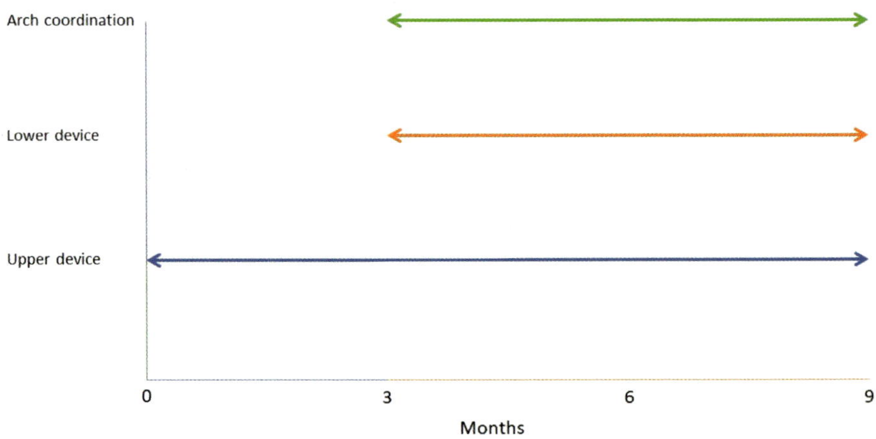

Table 4: The upper device is worn for 1–3 months (blue line) prior to provision of lower device at month 3 (orange line), at which time arch re-coordination commences, and finishes at month 9 (green line) in this hypothetical example.

Clinical algorithm

During treatment planning, once the treatment objectives have been delineated, the question becomes, which device will permit the achievement of the goals required for craniofacial correction? To answer this question, a clinical algorithm (Table 5) can be useful and has been successfully deployed as discussed below. In determining the device design, the first question to ask is, is the maxilla abnormal? If so, biomimetic oral appliance therapy may be indicated. In traditional dental/orthodontic training, less emphasis is placed on midfacial morphology and much more attention is given to tooth position. In the cranio-caudal gradient of human development, however, teeth are downstream from the skeletal tissues, soft tissues and functional spaces. In fact, the teeth will erupt into whatever space(s) is left and sometimes become unerupted, impacted, or even absent if there is insufficient space available for development at the outset. **Primary assessment of tooth position leads to an optical illusion**, in effect. Thus, for decades it was believed that Class II cases exhibit maxillary protrusion and/or protruded maxillary incisors whereas more modern techniques

Is the maxilla abnormal?	Yes	Consider Acrylic-based, Wireframe or Hybrid device
	No	Not suitable for PACE therapy
Is the vertical deficient?	Yes	Consider Acrylic-based or Hybrid device
	No	Consider Wireframe appliance
Is the patient a mouth breather?	Yes	Consider Wireframe appliance
	No	Consider Acrylic-based or Hybrid device
Is recapture of premolar spaces needed?	Yes	Consider Acrylic-based appliance with Y-split and 3-way screw
	No	Consider Acrylic-based appliance with sagittal split and transverse screw
Has a diagnosis of OSA been made?	Yes	Add pharyngeal stent or use mRNA appliance
	No	No pharyngeal stent needed. This extension is not used in pediatric cases

Table 5: Clinical algorithm for device selection.

of craniofacial analysis reveal that the midface is often hypoplastic and the maxillary incisors are retroclined even in Class II cases. These findings mean that retractive orthodontics may be inappropriate in certain cases and, if so, might exclude the extraction of healthy premolar and wisdom teeth. To avoid such pitfalls, it's essential to assess maxillary morphology in 3D space. For example, does the maxilla have a high vault? If so, there is a good chance that the tongue does not lie on the palate at rest, and that nasal breathing might be impeded, since the roof of the mouth is the floor of the nose. Another feature to look for is the presence of torus palatinus. These bony exostoses are most often found in the midline of the palate and represent bone formation even in adults, since tori are known to grow larger with age. The localization of these palatal tori belies their *raison d'etre*. As mentioned earlier, the primary purpose of (craniofacial) sutures is to make bone. The palatal tori invariably lie directly below the midpalatal suture (Fig. 22) and, as noted previously, sutural stretch leads to bone deposition. Therefore, the presence of palatal tori leads to an abnormal maxillary morphology, secondary to chronic stretching of the midpalatal suture, for example from nocturnal bruxing, grinding, and/or clenching. This abnormal behavior may be an ineffectual attempt to relieve upper airway compromise and will be further discussed in a later chapter. Suffice to say that large midpalatal tori are, presumably, taking up valuable tongue space and likely displacing the tongue into the floor of the mouth during sleep, which predisposes to upper airway obstruction. Thus, the morphology of the maxilla needs to be assessed in the vertical axis, and this includes its anterior aspect, most often noted as a 'gummy smile'.

As noted in Chapter 3, the human face preferentially grows downward and forward (Enlow and Hans 1996), secondary to klinorhynchy (Davidson, 2003). In the absence of tongue support, the face will predominantly grow vertically downward, producing vertical maxillary excess and sometimes a 'gummy smile' (Fig. 1; Harris and Singh, 2013). This abnormal growth trajectory needs to be reduced and improved. In addition, however, there may be an antero-posterior deficiency of the maxilla. Most commonly this can appear clinically as an anterior crossbite, assuming the cranial base and mandible exhibit a Class I phenotype. An anterior deficiency of the maxilla might also manifest as anterior crowding, while a posterior deficiency of the maxilla might be seen as end molar impaction, typically involving the maxillary third molars, which may be partially erupted, impacted, or even absent. Similarly, transverse deficiencies in the posterior region might be apparent as a unilateral or bilateral posterior crossbite, with or without a midline discrepancy, as the mandible attempts to articulate with a narrow maxilla. In the first edition of this book, we referred to induced maxillary morphogenesis. This technique is a clinical attempt to restore midfacial bone volume to accommodate 16 maxillary teeth, if possible (Fig. 63). In fact, Singh *et al.* (2014) were the first to demonstrate that maxillary bone volume can be increased in adults without surgery, while others (Nada *et al.*, 2012) achieved similar but less favorable results. For example, Singh *et al.* (2014) reported that the mean transpalatal bone width increased from approx. 33.5mm to 36mm after biomimetic oral appliance therapy in adults, while the mean midfacial bone volume increased from 17.4cm^3 to 19cm^3 after approx. 18 months of therapy. In contrast, Nada *et al.* (2012)

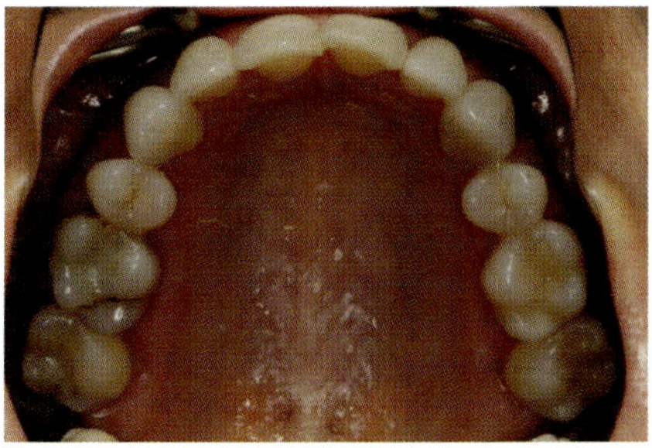

Figure 63a: Intra-oral photograph of an adult showing missing first premolars prior to treatment. Courtesy: Dr Gary Sacher

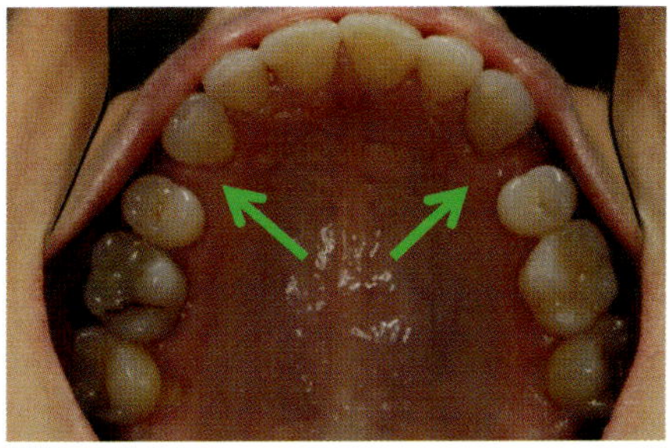

Figure 63b: Intra-oral photograph of same adult showing recapture of first premolar spaces during treatment.

used surgical transpalatal distraction osteogenesis (surgically assisted rapid maxillary expansion) for 22 months. The distances between the posterior alveolar segments of the maxilla increased, indicating lateral expansion, but the anterior maxillary region showed posterior displacement/retrusion of the anterior alveolar region. Therefore, midfacial morphology can be attenuated even in adult cases, and a non-surgical approach might be preferable instead.

Abnormalities of the maxilla often do not exist in isolation. Thus, a case may show perturbation of the vertical dimension allied with an increased overbite or deep bite. In these cases, the device design selected most likely will have occlusal pads/occlusal coverage to recapture the vertical dimension and improve the overbite to WNL. The effect of the occlusal coverage is to distract the condyle away from the glenoid fossa in the same way as TMJ orthotics. In accord with the spatial matrix hypothesis, this change in the position of the mandible results in a change in the pattern of gene expression, and subsequently alterations occur at the TMJ, which permit recapture of the vertical dimension of the occlusion. Note that during this phase, the occlusal acrylic of the upper device is periodically ground down to permit the lower posterior segments to upright and supra-erupt into the new spatial matrix so that major changes in the occlusion are not precipitated. Once the acrylic has been completely ground through, the teeth ought to be close to their final finishing positions, and this may be augmented by the use of fixed appliances (Fig. 97) or clear trays, etc. to optimize the cusp-fossa relationships, if indicated.

Another parameter to consider is whether the patient is a habitual mouth-breather. Sometimes, these cases find it difficult to tolerate a device in the mouth that covers the palate and encroaches on tongue space. Some of these patients may also have a hypersensitive gag reflex and/or nasal obstruction. In these instances, a device is selected that gives sufficient tongue space, such as a **Wireframe or Hybrid appliance**. The omega loops of these devices are activated by the tongue, which is encouraged to sit on an anterior plane and thereby activate 3D axial springs that are attached in the anterior region of the device. On the other hand, to recapture premolar spaces, an acrylic-based device is preferred with a Y-split design and 3-way screw system. Most often distal stops are placed on the second premolars and by using a gradual concentric pattern of development, the first premolar spaces can be recaptured to a greater or lesser extent even in adult patients (Fig. 63).

In this situation, the screw may reach the limit of its travel and, given tissue remodeling, the device may need to be relined and the screw re-set or an entirely new device may need to be fabricated since up to 7mm of functional, mesio-distal space needs to be regained on either side of the arch. Furthermore, some of these cases may have a diagnosis of OSA. If so, it's important to prevent upper airway collapse during sleep. This requirement can be achieved using different device components. First, it's possible to add a pharyngeal stent to the distal border of the device (Fig. 52b). This extension has a roller ball at its distal-most aspect. The stent is positioned to lie midway between the posterior aspect of the tongue and the soft palate/uvula, so that when the patient is standing or sitting upright, the stent is not touching any tissues. When the patient lies down, however, the tongue falls back, rolls forward off the rollerball and ends up sitting in the palate, thus opening the airway and activating the 3D axial springs as noted above. Positioning of the pharyngeal stent is crucial and if the 'sweet spot' can't be located, the gag reflex might be invoked. As an alternative, therefore, a screw-fin mechanism is used to posture the mandible forward while sleeping, similar to a MAD except that both the upper and lower components of this device (mandibular Repositioning Nighttime Appliance: mRNA appliance) have some six degrees of freedom, being adjustable in the antero-posterior, medio-lateral, and infero-superior planes, as well as the option of anterior re-positioning of the mandible in cases diagnosed with OSA. Note that in pediatric cases, neither a pharyngeal stent nor a MAD is used since it has been shown that palatal expansion is curative in certain cases of pediatric OSA (Camacho *et al.*, 2017).

Another constraint that influences the mode of treatment is the severity of the case. During triage, one can classify a case as being mild, moderate, comprehensive, severe, or complex. The mild/moderate categories constitute the vast majority of cases that are suitable for biomimetic oral appliance therapy. In these cases, the arches might not be very crowded, and a diagnosis of mild-moderate OSA may coexist. Despite this, no case can be regarded as being easy. The classification relates to the structural complexity of the case, and not to other factors that might lead to clinical success. One of these factors is patient compliance. In the absence of excellent patient cooperation, the treatment protocol is unlikely to succeed. Proffit (2005) considers that a device needs to be in a patient's mouth for at least 8hrs to have any clinical effect. After all, the patient's tissues are doing the correction by responding to appropriate signals from the device, but, if the device is not worn for prolonged periods of time, no clinical effect can be expected. In the biomimetic PACE protocol, device wear for 12-16hrs. is recommended, partly in line with circadian rhythm. For children the device can be worn after school, during the evening and at nighttime while sleeping. Proffit and Frazier-Bowers (2009) have shown that post-emergent premolars erupt during the early evening, presumably in preparation for deciduous tooth exfoliation during the late evening or at night during sleep (which coincides with the tooth fairy myth and the finding of a newly shed tooth the following morning). Moreover, it is known that human growth hormone peaks during stage N3 sleep at night. Therefore, wearing a device during the evening and at nighttime during sleep might also benefit adults who are undergoing induced maxillary morphogenesis.

Apart from mild-moderate cases, other cases can be described as being comprehensive, severe or complex. Comprehensive cases are those where some additional features need to be addressed. For example, a patient may present with a 'reduced' archform. This reduction is most commonly due to the extraction of healthy premolar or wisdom teeth for orthodontic reasons during childhood. It is not uncommon for some of these adults to be diagnosed with SDB in middle-age, especially if they have gained weight over the years. One treatment goal in these cases is to recapture the maxillary first premolar spaces, to provide sufficient functional space for breathing. Experience has shown that with excellent patient compliance and good device adjustments, regaining the maxillary premolar spaces in adults is not impossible (Fig. 8 and Fig. 63). However, these newly reformed spaces that represent bone volume will now require appropriate restorative reconstruction (Fig. 11). Classically, single-tooth implants would be the favored choice of treatment, but some may decide upon less expensive options, such as veneers, crowns, and bridges, etc. (Singh *et al.*, 2011). Therefore, these structural and cosmetic concerns need to be discussed prior to commencing any biomimetic oral appliance therapy. But, apart from esthetic considerations, loss of premolar teeth can have other functional consequences. Some patients find it difficult to tolerate a device in the mouth, especially if it takes up valuable functional space. These patients may find it difficult to comply with treatment requirements; and these issues need to be identified and addressed if a successful treatment outcome is to be achieved. For example, in the case of a habitual mouth-breather, the aim is to convert that individual into a nasal breather. Assuming that overt nasal obstruction is absent, then the principles of physics come into play. The nasal cavity is smaller than the oral cavity and communicates with it behind the soft palate. Let's assume that a device is provided that has occlusal coverage, which increases the vertical dimension of occlusion with an appropriate bite registration. In other words, the volume of the oral cavity has been increased while the pressure has been decreased. Assuming now that the patient is able to form a lip seal with the device in situ, physics dictates that the patient will suck air in through the nose, since the nasal cavity now has a relatively high air pressure, and thus the patient may experience a form of nasal breathing. Despite the mechanics, nasal breathing is subject to physiologic control, such as the nasal cycle. In subjects that demonstrate this pattern clearly, this behavior indicates that nasal breathing proceeds through one side preferentially for, say 30-90mins. After that time, the other side is predominantly used for breathing. However, if nasal obstruction exists, the cycle will be perturbed. During wakefulness, if an individual is unable to breathe through one side of the nose, they will resort to mouth-breathing during the day, but they will be in jeopardy during the night. For example, if a patient is sleeping in the supine position, nasal breathing will proceed through the unobstructed side. When the cycle switches to the obstructed side, the patient will subconsciously attempt to mouth breathe; but if the tongue is obstructing the upper airway, after a period of 10 seconds of airflow cessation the first episode of apnea will be recorded.

Severe cases largely represent a quantitative, not a qualitative, change in need; in other words, more of the same treatment is indicated. Consequently, a severe case often requires more treatment time and effort, and may require more than one device, or the device might need to be relined/rebased and the components re-set to achieve the desired result. Furthermore, patient compliance needs to be paced so that the patient doesn't undergo 'burn-out' part way through treatment. On the other hand, complex cases are those that have some additional requirements that need to be addressed: such as a history of surgery for trauma; a congenital anomaly, e.g. cleft lip and/or palate; or congenital absence of teeth, such as lateral incisors, etc. These features add a degree of complexity to the treatment plan since the behavior of the tissues and tissue response cannot be easily gauged. For example, it is imperative to determine whether a patient has been previously diagnosed with OSA when considering biomimetic oral appliance therapy. This information can help to design a device that can attempt to address the site and severity of the obstruction. Mallampati (1983) was the first to classify the aperture of the upper airway for anesthesia. However, this static classification does not indicate the clinical behavior of the upper airway. I first suggested that it would be useful to ask a patient to make the "Aaaah" sound for about 10 seconds to assess the functionality of the Mallampati score. Surprisingly, some subjects can change a Mallampati Class IV to a Class I on phonation while others show little or no improvement (Fig. 52). Therefore, some mechanism is needed to maintain the patency of the upper airway during sleep in these cases.

Plastic surgeons have long used pharyngoplasties in the past to alleviate functional deficits associated with a cleft palate that extends into the soft palate/uvula regions. Prior to that technology, obturators were used to help avoid velopharyngeal incompetence associated with clefts of the secondary palate, extending into the velar region. Using these methods as a starting point, Singh *et al.* (2009) showed that a stent extending from the distal aspect of an oral appliance could help maintain upper airway patency. Moreover, while a previous idea was to use a 'tail' to depress the tongue, my concept was one of a pharyngeal stent that would prevent the critical collapsing pressure of the upper airway being reached, by maintaining the diameter of the lumen of the upper airway. Some clinicians were initially reticent in trying out a pharyngeal stent as an extension for the prevention of OSA. The fear was based on the idea of initiating the gag reflex. This protective reflex is transmitted via the IX cranial nerve, the glossopharyngeal nerve. Its purpose is to prevent foreign particles from being inhaled. As such, it is located at the opening of the oropharynx, as demarcated by the circumvallate papillae of the tongue. Thus, a pharyngeal stent that is positioned too far anteriorly and touches the tongue is likely to elicit the gag reflex. On the other hand, if the stent is extended to pass behind the tongue, midway between the soft palate/uvula

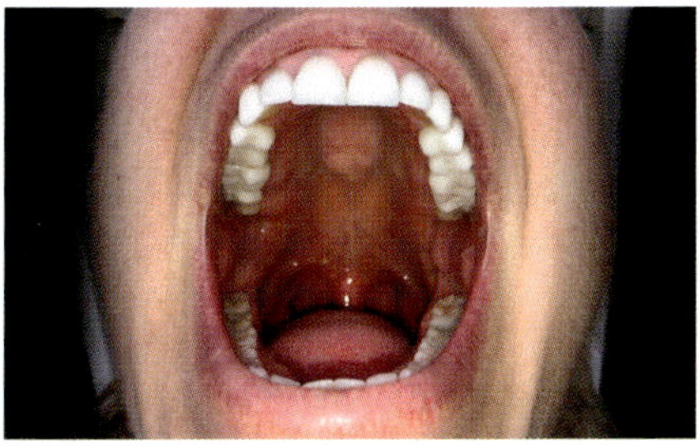

Figure 64a: Intra-oral view showing Mallampati Class 2 oropharyngeal airway aperture. Courtesy: Dr Tammarie Heit

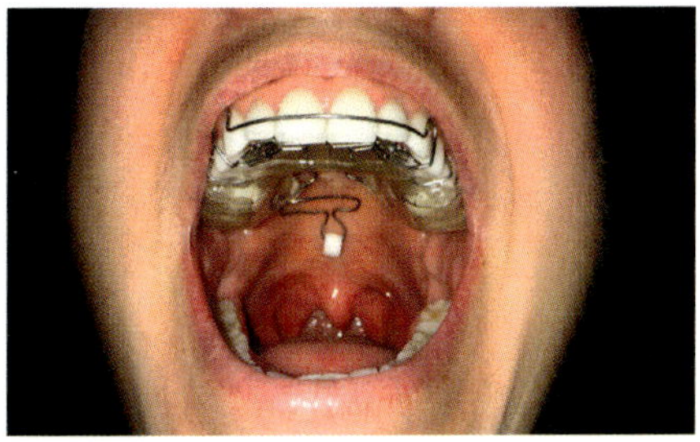

Figure 64b: Intra-oral view showing pharyngeal stent in the same patient that has improved the airway to Mallampati Class 1.

and the dorsal surface of the tongue, without touching any tissues in the sitting or standing positions, then the gag reflex is unlikely to be activated (Fig. 64). Despite these precautions, some patients have a hypersensitive gag reflex while others, notably those on long-term CPAP use, appear to be desensitized in the oropharyngeal region and are more readily able to accept a pharyngeal stent.

For hypersensitive individuals, further steps are required to ensure successful habituation to the pharyngeal stent. In these cases, erbium laser therapy can be used transiently shrink the oropharyngeal tissues (Frelich *et al.*, 2019). While the mechanism by which cold lasers affect tissue-shrinkage is still being debated in the literature, empirically, it can be surmised that the laser energy imparted to the tissues enhances collagen cross-linking. If so, the tissues would shrink or become 'tighter'. Fig. 65 shows a clinical example of this phenomenon. However, tissue rebound and relapse will likely occur at a later date. Nevertheless, this slow recovery ought to provide sufficient time for the patient to adapt to the pharyngeal stent with little or no discomfort. Moreover, the design and materials used in pharyngeal stent fabrication permit adaptability. First, the stent can be elongated, shortened and bent to optimally follow the tissue contours; in addition, the roller ball at the end of the extension ensures that both the tongue and uvula will glide past the stent, lubricated by saliva without causing

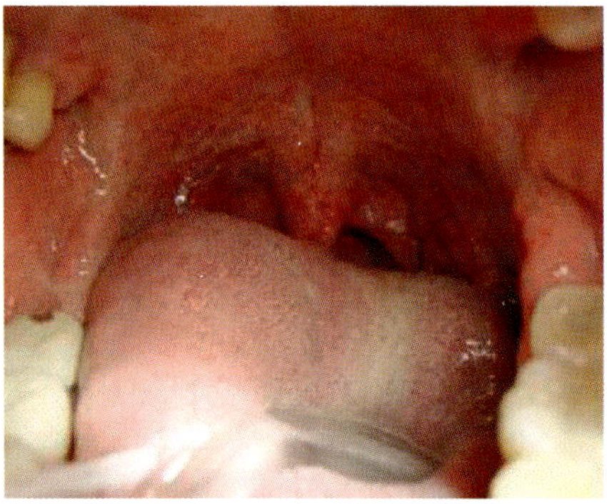

Figure 65a: Pre-operative intra-oral view showing oropharyngeal airway aperture. Courtesy: Dr Sang Min Lee

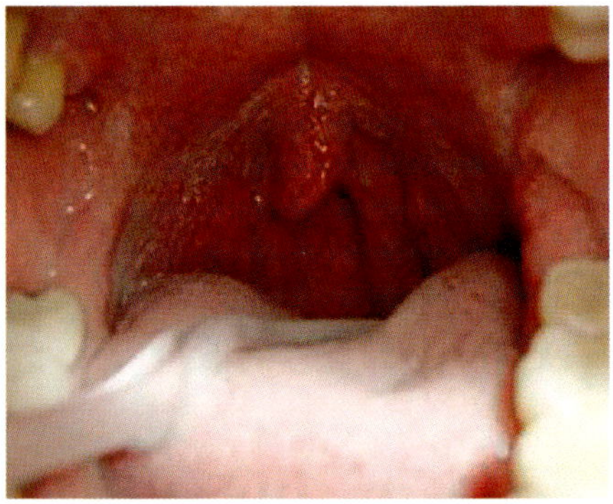

Figure 65b: Post-operative intra-oral view after erbium laser therapy to shrink soft palate and uvula to prevent gag reflex.

any tissue discomfort. Therefore, the design, materials, and protocol of biomimetic oral appliance therapy is uniquely developed to target and enhance the functional spaces of the upper airway.

In non-syndromic patients with midfacial hypoplasia, it is possible that the vertical dimension of occlusion might also be perturbed. It is well known that when the mandible is advanced, the vertical separation of the upper and lower arches will change, partly due to the curve of Spee. In cases where there is a vertical anomaly, the patient presents with a deep bite and the overbite is increased, sometimes to an alarming extent. In these cases, vertical control of the functional spaces is critical. Here, the device can be used to reposition the mandible antero-inferiorly. In so doing, the excessive degree of vertical overlap is relieved immediately. The upper device design now includes occlusal coverage or pads to guide or maintain the mandibular position. These occlusal pads play a pivotal role in correction. First, by separating the maxilla from the mandible, the midface is free to develop in 3D space, while simultaneously the mandible is free to move in 3D space. When the device is removed, re-coordination/re-equilibration occurs as the tissues remodel in an effort to maintain homeostasis. Studies in Rhesus macaque monkeys (McNamara and Bryan, 1987) investigated long-term changes associated with mandibular repositioning. These studies indicated that adaptations occurred in both

TMJs and the overall mandibular length increased. These findings are in accord with the spatial matrix hypothesis (Singh, 2004). However, doubt was expressed whether these types of changes occurred in humans, and if so, what were the underlying mechanisms. Put simply, stem cell differentiation in the condylar region leads to the deposition of cartilage, which in turn is converted into bone. This series of events would account for changes both at the TMJs and the mandible (Learreta, 1999). For example, when a lower orthotic is used for the treatment of TMD, long-term use (> 12 weeks) is avoided since a posterior open bite can be induced as the posterior segments undergo intrusion. Once the TMJ/mandibular position has been established by orthotic use, phase 2 of treatment is initiated often involving fixed orthodontic appliances to provide the final occlusal finishing. In the biomimetic approach adopted here, occlusal coverage of the lower posterior segments is not advocated. Instead, the occlusal coverage is transferred to the upper device, which repositions the mandible while midfacial development proceeds simultaneously. Thus, maxillo-mandibular correction is attempted while addressing upper airway issues, although final orthodontic finishing (Fig. 97) may still be required to a greater or lesser extent. As to the question of whether mandibular growth can be effected in humans, Singh and Clark (2001) studied mandibular growth in children and teenagers following Twin-Block appliance therapy, a type of mandibular advancement device. Even after correcting for natural growth, using finite-element scaling analyses, an approx. 30% increase in growth at the condylar neck was demonstrable. These mandibular changes helped correct the vertical dimension of occlusion/improve the overbite as evidenced by size increases at the labiomental groove (Singh and Clark, 2003), but these mandibular changes came at a price paid by the midfacial structures since maxillary retrusion was evident in the attainment of a normal overbite and overjet relationship (Singh and Hodge, 2002). Therefore, the design of the Twin Block appliance needed to be improved in order to attempt craniofacial correction in adults as well as pediatric cases.

Finally, as an integral part of treatment planning, one has to estimate the approx. treatment time. Some orthodontic treatment plans can extend for 2–5 years followed by life-long use of retainers. While those plans might be appropriate for some, the biomimetic approach suggests that treatment time for the upper arch typically varies between 9 and 12 months, assuming 12-16 hrs. of wear time (in the late afternoon, early evening, and all night long). Following the cranio-caudal gradient of human development, after about 1–3 months of upper device wear, a device for the lower arch is typically implemented (Table 4). Depending on the severity of the condition, 12 months of lower appliance therapy (with 12-16hrs of wear time) is not uncommon. Thus, the treatment time is currently at about 21 months since the upper and lower device timings overlap after the first 1–3 months. During this time, the aim also includes arch re-coordination. In some protocols (e.g. mandibular advancement devices) little or no attention is paid to the upper arch, and arch coordination is either ignored (Korngut, 2010) or the default result with side-effects is accepted. In contrast, during biomimetic oral appliance therapy an integrated phase of approx. 12 months is set aside for arch re-coordination; this phase coincides with the wearing of the lower device. Thus, the overall treatment time averages about 15-21 months in a typical case. In more severe cases, an additional 3–6 months of orthodontic finishing may be indicated (Fig. 97). These tooth alignments can be achieved with either a system of clear tray aligners or fixed orthodontic appliances with the use of vertical elastics for anterior coupling or cross-arch elastics for interocclusal detailing. In all cases, oral myofunctional therapy is recommended since the tongue can act as a natural retainer, while occasional nighttime appliance wear will act as an anti-ageing device. The next chapter reviews device design, adjustments, and case finishing.

References

ada.org/en/press-room/news-releases/2017-archives/october/ada-adopts-policy-on-dentistry-role-in-treating-obstructive-sleep-apnea

Angle EH. Malocclusion of teeth. 1907, 7th edition. Philadelphia, USA: SS White Dental Manufacturing Company.

Armijo BS, Brown M, Guyuron B. Defining the ideal nasolabial angle. *Plast Reconstr Surg*. 2012;129(3):759–764.

Baccetti T, Franchi L, McNamara JA Jr. The cervical vertebral maturation (CVM) method for the assessment of optimal treatment timing in dentofacial orthopedics. *Seminars Orthod*. 2005;11:119–129.

Banabilh SM, Suzina AH, Dinsuhaimi S, Singh GD. Cranial base and airway morphology in adult Malays with obstructive sleep apnoea. *Aust Orthod J*. 2007;23(2):89–95.

Banabilh SM, Suzina AH, Dinsuhaimi S, Singh GD. Craniofacial obesity in patients with obstructive sleep apnea. *Sleep Breath*. 2009;13(1):19–24.

Banabilh SM, Suzina AH, Mohamad H, Dinsuhaimi S, Samsudin AR, Singh GD. Assessment of 3-D nasal airway morphology in Southeast Asian adults with obstructive sleep apnea using acoustic rhinometry. *Clin Oral Investig*. 2010;14(5):491–498.

Bench R W. Growth of the cervical vertebrae as related to tongue, face, and denture behavior. *Am J Orthod*. 1963;49:183–214.

Bookstein FL. Reconsidering "The inappropriateness of conventional cephalometrics". *Am J Orthod Dentofacial Orthop*. 2016;149(6):784–797.

Brennick MJ, Pack AI, Ko K, Kim E, Pickup S, Maislin G, Schwab RJ. Altered upper airway and soft tissue structures in the New Zealand Obese mouse. *Am J Respir Crit Care Med*. 2009;179(2):158–169.

Burwell RG, Dangerfield PH, Freeman BJ. Concepts on the pathogenesis of adolescent idiopathic scoliosis. Bone growth and mass, vertebral column, spinal cord, brain, skull, extra-spinal left-right skeletal length asymmetries, disproportions and molecular pathogenesis. *Stud Health Technol Inform*. 2008;135:3–52.

Camacho M, Chang ET, Song SA, Abdullatif J, Zaghi S, Pirelli P, Certal V, Guilleminault C. Rapid maxillary expansion for pediatric obstructive sleep apnea: A systematic review and meta-analysis. *Laryngoscope*. 2017;127(7):1712–1719.

Carberry JC, Jordan AS, White DP, Wellman A, Eckert DJ. Upper airway collapsibility (Pcrit) and pharyngeal dilator muscle activity are sleep stage dependent. *Sleep*. 2016;39(3):511–521.

Celenk M, Farrell ML, Eren H, Kumar K, Singh GD, Lozanoff S. Upper airway detection and visualization from cone beam image slices. *J Xray Sci Technol*. 2010;18(2): 121–135.

Chaplain MAJ, Singh GD, McLachlan JC (eds.) "On Growth and Form: Spatio-Temporal Patterning in Biology". England: John Wiley and Sons Publishers, 1999. ISBN: 0–471-98451–5.

Chapman C, Singh GD. Combined effect of a biomimetic oral appliance and atlas orthogonist cervical adjustment on leg lengths in adults. *Annals Vert Sub Res*. 2013:46–50.

Cooper BC, Cooper DL, Lucente FE. Electromyography of masticatory muscles in craniomandibular disorders. *Laryngoscope*. 1991;101(2):150–157.

Corruccini RS, Flander LB, Kaul SS. Mouth breathing, occlusion, and modernization in a north Indian population. An epidemiologic study. *Angle Orthod*. 1985;55(3):190–196.

Davidson TM. The great leap forward: The anatomic basis for the acquisition of speech and obstructive sleep apnea. *Sleep Med*. 2003;4(3):185–194.

Enlow DH, Hans MG. Essentials of facial growth. Philadelphia: Saunders, 1996.

Fletcher EC. Obstructive sleep apnoea and cardiovascular morbidity. *Monaldi Arch Chest Dis*. 1996;51(1):77–80.

Fonder AC. The Dental Distress Syndrome (Part One). *Stress*. 1980;1(1).

Fonder AC. The Dental Distress Syndrome (Quantified). *Quantum Med*. 1988;1(1).

Frelich H, Ścierski W, Markón M, Frelich J, Frelich H, Maciej M. Minimally invasive erbium laser treatment for selected snorers. *Lasers Med Sci*. 2019;34(7):1413–1420.

Gao YY, Wang HJ, Wu Y. Superficial punctate keratopathy in a pediatric patient was related to adenoid hypertrophy and obstructive sleep apnea syndrome: A case report. *BMC Ophthalmol*. 2018;18(1):55.

Garrett-Bakelman FE, Darshi M, Green SJ, Gur RC, Lin L, Macias BR, McKenna MJ, Meydan C *et al*. The NASA twins study: A multidimensional analysis of a year-long human spaceflight. *Science*. 2019;364:eaau8650.

Gribel BF, Gribel MN, Frazäo DC, McNamara JA Jr, Manzi FR. Accuracy and reliability of craniometric measurements on lateral cephalometry and 3D measurements on CBCT scans. *Angle Orthod*. 2011;81(1):26–35.

Harris WG, Singh GD. Resolution of 'gummy smile' and anterior open bite using the DNA appliance™: Case Report. *J Amer Orthod Soc*. 2013;13(4):30–34.

Heit T, Sebastian J, Singh GD. A novel combined protocol for the resolution of severe obstructive sleep apnea. *J Sleep Disord Ther*. 2016;5(5):251–254.

Herulf M, Lundberg JO, Weitzberg E. Nostril widening improves arterial oxygenation: a role for nasal nitric oxide? *Respir Med*. 1999;93(2):134–135.

Huggare J. The first cervical vertebra as an indicator of mandibular growth. *Eur J Orthod*. 1989;11(1):10–16.

Korngut R. Case study: A persistent positive outcome treating OSA with a MAD following the treatment protocol. *Dialogue*. 2010;1:26–27.

Lam B, Ip MS, Tench E, Ryan CF. Craniofacial profile in Asian and white subjects with obstructive sleep apnoea. *Thorax*. 2005;60(6):504–510.

Lamparski D. Skeletal age assessment utilizing cervical vertebrae. Thesis, University of Pittsburgh, Pennsylvania, 1972.

Learreta JA. Regeneration ad integrum of the condyle head in a patient with temporomandibular disorders. *Cranio*. 1999;17(3):221–227.

Lilja-Kurlander E, Kurol J, Josefson E. Attitudes and satisfaction with dental appearance in young adults with and without malocclusion: *Swedish Dent J*. 2003;27(3):143–150.

Lilja-Maula L, Lappalainen AK, Hyytiäinen HK, Kuusela E, Kaimio M, Schildt K, Mölsä S, Morelius M, Rajamäki MM. Comparison of submaximal exercise test results and severity of brachycephalic obstructive airway syndrome in English bulldogs. *Vet J*. 2017;219:22–26.

López del Valle LM, Singh GD, Feliciano N, Machuca M del C. Associations between a history of breast feeding, malocclusion and parafunctional habits in Puerto Rican children. *PR Health Sci J*. 2006;25(1):31–34.

Lozanoff S, Jureczek S, Feng T, Padwal R. Anterior cranial base morphology in mice with midfacial retrusion. *Cleft Palate Craniofac J*. 1994;31(6):417–428.

Ludlow JB, Davies-Ludlow LE, Brooks SL. Dosimetry of two extraoral direct digital imaging devices: NewTom cone beam CT and Orthophos Plus DS panoramic unit. *Dentomaxillofacial Rad*. 2003;32:229–234.

Ludlow JB. A manufacturer's role in reducing the dose of cone beam computed tomography examinations: effect of beam filtration. *Dentomaxillofac Radiol*. 2011;40(2):115–122.

Lundberg JO. Nitric oxide and the paranasal sinuses. *Anat Rec* (*Hoboken*). 2008;291(11):1479–1484.

Mallampati SR. Clinical sign to predict difficult tracheal intubation(hypothesis). *Can Anaesth Soc J*. 1983;30(3):316–317.

Marklund M. Long-term efficacy of an oral appliance in early treated patients with obstructive sleep apnea. *Sleep Breath*. 2016;20(2):689–694.

McNamara JA Jr, Bryan FA. Long-term mandibular adaptations to protrusive function: An experimental study in Macaca mulatta. Am J Orthod Dentofacial Orthop. 1987;92(2):98–108.

McNamara JA Jr. Maxillary transverse deficiency. *Am J Orthod Dentofacial Orthop*. 2000;117(5):567–570.

Moya H, Miralles R, Zuñiga C, Carvajal R, Rocabado M, Santander H. Influence of stabilization occlusal splint on craniocervical relationships. Part I: Cephalometric analysis. *Cranio*. 1994;12(1):47–51.

Moyers RE, Bookstein FL. The inappropriateness of conventional cephalometrics. *Am J Orthod*. 1979;75(6):599–617.

Nada RM, Fudalej PS, Maal TJ, Bergé SJ, Mostafa YA, Kuijpers-Jagtman AM. Three-dimensional prospective evaluation of tooth-borne and bone-borne surgically assisted rapid maxillary expansion. *J Craniomaxillofac Surg*. 2012;40(8):757–762.

Nashi N, Kang S, Barkdull GC, Lucas J, Davidson TM. Lingual fat at autopsy. *Laryngoscope*. 2007;117(8):1467–1473.

Obelenis Ryan DP, Bianchi J, Ignácio J, Wolford LM, Gonçalves JR. Cone-beam computed tomography airway measurements: Can we trust them? *Am J Orthod Dentofacial Orthop*. 2019;156(1):53–60.

Parsons TE, Downey CM, Jirik FR, Hallgrimsson B, Jamniczky HA. Mind the gap: genetic manipulation of basicranial growth within synchondroses modulates calvarial and facial shape in mice through epigenetic interactions. *PLoS One*. 2015;10(2):e0118355.

Proffit WR, Fields HW Jr. Contemporary Orthodontics. St. Louis: Mosby, 2000, pp. 296–310.

Proffit WR, Frazier-Bowers SA. Mechanism and control of tooth eruption. *Orthod Craniofac Res*. 2009;12(2):59–6.

Proffit WR. Contemporary Orthodontics, 3rd edition. Elsevier, 2005.

Sabino CV, Holowaychuk M, Bateman S. Management of acute respiratory distress syndrome in a French Bulldog using airway pressure release ventilation. *J Vet Emerg Crit Care* (*San Antonio*). 2013;23(4):447–454.

San Román P, Palma JC, Oteo MD, Nevado E. Skeletal maturation determined by cervical vertebrae development. *Eur J Orthod*. 2002;24(3):303–311.

Sanders AE, Essick GK, Fillingim R, Knott C, Ohrbach R, Greenspan JD, Diatchenko L, Maixner W, Dubner R, Bair E, Miller VE, Slade GD. Sleep apnea symptoms and risk of temporomandibular disorder: OPPERA cohort. *J Dent Res*. 2013;92(7 Suppl):70S-77S.

Saunders NC, Birchall MA, Armstrong SJ, Killingback N and Singh GD. Morphometry of paranasal sinus anatomy in chronic rhinosinusitis: a pilot study. *Arch Otolaryngol Head Neck Surg*. 1998;124(6):656–658.

Shapira IL. TMJ alias, The Great Imposter, has a co-conspirator: poor sleep. *Cranio*. 2013;31(1):1–2.

Singh GD, Chandrashekhar R. Breath of life: Complexity and heterogeneity in the integration of etiologic components associated with sleep disordered breathing. In: LeFebvre E and Moreau R (eds.) Snoring: Symptoms, Causes, Diagnosis and Treatment. New York, USA: Nova Science Publishers, 2009, pp. 109–126.

Singh GD, Chapman C, Preble M. Craniofacial changes after combined atlas-orthogonal and biomimetic oral appliance therapy. *Annals Vert Sub Res*. 2014;4:112–118.

Singh GD, Clark WJ. Localization of mandibular changes in patients with Class II division 1 malocclusions treated using Twin Block appliances: finite-element modeling. *Am J Orthod Dentofacial Orthop*. 2001;119(4):419–425.

Singh GD, Clark WJ. Soft tissue morphometry of subjects with Class II division 1 malocclusions treated using Twin Block appliances: finite-element scaling analysis. *Euro J Orthod*. 2003;25(3):225–230.

Singh GD, García AV, Hang WM. Evaluation of the posterior airway space following Biobloc therapy: Geometric morphometrics. *Cranio*. 2007;25(2):84–89.

Singh GD, Heit T, Preble D, Chandrashekhar R. Changes in 3D nasal cavity volume after biomimetic oral appliance therapy in adults. *Cranio*. 2016;34(1):6–12.

Singh GD, Heit T, Preble D. Changes in 3D midfacial parameters after biomimetic oral appliance therapy in adults. *J Ind Orthod Soc*. 2014;48(2):104–108.

Singh GD, Hodge MR. Bimaxillary morphometry in patients with Class II division 1 malocclusion treated with Twin Block appliances. *Angle Orthod*. 2002;72(5):402–409.

Singh GD, Johnston J, Ma W, Lozanoff S. Cleft palate formation in fetal Br mice with midfacial retrusion: tenascin, fibronectin, laminin, and type IV collagen immunolocalization. *Cleft Palate Craniofac J*. 1998;35(1):65–76.

Singh GD, Jung SC, Chandrashekhar R. Resolution of pediatric chronic rhinitis using biomimetic oral appliance therapy: a case report. *Open J Clin Med Case Rep*. 2016;2(4):1082.

Singh GD, Keropian B, Pillar G. Effects of the Full Breath Solution appliance for the treatment of obstructive sleep apnea: A preliminary study. *Cranio*. 2009;27(2):109–117.

Singh GD, Kim HN, Kim SH, Wang L. 3D craniofacial and upper airway changes after biomimetic oral appliance therapy in Korean adults. J Otorhinolaryngol Head Neck Surg. 2020 (submitted).

Singh GD, Kim HN. Changes in pneumatization of the maxillary air sinuses in Korean adults following biomimetic oral appliance therapy. *World J Otorhinolaryngol Head Neck Surg*. 2020. doi.org/10.1016/j.wjorl.2020.07.007.

Singh GD, Kim KY. Facial enhancement using biomimetic oral appliance therapy in adults. *Dent Oral Craniofac Res*. 2016;2(4):313–317.

Singh GD, Kim SH. Short term changes in upper airway morphology and sleep architecture using biomimetic oral appliance therapy. *Chest*. 2019;155(4):1A.

Singh GD, Krumholtz J. Epigenetic Orthodontics in Adults. *Appliance Therapy Group*, USA, 2009.

Singh GD, Krumholtz J. Epigenetic Orthodontics in Adults. *Appliance Therapy Group*, USA, 2009.

Singh GD, Levy-Bercowski D, Santiago PE. 3-D effects of nasoalveolar molding in patients with orofacial clefts: geometric morphometrics. *Cleft Palate Craniofac J*. 2005;42(4):403–409.

Singh GD, Levy-Bercowski D, Yañez MA, Santiago PE. Three-dimensional facial morphology following surgical repair of unilateral cleft lip and palate in patients after nasoalveolar molding. *Orthod Craniofac Res*. 2007;10(3):161–166.

Singh GD, Liao F. Long term changes in upper airway volume and sleep architecture using biomimetic oral appliance therapy. *Am J Respir Crit Care Med*. 2019;199:A5533.

Singh GD, McNamara JA Jr, Lozanoff S. Allometry of the cranial base in prepubertal Korean subjects with class III malocclusions: finite element morphometry. *Angle Orthod*. 1999;69(6):507–514.

Singh GD, McNamara JA Jr, Lozanoff S. Craniofacial heterogeneity of prepubertal Korean and European-American subjects with Class III malocclusions: Procrustes, EDMA, and cephalometric analyses. *Int J Adult Orthodon Orthognath Surg*. 1998;13(3):227–240.

Singh GD, McNamara JA Jr, Lozanoff S. Finite-element morphometry of soft tissue morphology in subjects with untreated Class III malocclusions. *Angle Orthod*. 1999;69(3):215–224.

Singh GD, McNamara JA Jr, Lozanoff S. Finite-element morphometry of soft tissues in prepubertal Korean and European-Americans with Class III malocclusions. *Arch Oral Biol*. 1999;44(5):429–436.

Singh GD, McNamara JA Jr, Lozanoff S. Midfacial morphology of Koreans with class III malocclusions investigated with finite-element scaling analysis. *J Craniofac Genet Dev Biol*. 2000;20(1):10–18.)

Singh GD, Olmos S. Use of a sibilant phoneme registration protocol to prevent upper airway collapse in patients with TMD. *Sleep Breath*. 2007;11(4):209–216.

Singh GD, Wendling S, Chandrashekhar R. Midfacial development in adult obstructive sleep apnea. *Dent Today*. 2011;30(7):124–127.

Singh GD. Digital diagnostics: Three-dimensional modelling. *Br J Oral Maxillofac Surg*. 2008;46(1):22–26.

Singh GD. On Growth and Treatment: The spatial matrix hypothesis. In: Ribbens KA and McNamara JA Jr (eds.) Growth and treatment: A meeting of the minds. Craniofacial Growth Series, Ann Arbor, USA. 2004;41:197–239.

Singh GD. Spatial matrix hypothesis. *Brit Dent J*. 2007;202(5):238–239.

Singh GD. The significance of occlusal changes. *J Dent Sleep Med*. 2015;2(2):57.

Sutherland K, Cistulli P. Mandibular advancement splints for the treatment of sleep apnea syndrome. Swiss Med Wkly. 2011;141:w13276.

Talley RL. TMJ and OSA are sisters. *Cranio*. 2019;37(5):273–274. doi: 10.1080/08869634.2019.1641910.

Tomooka K, Tanigawa T, Sakurai S, Maruyama K, Eguchi E, Nishioka S, Miyoshi N, Kakuto H, Shimizu G, Yamaoka D, Saito I. Scalloped tongue is associated with nocturnal intermittent hypoxia among community-dwelling Japanese: The Toon Health Study. *J Oral Rehabil*. 2017;44(8):602–609.

Vrcek I, Ozgur O, Nakra T. Infraorbital Dark Circles: A Review of the Pathogenesis, Evaluation and Treatment. *J Cutan Aesthet Surg*. 2016;9(2):65–72.

Watanabe T, Isono S, Tanaka A, Tanzawa H, Nishino T. Contribution of body habitus and craniofacial characteristics to segmental closing pressures of the passive pharynx in patients with sleep-disordered breathing. *Am J Respir Crit Care Med*. 2002;165(2):260–265.

Weiss TM, Atanasov S, Calhoun KH. The association of tongue scalloping with obstructive sleep apnea and related sleep pathology. *Otolaryngol Head Neck Surg*. 2005;133(6):966–971.

Willems G, De Bruyne I, Verdonck A, Fieuws S, Carels C. Prevalence of dentofacial characteristics in a Belgian orthodontic population. *Clinical Oral Invest*. 2001;5(4):220–226.

Witzel MA, Posnick JC. Patterns and location of velopharyngeal valving problems: atypical findings on video-nasopharyngoscopy. *Cleft Palate J*. 1989;26(1):63–67.

Chapter 6

Biomimetic Oral Appliance Designs

Synopsis: This chapter first discusses the requirements of a biomimetic oral appliance. Next, it describes actual biomimetic device components and designs, and briefly touches on protocol and adjustments. Device selection, indications and contra-indications are included. As well, an overview of various bite registration procedures is provided. Although special emphasis is placed on achieving enhancement of the upper airway for sleep and breathing, case finishing must address the chief concerns of each patient, which vary from orthodontic concerns, pain issues, esthetic considerations as well as sleep-related breathing disorders.

Requirements of a biomimetic oral appliance

According to the spatial matrix hypothesis (Singh, 2004), four tissue groups need to be addressed for craniofacial correction. These include: the hard tissues (bones of the jaws, the cervical vertebrae, etc.), soft tissues (muscles of the face and mastication, including the tongue), dental tissues (deciduous and permanent teeth, including the third molars), and functional spaces (such as the upper airway and TMJ spaces). Currently, there is a plethora of dental, orthodontic, and oral sleep appliances, including oral orthotics and mouthguards that were historically introduced and are still available. Each appliance makes general and/or specific claims, some of which are/are not supported by the peer-reviewed medical, dental and orthodontic literature. In addition, in each device category, there are subdivisions, such as removable, functional, and fixed orthodontic appliances. In turn, some but not all of these appliances are recognized by regulatory bodies, such as the US Food and Drug Administration (FDA), and verified as being relatively safe for the conditions that they attempt to address with low or moderate risks, including side-effects. For example, numerous oral appliances are categorized as mandibular advancement devices (MADs), which are cleared by the FDA for the treatment of mild to moderate obstructive sleep apnea (OSA) in adults. In this case, several appliances are putatively designed to deliver the same treatment effect. In that context, what is the need for yet another set of devices?

Prior to the introduction of the Daytime-Nighttime Appliance (DNA appliance®) system, and after the publication of the first edition of this book, I reviewed 148 appliances (Singh and Clark, 2001; Singh and Thind, 2003; Veis and Christian, 2004; Singh *et al.*, 2005; Singh *et al.*, 2007; Singh and Abramson, 2008; Singh *et al.*, 2009; Singh *et al.*, 2009) and noted that some of the findings were rather interesting. I was able to assess the advantages, deficiencies, and risks of various appliances; and since the unifying principle on how various oral devices work had been predicted in the spatial matrix hypothesis (Singh, 2004), I only then started working on a family of devices that would be relatively comfortable to wear and relatively easy to adjust. This means that the materials, designs and protocols would have to be based on the evidence available in the medical, dental, and orthodontic literature that described the effects of a particular approach or technique on the hard tissues, soft tissues, dental tissues, and functional spaces in the craniofacial region, in accord with the spatial matrix hypothesis.

In one early study, we evaluated 3D changes in nasal morphology in babies born with unilateral cleft lip and palate who were treated with a presurgical nasoalveolar molding (NAM) appliance to correct the nasolabio-alveolar deformity (Singh *et al.*, 2005). The treatment goal was to permit these babies to breathe through the nose and feed through the mouth. A follow-up study (Singh *et al.*, 2007) showed that the facial development in these children was virtually indistinguishable from a control group of non-cleft children. **Therefore, one aspect of biomimetic oral appliance design is to restore nasal function and enhance nasal symmetry, to improve the ability to breathe through the nose**. This feature was addressed in adults in a further study (Singh and Abramson, 2008). To determine nasal airway patency, acoustic rhinometry was undertaken before and after the placement of a nasal dilation appliance. Size and shape changes were found, suggesting that an oral appliance can have the ability of intra-oral nasal dilation, especially in the management cases where nasal obstruction is demonstrable, such as SDB, snoring, upper airway resistance syndrome, obstructive sleep apnea, and similar conditions. The two issues of external morphologic nasal symmetry and internal nasal architecture were addressed in several other studies using biomimetic oral device designs. Harris and Singh (2013) and Singh and Cress (2013) reported improved soft tissue nasal symmetry in adult patients (Fig. 1 and Fig. 12) while Singh *et al.* (2016) and Singh and Kim (2020) showed an enhancement in nasal airway volume by approx. 2–3cm^3 measured in 3D CBCT scans of adults treated with biomimetic oral appliance therapy.

The floor of the nose is the roof of the mouth and if the nasal airway is deficient then the upper arch might also reflect this. Banabilh *et al.* (2009) studied upper arch morphology in over 100 Asian adults that had been tested for OSA with an overnight sleep study in a university hospital ENT department. Finite-element analysis (FEM) showed that the upper arch was narrower in the transverse plane in patients with OSA, while the lower arch was shorter in the antero-posterior plane compared to matched controls. Specifically, we reported that concentric arch collapse appeared to be an etiological factor associated with OSA in adults. **Therefore, another feature that needs to be addressed by a comprehensive oral device is midfacial hypoplasia and mandibular retrognathia**. In that latter respect, the Twin-block appliance (TBA) is currently favored in cases of mandibular retrognathia in children with or without a diagnosis of OSA. Therefore, a study was performed to assess changes in midfacial and mandibular morphology in pediatric cases with Class II malocclusions exhibiting an increased overjet treated using a TBA. The lateral cephalographs of 100 patients aged 7–16 years were compared (Singh and Hodge, 2002). The results, after correcting for size, using geometric morphometric analyses indicated that midfacial distances proportionately decreased in cases treated with TBA. Furthermore, after scaling to equivalent size, graphical analysis showed antero-posterior compression of the midface in the region of prosthion, i.e. posterior displacement of prosthion or midfacial retrusion. Thus, supposed improvements in facial balance following TBA treatment were associated with a relative restriction of anterior growth within the midface, by exerting a growth-inhibitory effect on the maxilla — the so-called 'headgear effect'. In adults, Singh and Thind (2003) studied patients with Class II malocclusion treated with headgear and a Teuscher appliance (HATA). Pre- and post-treatment cephalographs were tested using FEM to localize and quantify any differences. Traditional cephalometry again showed that the angle SNA decreased while the angle SNB increased, as expected but the question remains: How was this net effect attained? FEM revealed increased size in the mandibular ramus and body, while the lip region was diminished (approx. 20% in females). Thus, in the attainment of facial balance, both male and female patients treated for Class II malocclusion using HATA exhibit antero-posterior restraint of the maxilla, which is associated with overall changes in the soft tissue profile. It can be speculated that while the orthodontic concerns of an increased overjet have been addressed, these types of protocols may elevate the risk of children and adults developing SDB through nasal obstruction, especially if they become obese. **These findings when re-examined in the current context suggest that separation of maxillary development and mandibular repositioning is a requirement for biomimetic devices that attempt craniofacial correction.**

In addition to the above, controversy exists regarding maxillary bone growth changes in adults; some claim that the craniofacial sutures are synostosed in adulthood, but other studies, especially in forensic medicine refute this assertion. For example, sutural width measurement is used by forensic pathologists to estimate the age at death of victims in certain cases (Masset, 1989). Using a different approach to determine sutural synostosis in adults, we investigated the link between bruxism and temporal bone mobility associated with multiple sclerosis (Williams *et al.*, 2011). To quantify the degree of sutural movement at the temporo-parietal (squamosal) suture during clenching, an ultrasonic pulsed phase locked loop technique was used. For the control subjects the average movement was found to be 0.27mm, which represents the normal sutural width of approx. 0.25mm (100–400µm; 250µm on average). In patients with multiple sclerosis the movement was 1.7mm. Therefore, although this particular study found marked displacement of the temporal bones in patients with multiple sclerosis, the control subjects showed a normal range of sutural widths consistent with sutural homeostasis. However, previous studies on craniofacial suture behavior, such as that during palatal expansion, have relied on 2D cephalometric analyses, which may be unable to capture 3D phenomena. In one study, the midpalatal sutural width was measured along with overall upper arch width in children. The researchers were unable to explain how the palate got wider without the width of the midpalatal suture showing any significant change in width (Vizzotto *et al.*, 2008). We now suspect that these clinical findings can be explained by sutural homeostasis as discussed previously. Heit *et al.* (2014) investigated 2D and 3D midfacial bone parameters in 'non-growing' adults that had been diagnosed with midfacial hypoplasia. Instead of using a standard palatal expander, a biomimetic oral device was used. We found that the mean transpalatal bone width increased statistically from 33.5mm to 35.8mm, while the mean midfacial bone volume increased significantly from 17.4cm^3 to 19.1cm^3 ± 2.6 after biomimetic oral appliance therapy. **Therefore, biomimetic device design must include components that take advantage of potential sutural osteogenesis** as a basis for induced maxillary morphogenesis.

In addition, it has been shown that when the spatial position of the mandible is changed, the pattern of gene expression is also changed

(Fuentes *et al.*, 2003). Thus, a biomimetic oral device has occlusal coverage that permits changes in mandibular position. There is some debate as to whether the occlusal coverage ought to be symmetric or unilateral. In a study in rats (D'Attilio *et al.*, 2005), it was found that the introduction of an asymmetric interference of the occlusion produced a disruption of systemic posture, as confirmed by radiographs, and that removal of the interference resulted in normalization of the spinal alignment. For these and other reasons, the **use of a unilateral bit block ought to be avoided**, although some intransigents still attempt this approach, perhaps unaware of its potential risks. Therefore, a biomimetic oral device has symmetric occlusal coverage or bilateral posterior occlusal stops. However, changes in the midface need to be coordinated with the mandible. Thus, in addition to upper devices, a set of lower biomimetic oral devices that follow the same principles is also needed. These lower devices may have an acrylic baseplate, a wire framework and/or may incorporate a 'screw-fin' mechanism (mRNA appliance®) that stabilizes the mandible in a forward position similar to other mandibular advancement devices. The difference in this protocol is that the upper acrylic-based or wireframe devices are worn for approx. 12–16hrs in total, whereas the lower component of the mRNA appliance is typically worn for approx. 8hrs only during sleep.

Another essential difference between mandibular advancement device therapy and biomimetic oral appliance therapy is that the midface is all but ignored in the former but comprehensively addressed in the latter. Not surprisingly, therefore, there is much controversy in dental sleep medicine concerning 'bite changes' that occur as a side effect of MAD therapy. To address this concern a biomimetic oral device must address dental (tooth) tissues. As mentioned earlier, ultra-light forces are thought to be detected by stretch-sensitive genes that are found in stem cells distributed in the craniofacial region, such as the periosteum covering the underlying bones, and localized at various sutures within the craniofacial architecture (Ansari *et al.*, 2017). Furthermore, El-Bialy *et al.* (2004) have shown root resorption repair using ultrasound in orthodontic patients. In fact, orthodontists have been using a variety of finger springs, flap springs, coiled springs, etc. for tooth alignment for centuries. However, I noticed that these springs have limited contact with the tooth surfaces; they simply act as spring levers that predominantly tip the anterior teeth. Bearing in mind my research background in craniofacial, molecular, and genetic biology, I soon realized that this design was deficient and patented my 3D axial springs™, which have a compressible 3D design and, being fabricated from a super-elastic nickel-free alloy, have the capability of exerting cyclic, intermittent signals, which can enhance bone development, as discussed earlier and, therefore, tooth alignment. Thus, the biomimetic oral device uses 3D axial springs, which are fabricated from a super-elastic, nickel-free alloy. One of the properties of this material is cyclic, intermittent signals (ultra-light forces). In addition, the Wireframe device has midline anterior and posterior omega loops (see below), which are also formed from the same super-elastic, nickel-free alloy as the 3D axial springs, to gently stretch the overlying midfacial sutural system and periosteum.

When using the PACE protocol, consideration is also given to the other facial components, such as the soft tissues of the face and neck. During craniofacial correction, the goal of biomimetic oral devices is to normalize the overbite and overjet relations to within normal limits (WNL) of the soft tissue facial profile. In order to address this requirement, a study was performed on Korean adults using biomimetic oral appliance therapy (Singh and Kim, 2016). Craniofacial parameters were measured on standardized lateral photographs, and the mean configurations were subjected to statistical and geometric morphometric analyses. The results showed that the labiomental angle statistically improved from 126° to 134° (similar to the findings in the pediatric studies; Singh and Clark, 2003). Moreover, the thyromental angle improved significantly from 126.5° to 118.5° ($p < 0.01$). Therefore, this study supports the notion that the PACE protocol may enhance not only maxillo-mandibular relations, but also decreases the risk of SDB in adults since a smaller thyromental angle is associated with a lower severity of OSA (Lam *et al.*, 2005).

Bearing in mind the above, **another principle of biomimetic oral appliance therapy is enhancement of the upper airway**. In one of the first studies of its kind, we assessed the response of the upper airway following palatal expansion in children (Singh *et al.*, 2007). The pre- and post-treatment lateral cephalographs of children (aged approx. 13yrs) were compared after about 21 months of treatment. Using pseudo-colored FEM, a 30% increase in nasopharyngeal airway area was found above and behind the soft palate. In addition, a 23% increase in oropharyngeal airway area was located behind the base of the tongue allied with a 9% increase in hypopharyngeal area near the hyoid bone. It was concluded that morphologic airway improvements are associated with oral appliance therapy in actively growing patients. This finding is now attributed to 'palatal expansion' in the medical literature since numerous studies on children have verified both the morphologic and functional upper airway improvements. However, the effect of this approach on adults was unknown until Singh and Krumholtz (2009) showed that 'palatal expansion' in adults had very similar effects. Using pseudo-colored FEM, we found a 22% increase in nasopharyngeal airway area located above and behind the soft palate as well as a 16% increase in oropharyngeal airway area behind the base of the tongue with a 13% increase in hypopharyngeal area near the level of the hyoid bone. Therefore, I first suggested that midfacial development might be a potential solution in cases of both adult and pediatric OSA, as alluded to earlier in this book. However, other approaches that prevent collapse of the upper airway in adults are also needed. In one study (Singh *et al.*, 2009) we investigated the effects of a 'tail' extending from the back of an oral appliance that depressed the tongue during sleep. The idea originated from the historical use of obturators utilized in the treatment of cleft palate cases, especially those with a cleft soft palate. In adults diagnosed with OSA, use of the device during sleep resulted in the AHI falling by 73% and the SaO_2 improving from 84% to 89%. It was concluded that a 'tail' added to an oral appliance is an effective approach in the management of OSA, but similar to MADs and CPAP, an extension used to depress the tongue represents a life-time of overnight use. On the other hand, a biomimetic oral device or protocol that mimics natural behavior should not require lifelong wear, thus it was further concluded that an extension added as a pharyngeal stent to a biomimetic oral appliance might be an alternative approach in the management of OSA. Thus, although further studies are ongoing, **the biomimetic approach attempts to target the site and severity of craniofacial issues in both adult and pediatric sleep disordered breathing**. In addition to these changes in design and materials, all subjects are instructed to wear the biomimetic oral device during the late afternoon, early evening and at night time (ideally for approx. 12–16hrs in total), but not during the daytime and not while eating, partly in line with the circadian rhythm of tooth eruption (Proffit and Frazier-Bowers, 2009), although this has only been demonstrated in premolar teeth in young patients. Nevertheless, it is known that human growth hormone peaks during stage N3 sleep at night in adults. Therefore, the epigenetic-pneumopedic protocol adopted is in line with the circadian rhythm as far as possible. In fact, biomimetic oral appliance therapy is based on a family of devices that share specific components, materials and protocol. It is not a series of appliances like clear tray aligners, but rather a suite of devices that are customized to meet the patient's requirements as outlined in the diagnostic process discussed in the previous chapter. This suite of biomimetic oral appliances includes the Daytime-Nighttime Appliance (DNA appliance®) as well as the mandibular Repositioning Nighttime Appliance (mRNA appliance®) prescribed as:

- Upper and/or lower acrylic-based DNA appliance®
- Upper and/or lower Wireframe DNA appliance®
- Upper Hybrid DNA appliance®
- Acrylic-based or Wireframe mRNA appliance®

All of these designs can be extended with a pharyngeal stent in cases diagnosed with OSA, and all of these biomimetic oral devices are either FDA registered and/or FDA cleared for mild-moderate OSA at the time of writing.

3D axial springs™

One unique feature in all biomimetic oral appliances are the (patented) 3D axial springs™. These springs are different from traditional orthodontic finger-springs in several different ways. First, the design of the springs is a 3D configuration of loops and this means that the springs are compressible in the vertical axis (Fig. 66). It is a well-known orthodontic principle that the more wire in the spring loops, the lighter the force, and the longer the distance over which it will be effective. Thus, each 3D-axial spring has five loops, but if the clinical crown height is short, for example in deciduous teeth, this can be reduced to three loops. On swallowing, the opposing teeth gently come into contact with the device and a light force is exerted, which compresses the springs momentarily. This compression represents potential energy and when the force is released, the potential energy is dissipated as kinetic energy in the form of vibration (Fig. 67). This response is undetected by the human eye and causes no intra-oral pain or discomfort. The reason for the vibrational response is the nature of the spring's material, which is a nickel-free, super-elastic alloy. It is known that these materials transmit uniform, low magnitude pressures to the teeth (Niinomi *et al.* 2012) with the subject activating a mild force on biting.

Second, unlike orthodontic finger-springs, the 3D axial springs are adapted to the palatal surfaces of the anterior teeth (Fig. 66a). This design

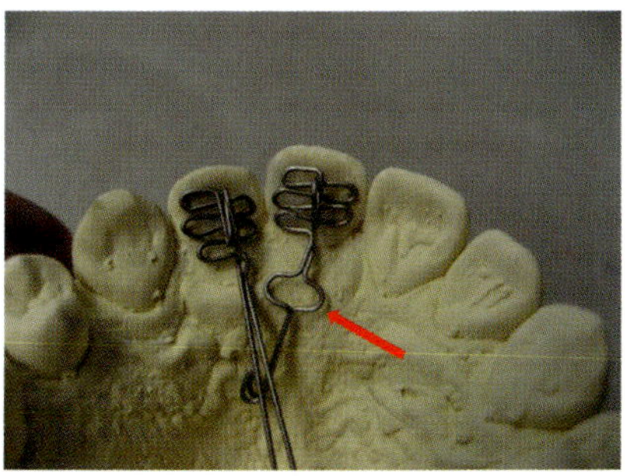

Figure 66a: 3D axial springs shown on study model with the one on the right showing a 'C loop' (arrow).

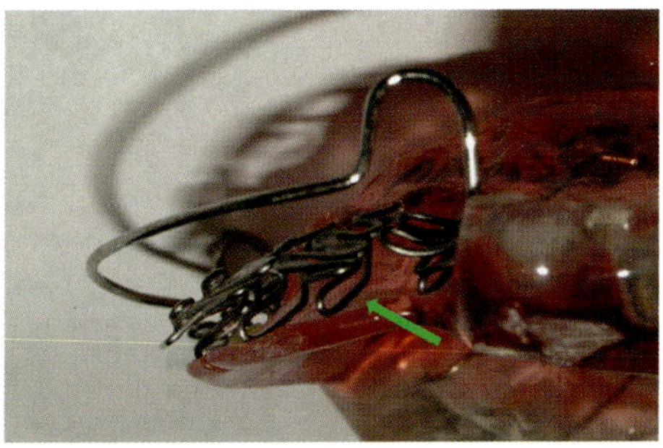

Figure 66b: 3D axial springs shown in an upper device. The heads of the springs clearly show a vertical spring loop (arrow).

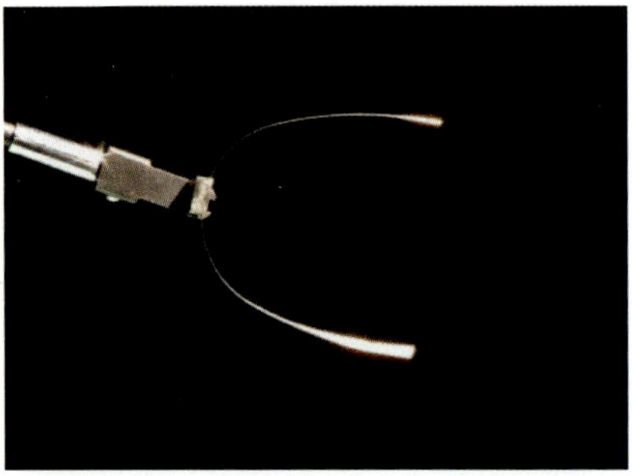

Figure 67a: Super-elastic wire showing vibrational response at its two free ends but not at the fixed point.

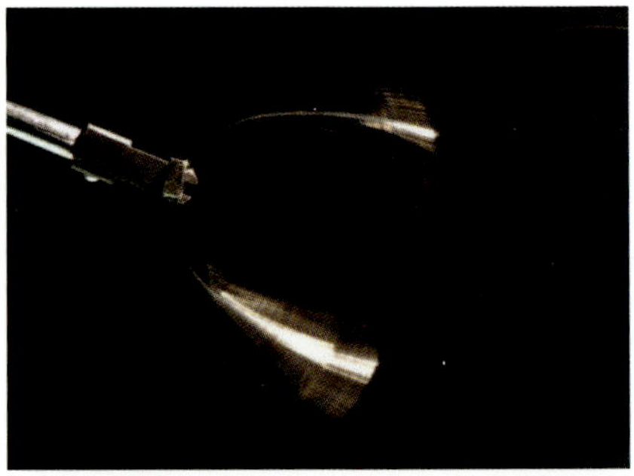

Figure 67b: Super-elastic wire showing frozen vibrational motion using a high shutter speed camera.

means that instead of exerting a single point of force like a finger-spring, the 3D axial springs dissipate the signal over a larger surface area. In effect, the wire material produces cyclic, intermittent signals (ultra-light forces). As mentioned earlier, these ultra-light forces are detected by stretch-sensitive stem cells that are found in the periodontium (Jia *et al.*, 2019), distributed in other craniofacial regions such as the periosteum covering the underlying bones, and localized at various sutures within the craniofacial architecture (Zhao *et al.*, 2015). Earlier, O'Neal *et al.* (1994) reviewed the regenerative capacities of the periodontium, while Basdra and Komposch (1997) characterized isolated fibroblasts from the human periodontium. They indicated that these cells exhibit phenotypic characteristics consistent with osteoblasts, suggesting that they have the potential to differentiate into osteoblasts and deposit bone. Furthermore, Kopher *et al.* (2003) have shown that intermittent stretch of sutures results in new bone formation in rabbits, while Williams and Murphy (2008) have shown *de novo* woven bone formation in adults in response to ultra-light forces. Therefore, the 3D axial springs may enable bone formation, likely in conjunction with gentle stretch of the overlying midfacial periosteum and sutural system from the remainder of the particular device design.

In addition, teeth in contact with the 3D axial springs can simultaneously be orthodontically aligned/advanced, particularly in those cases incorporating a C loop 3D axial spring design (Fig. 66a). In this new generation of biomimetic oral appliances, the 3D axial springs typically have a mesio-distal width of 6mm for upper anterior teeth, 5mm for lower anterior teeth, and 8mm for posterior teeth. Classically, the 3D axial springs are only found on the anterior six upper and lower teeth. The reason for this design is twofold. First, the premaxillary-maxillary suture undergoes synostosis in the deciduous dentition, which means antero-posterior bone formation is less prominent in this region since the human face does not grow forward *per se*. This mode of development also means that crowding is more likely to occur in the anterior region of the arch. Second, in the mandible, the midline mandibular symphysis undergoes ossification, and thus the periodontium is the predominant bone-forming mechanism during the eruption of permanent maxillary and mandibular anterior teeth. Further distally, in the maxilla the midpalatal suture can be used for bone formation, while the condyles provide that ability in the mandible. Therefore, 3D axial springs are most often found on the anterior six teeth. However, if an isolated posterior tooth is palatally or lingually displaced or in crossbite then an additional 3D axial spring can be placed on that particular tooth to help in its orthodontic alignment. In any case, the baseplate of the device should only extend as far as the first loop of the 3D axial springs. The 3D axial springs should not be entrapped by acrylic and should be free to vibrate. In addition, the stem or tail of the spring should be embedded closer to the fitting surface of the device and away from the polished surface since adjustments to the device's fitting surface will be made to permit the remodeling process.

Device designs

Acrylic-based DNA appliance®

In the acrylic-based upper device, the baseplate extends as far anteriorly as the first loop of the 3D axial springs (Fig. 68) and it may extend distally to the last standing tooth or it might be extended only as far as the mesial

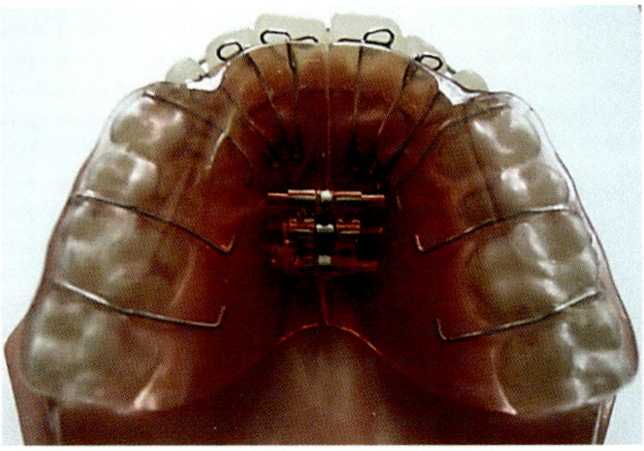

Figure 68a: Upper acrylic-based design showing sagittal split with baseplate extending to first loops of springs.

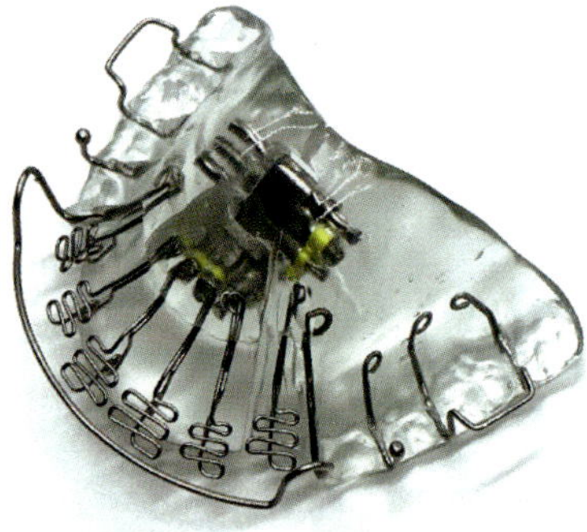

Figure 68b: Upper acrylic-based design showing Y-split and 3-way screw with baseplate extending to second molars.

aspect of the second maxillary molars. In this latter design, the clinician is using the second molars as an initial guide on how much development might be needed in the medio-lateral axis in a specific case. If the upper archform is narrow transversely, a mid-sagittal split with a transverse screw can be used (Fig. 68a) to increase the transpalatal bone width. More commonly, in a tapered archform, in order to achieve concentric development, a Y-split design of the acrylic baseplate distal to the maxillary lateral incisors or cuspids (Fig. 68b) might be deployed. In the former, the split lies above the original site of the premaxillary-maxillary suture. Although most believe that this suture is invariably synostosed during the primary dentition, others (e.g. Trevizan and Consolaro, 2017) believe that the premaxilla is an independent bone that becomes semi-independent and is finally fully integrated into the maxilla. Until that time, the premaxillary-maxillary suture may be used orthopedically to influence anterior facial growth. Therefore, in conjunction with a Y-split design, a 3-way expansion screw might be placed anteriorly, especially if reduction of a 'gummy smile' through anterior bone remodeling is anticipated. Alternatively, separate antero-posterior (AP) and transverse (TV) expansion screws might be utilized, if sufficient space permits, for differential development of the AP and TV axes, especially if the premolar spaces need to be re-captured. In these cases, a mesial 'stop' is placed on the last standing premolar so that the space regained is localized to the premolar region. In cases where asymmetric development is indicated, say in the case of a unilateral missing premolar, a cruciform split can be used, incorporating two separate anterior screws with an additional TV screw further distally.

It is important to note that the change in spatial relations initiates the remodeling process, in accord with the spatial matrix hypothesis. The role of the screw(s) is to keep up with the changes, and to maintain gentle tension when the device is being worn. **Unlike other palatal expansion protocols, the screw(s) are not used as the primary driver for expansion**, and over-expansion must be avoided at all times. With gradual tissue response, it's imperative to not impede bone remodeling. Thus, unlike some other palatal expanders, the fitting surface acrylic does not contact the mucosa of the hard palate and a separation exists between the palate and the device. This space becomes filled with saliva during device wear. As the patient swallows this saliva, a relative negative pressure is created and the patient 'sucks' on the device. This suction effect is well known in dental prosthetics when complete dentures are worn. The effect of this suction is that it pulls on the oral mucosa and the underlying mucoperiosteum, which in turn gently stretches the midpalatal suture, thereby encouraging the remodeling process.

Changes in the spatial position of the mandible are associated with changes in gene expression (Fuentes *et al.*, 2003). For example, if an occlusal restoration is 100μm (0.1mm) too high, a patient will be able to detect this occlusal change. Thus, even subtle changes in mandibular position may be sufficient to kick start the remodeling process. Therefore, for the remodeling process to be initiated it is not unusual to use (minimal) occlusal coverage of the upper arch (Fig. 68) to reposition mandible close to its optimal position as a starting point, using an appropriate bite registration. Generally speaking, the occlusal pads need to have a smooth and even surface with no occlusal interference so that that the midface is free to develop in 3D space while the mandible is free to move in 3D space. The device's occlusal coverage represents the initial bite registration, but also the approximate (physiologic) finishing positioning of the mandible. At the delivery appointment, it's unlikely that much occlusal grinding will be required, especially if the device has been fabricated following the bite registration provided. However, as treatment proceeds, this step may become increasingly important, as outlined below. This means that any occlusal acrylic will need to be reduced and/or removed throughout treatment. Using selective grinding, it's important to equilibrate the occlusal pads and gradually reduce/remove the occlusal acrylic to permit the lower teeth to track the subtle changes in occlusion as treatment progresses.

In order to ensure anterior bone remodeling/development, a round labial bow is used as a lip bumper. This labial bow is used to keep the upper lip away from the anterior teeth, forming a new spatial matrix. The lip musculature will be activated, sometimes producing esthetic changes. In fact, in cases where lip development is sought, an additional sleeve is sometimes placed on the labial bow. On the other hand, the labial bow should not be in contact with the labial surfaces of the anterior teeth, otherwise it will simply be acting as a retainer by preventing tooth movements. Tooth movements are secondary to functional space, appropriate signaling, and clinical guidance. As noted in Chapter 4, mechanically induced inflammation permits orthodontic tooth movements (Roberts and Hartsfield, 2004). In contrast, force is not a pre-requisite for biomimetic tooth movement. In this case, the non-inflammatory pathways of tooth movement, such as passive eruption, mesial drift, and 'relapse' are invoked for craniofacial correction, likely secondary to bone remodeling. Thus, the labial bow may contact a specific tooth if no tooth movement is desired. Typically, the labial bow extends from the distal aspects of the canines with a 0.5mm to 1mm gap from the labial surfaces of the teeth unless contact is due to the position of a tooth. In other cases, a short labial bow, extending from the distal aspect of the lateral incisors might be more preferable. In some cases where the teeth are well-aligned, a wrap-round labial bow that extends from the molar regions might be appropriate. In all cases, acting somewhat to Frankel's vestibular shields (Aytan *et al.*, 1989),

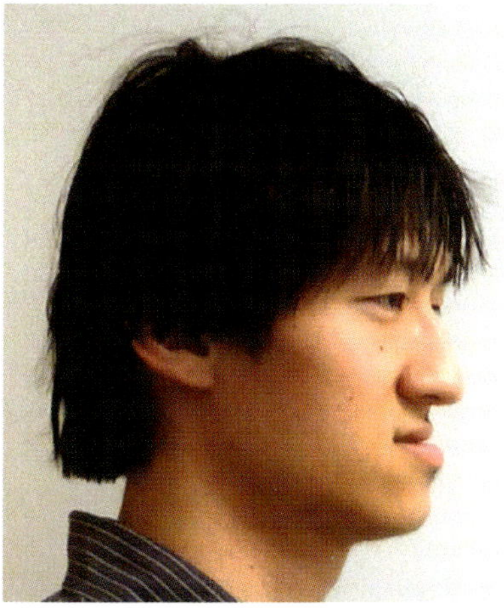

Figure 69a: Pre-treatment lateral photograph of adult showing midfacial deficiency. Courtesy: Dr Lihua Zhang

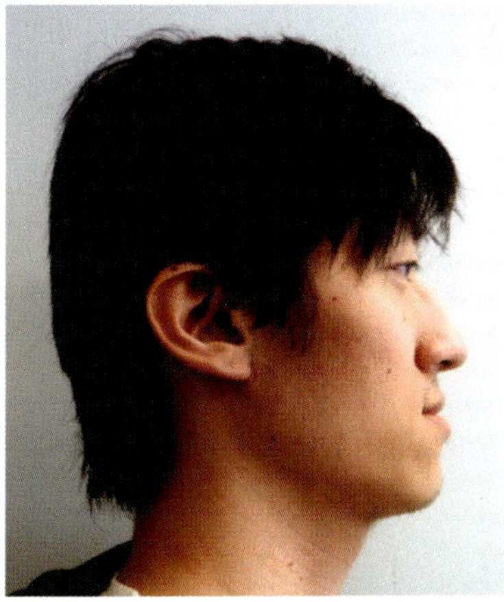

Figure 69b: Post-treatment lateral photograph of same adult showing midfacial development in the sagittal plane.

the labial bow keeps the lips and cheeks away from the teeth, forming a new spatial matrix into which development can occur.

In order to be retentive, clasps are needed to attach the device to the teeth. Classically, Adams clasps are sufficient but in some cases ball clasps are preferred. In cases where additional retention is required, delta clasps can be used and, if retention is an issue, then Crozat clasps can be used; making the device removable, at least in name. Note that the device only touches the patient's tissues in two places: at the clasps and at the 3D axial springs. This design ensures comfort for the patient, but each biomimetic oral appliance has six degrees of freedom: six for the teeth and six for the bone, making it unique. For bone development in the antero-posterior plane, 3D axial springs are placed on the anterior six teeth. Clinical cases show the extent of AP midfacial development (Fig. 69), representing two degrees of freedom. Next, medio-lateral expansion at the midpalatal suture using a screw tension system increases transpalatal bone width (Fig. 70; Singh *et al.*, 2014), representing another two degrees of freedom. Finally, the occlusal

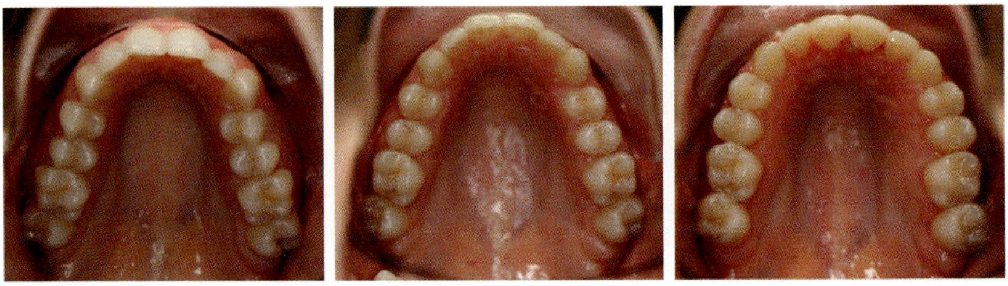

Figure 70: Pre-treatment (left), mid-treatment (middle), and post-treatment (right) intra-oral photographs of an adult case showing increased transpalatal bone width following biomimetic oral appliance therapy. Courtesy: Dr Tammarie Heit

pads permit condylar bone formation and correction of a deep overbite, giving a total of six degrees of freedom for the bone. Similarly, for the teeth, the 3D axial springs permit antero-posterior tooth movement. In addition, an increased inter-molar width accompanies an increased transpalatal bone width since the posterior teeth remain in homeostasis with bone remodeling (Fig. 70). Finally, supra-eruption of teeth in the inferior-superior plane provides a total of six degrees of freedom for the teeth.

Wireframe DNA appliance®

As noted above, biomimetic oral appliances are a suite of devices that are customized to meet a patient's requirements. However, some patients find it difficult to tolerate a device that has palatal coverage. These patients may be mouth-breathers, may have nasal obstruction, or may gag when a device covers the palate. In these cases, the same principles for craniofacial correction apply and the same materials are deployed but the device design has to be modified to meet the patient's concerns. Thus, in the Wireframe DNA appliance® design, the palatal acrylic and screw system is replaced with a double omega loop design instead. The device has an anterior or minor omega loop as well as a posterior or major omega loop (Fig. 71). The shape of the omega loops permits widening of the palate without using a screw system since the omega loops lie in a plane parallel to the palate.

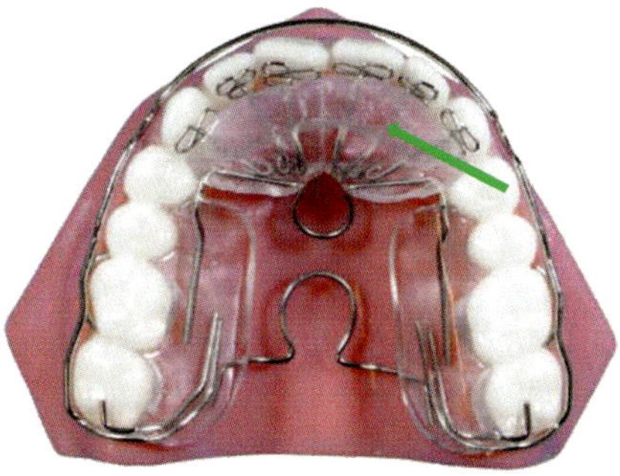

Figure 71a: Wireframe DNA appliance showing omega loops and anterior bite ramp/ tongue-trainer (arrowed).

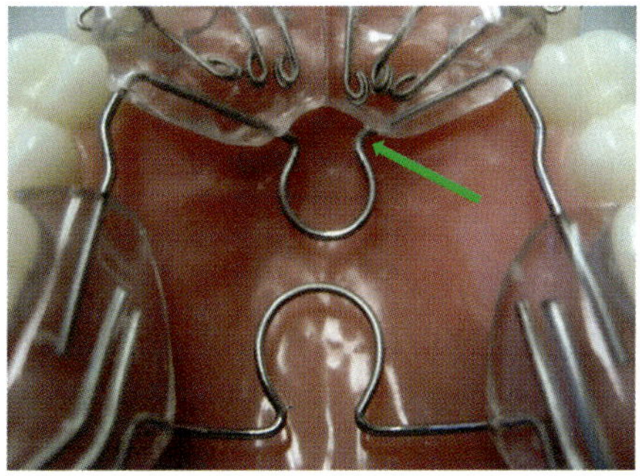

Figure 71b: Close-up of omega loops showing clearance for counter-loops (arrowed) of anterior omega loop.

In so doing, the space for the tongue is not encroached upon and the patient finds the device comfortable to wear. The wire used to construct the anterior and posterior omega loops is the same super-elastic, nickel-free wire as the 3D axial springs; however, the gauge of the omega loop wire is heavier. The activation of the device remains biomimetic. In other words, when the patient swallows, the tongue compresses the omega loops and upon release the vibrational response is thought to stimulate palatal remodeling. Both the anterior and posterior omega loops are adjusted periodically during treatment to keep up with the developmental changes. Note that in cases where additional anterior development is indicated, the use of two mini-omega loops can be added to help guide the anterior segments in a forward direction.

To encourage proper swallowing and tongue placement, a tongue-trainer (Fig. 71a) is used for myo-spatial correction. The tongue trainer is found in the anterior palatal region and serves at least two functions. First, it provides a smooth landing place for the tongue, and second, with the tongue sitting on the anterior region of the palate, the upper airway is opened, and breathing is enhanced. In addition, however, the tongue trainer also embeds the 3D axial springs as well as the anterior omega loop. Thus, when the tongue sits on the anterior ramp, the 3D axial springs are compressed and are activated upon release. If needed, the anterior acrylic can act as a bite plane, for example when the overbite is increased. In these cases, the anterior acrylic should be finished in balanced contact with the lower anterior teeth. Thus, it is not unusual for the lower anterior teeth to make light contact with the anterior bite ramp/tongue-trainer (Fig. 71a), and proactively compress the 3D axial springs, although ideally, a tripod of support should be attained. Note also that the acrylic of the tongue trainer extends as far anteriorly as the first loops of the 3D axial springs, and it is split in half in the midline so that palatal development can proceed in an unimpeded fashion. Moreover, it's important that the contra-loops (Fig. 71b) of the anterior omega loop are free from acrylic to permit its adjustments. In addition, the tongue-trainer is split bilaterally from the posterior acrylic that embeds the posterior omega loop, the cut being distal to the cuspids (Fig. 71a). Therefore, the tongue-trainer provides myo-spatial correction since the muscles of the tongue are trained to occupy a new spatial matrix for the upper airway, and muscle memory is used to maintain that correction. These components are predominantly acting on the anterior aspect of the palate similar to the AP component of a 3-way screw.

The posterior omega loop predominantly acts on the posterior aspect of the palate similar to the TV component of a 3-way screw. It is embedded in the distal portions of acrylic and separated from the anterior part of the device so that appropriate adjustments can be made somewhat independently. The posterior omega loop is approx. 3mm distal to the anterior or minor omega loop; not in contact with it for ease of adjustment, and it does not overlap the anterior omega loop. Minimal amounts of acrylic are used for retention of the wire components, which also include occlusal stops. These occlusal rests usually pass over the distal marginal ridge of the last standing molar or sometimes lie in the disto-palatal groove of the first permanent molar, depending on the case. Either way, the job of the distal stops is to 'trip' the mandible and prevent it from occluding in its habitual position. This change in the spatial position of the mandible is associated with changes in gene expression, which is thought to be a component of the corrective mechanism. The change in the spatial matrix is also aided by a wrap-round labial bow (Fig. 71a). The gauge of the labial bow wire is the same as that used in the acrylic-based design but in this case, it's soldered to the retentive C clasps that engage the mesial and distal undercuts of the first molar. If increased retention is required, a composite ledge or button can be bonded on to the buccal surface of the molars, to give the clasps a 'snap-on' fit. This technique avoids over-adjustment of the soldered C clasps that can fatigue or occasionally fracture with overuse. The wrap-round or circumferential labial bow keeps the lips and cheeks away from the tooth surfaces and provides space for the remodeling process and tooth movement as before.

Hybrid DNA appliance

The Hybrid DNA appliance is an upper device for patients that find it difficult to tolerate palatal coverage but may concurrently have a deep overbite, which requires recapture of the vertical dimension. In these cases, even though the same principles for craniofacial correction apply, the device design has to be modified to increase the vertical dimension, which cannot be easily done with the Wireframe appliance alone. Thus, the Hybrid DNA appliance® design largely follows the specification of the upper Wireframe design except that it has occlusal coverage on the posterior teeth (Fig. 72a). The occlusal pads

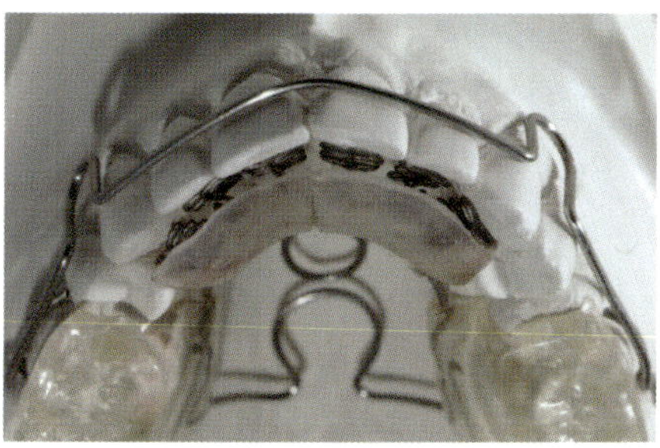

Figure 72a: Hybrid DNA appliance from palatal view showing occlusal pads, omega loops, and tongue-trainer.

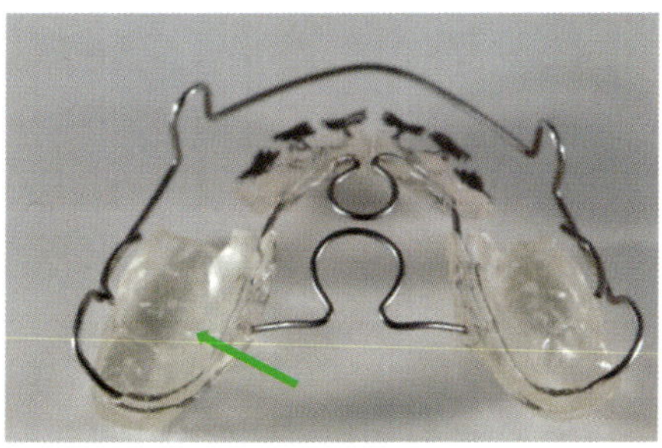

Figure 72b: Hybrid appliance showing fitting surface with occlusal pads (arrowed) and omegas loops.

may cover the molars only, or the bicuspids may also be included. Thus, in the Hybrid design (minimal) occlusal coverage of the upper arch (Fig. 72b) is used to reposition mandible close to its optimal position, using an appropriate bite registration. Again, the occlusal pads often have a smooth surface with no occlusal interferences so that that maxillary structures are free to develop three-dimensionally while the mandible is repositioned in 3D space.

The Hybrid appliance's occlusal coverage, indicated by the initial bite registration, also approximates the finishing positioning of the mandible. Thus, on insertion, little occlusal grinding is required but, as treatment proceeds, this step becomes increasingly important. At follow-up appointments, selective grinding is used to equilibrate the occlusal pads and permit the lower teeth to track the changes in occlusion. In addition, in these cases the anterior acrylic can be built up to act as a bite plane, so that the occlusal pads and anterior acrylic provide a tripod of support for the lower teeth.

Pharyngeal stent for OSA

Biomimetic oral devices target four craniofacial tissues for correction and these include the functional spaces, such as the upper airway. Therefore, in cases where obstruction of the retropalatal and/or retroglossal airway is demonstrable (for example, on a CBCT scan), the appliance design features the addition of a posterior midline extension for OSA. This pharyngeal stent takes the form of a wire loop extending from the distal-most aspect of the upper appliance (Fig. 73a). The extension curves away from the soft palate and extends behind the dorsal surface of the tongue, ending in a roller bead (Fig. 73b). In addition, a 'C loop' is incorporated into the extension so it can be lengthened or shortened, as well as being bent into the optimal position. The actual length of the pharyngeal stent varies as prescribed. First, the Mallampati score is used to classify the aperture of the upper airway. Since this static classification does not indicate the clinical behavior of the upper airway, I suggested that it would be useful to ask

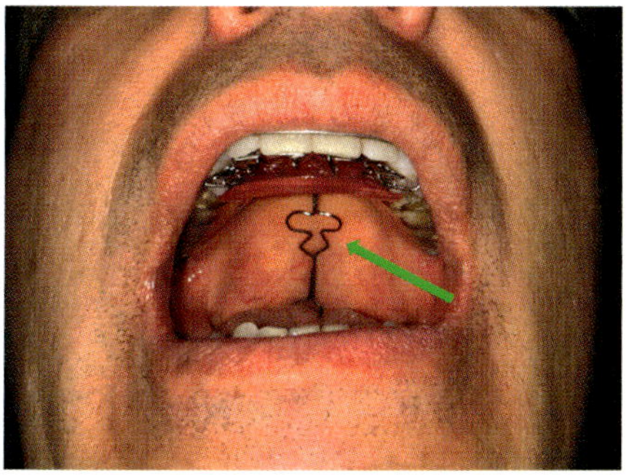

Figure 73a: Upper appliance showing pharyngeal extension with C loop (arrowed) for adjustability.

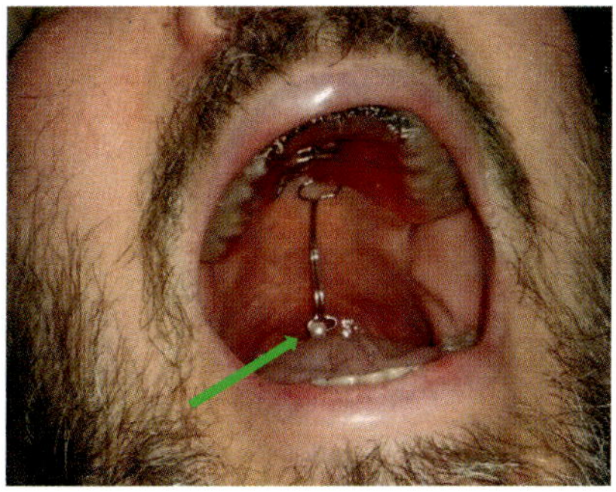

Figure 73b: Pharyngeal stent lying halfway between soft palate and tongue, showing roller ball (arrowed).

a patient to make the "Aaaah" sound for about 10 seconds to assess the functionality of the upper airway. For example, some patients can change a Mallampati Class IV to a Class I on phonation while others show little or no improvement. In these cases, a pharyngeal stent is needed to maintain the patency of the upper airway during sleep. Clinically, we simply ask the patient to say "Aaaaahhhh" and observe the behavior of the tongue and soft palate. Invariably, the Mallampati score changes and this response is used to estimate the approx. length and position of a pharyngeal stent. Thus, the desired length of the pharyngeal stent should always be part of the instructions received by the dental technicians fabricating the appliance.

On insertion, the stent should lie passively about halfway between the soft palate and the tongue (Fig. 73b). In the sitting or standing position, the stent does not contact any tissues and the patient may be unaware of the extension. If properly placed behind the tongue, the extension should not interfere with swallowing and if the patient finds it comfortable to wear, the gag reflex will not be initiated since the swallow reflex will predominate because of saliva flow. On first insertion, it's important to ascertain the ideal location for the stent, bearing in mind it may take 24–72hrs for the patient to habituate to this new spatial matrix. Often it is found that a correctly placed pharyngeal stent will improve the Mallampati score (Fig. 65) on placement, and this is one of the goals of the pharyngeal stent. On lying down, however, the tongue will fall back into the oropharynx where it will now contact the extension. In this case, the tongue will be guided forward to occupy its position on the anterior bite ramp/tongue trainer (Fig. 71a), thereby activating the device, as planned. In addition, with the tongue in this position, upper airway obstruction will be reduced and/or prevented since the airway is opened, and the patient should be able to tolerate the device easily. As well, on lying down the uvula may contact the extension. In this case, reflex contraction of the musculus uvulae will change the shape and/or position of the uvula. This little muscle maneuver will open the velopharyngeal isthmus, ensuring that nasal airflow can proceed behind the soft palate and into the hypopharynx. In fact, all the upper devices, be they acrylic-based, wireframed, or hybrids can be extended with a pharyngeal stent in cases diagnosed with OSA and upper airway obstruction. In recalcitrant cases, cold laser therapy can be used to shrink the tissues of the soft palate, uvula, and pillars of the fauces (Fig. 65). This technique temporarily prevents the gag reflex, and by the time the tissues rebound, most patients have acclimatized to the pharyngeal stent.

Lower acrylic-based DNA appliance®

Following 1–3 months of successful upper appliance therapy, it is essential to ensure that the lower arch maintains its coordination with developments in the upper arch. In order to achieve this, a lower device is invariably required. The lower acrylic-based DNA appliance® is somewhat similar to the upper, with six 3D axial springs acting on the lower anterior teeth (Fig. 74a). In addition, a TV screw is placed in the midline. The split in the acrylic lies above the former site of the mandibular symphysis although this is thought to synostose during the first postnatal year (Becker, 1986). Nevertheless, some are of the opinion that the hormone relaxin can affect the dentofacial sutures and similar structures, such as the mandibular symphysis, even in later life (Nicozisis *et al.*, 2000), while others believe that non-surgical mandibular expansion is feasible (Jäger *et al.*, 1990; Di Ventura

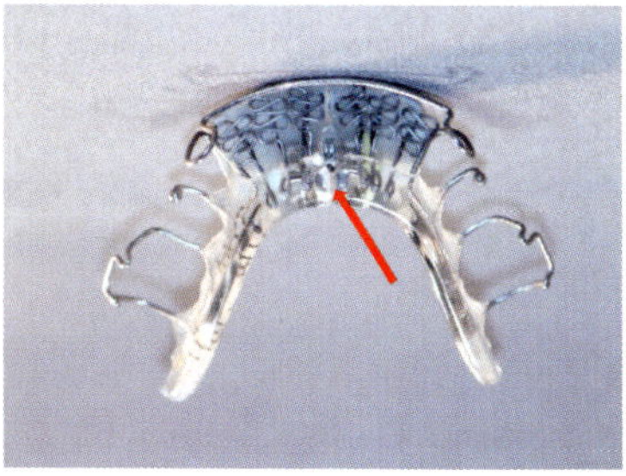

Figure 74a: Lower acrylic-based DNA appliance showing 3D axial springs and transverse screw in midline (arrow).

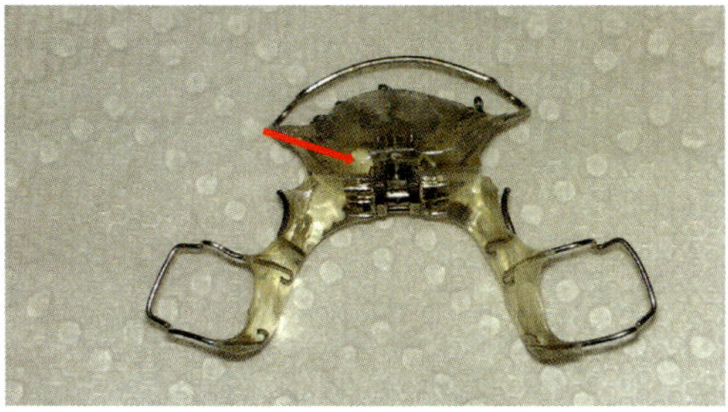

Figure 74b: Lower acrylic-based DNA appliance showing 3-way screw (arrow) for antero-posterior and transverse development.

et al., 2019). In some cases, severe lower anterior segment crowding is present (Fig. 50b and Fig. 51b). In these individuals a 3-way screw may be used if space is available (Fig. 74b). In other cases, a 3D axial spring may be omitted from the initial device until there is sufficient space. This spring can be added at a later date, especially if the device is re-lined or re-based after some development has been gained.

In order to change the spatial matrix, a labial bow is extended across the canine region, but it does not make contact with anterior teeth, keeping the lower lip at bay as described for the upper arch. For retention, Adams clasps are most often preferred on the molar teeth (Fig. 74). These clasps are used for retention of the device and do not impede bone remodeling or tooth movement. Importantly, the **lower device does not have any occlusal coverage**. Classically, the lower posterior teeth show developmental compensation and are lingually inclined. Following the cranio-caudal gradient of development, if the palate is narrow, the tongue adopts a lower posture and lies on the occlusal surfaces of the lower teeth. Over a period of time, the lower posterior segments become lingually inclined, sometimes showing 'cuspid drop-off' or a deep curve of Spee. In the biomimetic approach, the lower posterior segments are encouraged to upright and supra-erupt, especially if an increased overbite is diagnosed. Note that if a lower appliance with occlusal coverage is used, after a period of, say, 12 weeks, it is not unusual to find intrusion of the lower posterior segments and posterior open bite formation. This phenomenon most often occurs with (excessive) lower orthotic use. Therefore, no occlusal coverage is used in the lower acrylic-based DNA appliance® but adjustments, particularly in the disto-lingual flange region, may be needed as tissue remodeling progresses.

Lower Wireframe DNA appliance®

In some cases, only minor development of the lower arch is needed. In these cases, a lower Wireframe DNA appliance® may be indicated. The lower Wireframe DNA appliance is similar to the lower acrylic-based DNA appliance® since it also has the 3D axial springs on the lower six anterior teeth (Fig. 75a). These 3D axial springs have 5 loops if the crown length provides adequate space. For teeth with a short clinical crown height, fewer loops are acceptable; however, the head of each 3D axial spring needs to be in intimate contact with the lingual surface of each tooth. In some cuspids, the head of the spring needs to be curved or contoured to correspond to the lingual surface of a particular tooth. On lingually displaced teeth, 'C loops' can be integrated into the spring design. In this device, instead of a TV screw, an omega loop is placed in the midline (Fig. 75b) above the former site of the mandibular symphysis. This device design is only used if there is enough depth on the lower

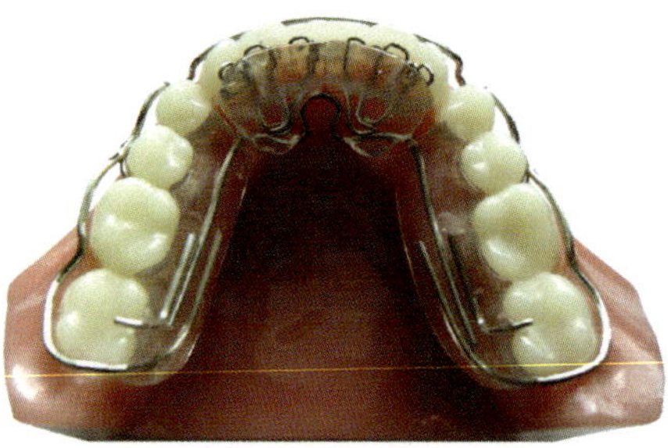

Figure 75a: Lower Wireframe appliance on model showing midline omega loop, 3D axial springs and occlusal stops.

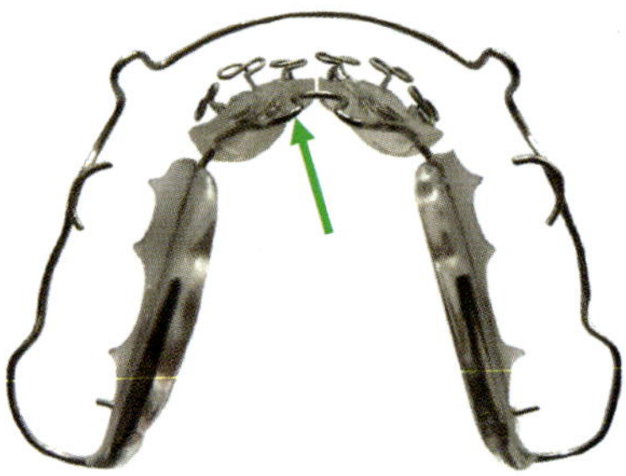

Figure 75b: Lower wireframe appliance viewed from below showing counter-loops (arrowed) of midline omega loop.

study model to accommodate all wire components as shown. The lingual omega loop is fashioned from 0.032-inch gauge super-elastic wire in the anterior portion of the appliance and is supported by acrylic, which has a mid-sagittal split, and has the 3D axial springs attached to it. The acrylic is trimmed back to the first loop of the spring, and approx. 50% of the legs of the springs are embedded into the acrylic to permit both spring adjustments and the vibrational response. The lingual omega loop is formed as an 'omega' with counter-loops (Fig. 75b), and not a 'U-shaped' loop, since the counter-loops must be free of acrylic for ease of adjustment. The legs of the omega loop (archform wire) are embedded in acrylic as illustrated in Figs. 75a and 75b. Only minimal amounts of acrylic are used for retention of the wire components since the nature of the wire does most of the work.

The posterior portions of acrylic have two further splits in the cuspid regions on both sides so that targeted adjustments can be made. The bilateral posterior acrylic is tightly festooned to the lingual aspect of the first and second molars, using minimal amounts acrylic. In the lower Wireframe DNA appliance, a wrap-around labial bow constructed of 0.036-inch stainless steel wire is used. It is ideally shaped in the anterior segment for guidance during tooth alignment. For device retention, C clasps are soldered onto the labial bow, and placed on the first molars and/or the second bicuspids. They are made of 0.30-inch gauge stainless steel wire. In addition, occlusal stops/rests made of the same wire are placed in the lingual groove (Fig. 75a) or sometimes on the distal marginal ridge of the second molars so that mandible cannot occlude in its habitual position. The lower Wireframe DNA appliance® is a light-weight device that is very comfortable to wear and is ideally suited to cases where a lot of development is not indicated.

mRNA appliance® design

A significant feature in biomimetic correction is that the mandible needs to change its original spatial relationship to putatively affect gene expression.

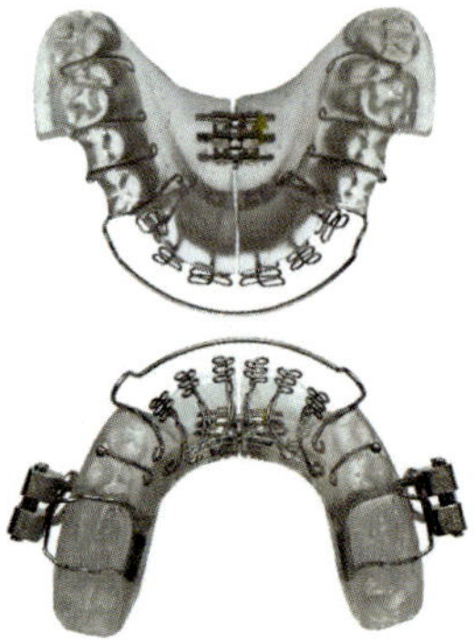

Figure 76a: mRNA appliance showing upper and lower components.

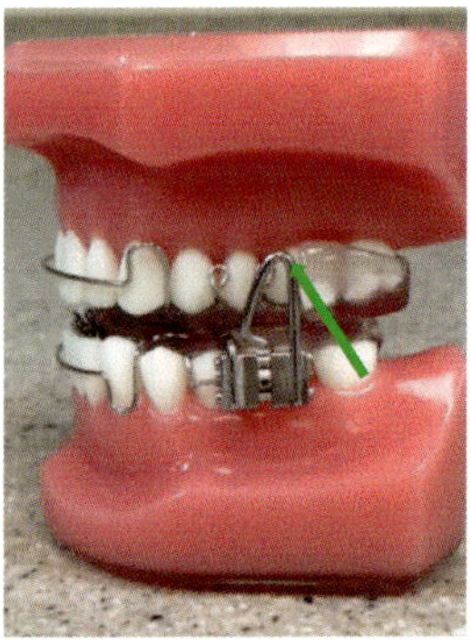

Figure 76b: mRNA appliance showing screw-fin engaging upper acrylic slot.

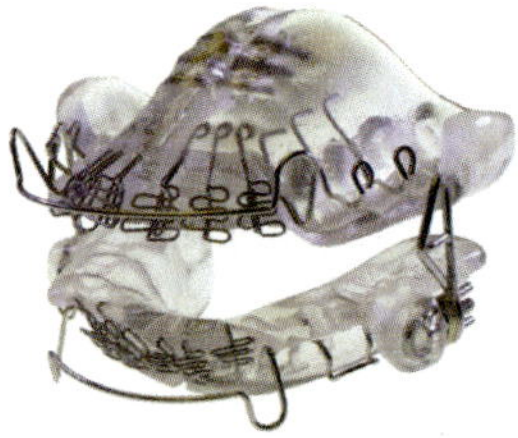

Figure 76c: mRNA appliance assembled for patient wear.

Not surprisingly, mandibular manipulation has taken various guises in dental and orthodontic history, starting with the original concept of 'jumping the bite' in children to the current-day mandibular advancement devices that are used for the management of mild/moderate OSA in adults. The mRNA appliance® integrates and enhances this latter approach since this design essentially has the same features as the upper and lower acrylic-based DNA appliances combined together (Fig. 76a) with the addition of a (patented) 'screw-fin' mechanism that permits mandibular advancement (Fig. 76b). Thus, the vertical flange of the 'screw-fin' mechanism of the lower component engages the acrylic slot of the upper component, and because of this unique design and functionality, it is advisable to use additional clasping for secure retention as shown in Fig. 76. In addition, in order to prevent breakages, especially in patients diagnosed with sleep bruxism, an occlusal table/coverage is provided in the lower component, specifically to embed the screw-fin mechanism that engages acrylic slots of the upper component (Fig. 76c). Thus, the screw-fin mechanism permits advancements of the mandibular component in 1mm increments, while the screw(s) in the maxillary component permit sutural stretch in 0.25mm increments. Note that periodic adjustments of the occlusal table/coverage of the lower component of the mRNA appliance are performed for patient comfort, as needed.

Although specific adjustments are detailed in the sections below, it's essential to selectively equilibrate and gradually reduce and/or remove the occlusal acrylic from the (internal) fitting surface of the lower component to permit the lower teeth to track any changes in the occlusion. Concurrently, it's important to monitor the response of the TMJs and mandible carefully. To surmise, the upper component of the mRNA appliance has all the features of an upper DNA appliance plus an acrylic slot to engage the 'screw-fin' mechanism. Similarly, the lower component of the mRNA appliance has all the features of a lower DNA appliance plus occlusal coverage and the 'screw-fin' mechanism. Note that the overall design is unique in many ways, having six degrees of freedom; especially since no other mandibular advancement device has a midline screw in the region of the former mandibular symphysis. These features aim to provide biomimetic correction following the circadian rhythm, since the lower component of the mRNA appliance is only worn during nighttime while asleep, whereas the upper component can be worn in the late afternoon and early evening prior to inserting the lower component of the mRNA appliance at night.

Bite registration

Following final impressions, which may be digital or manual, the jaw registration needs to be recorded, and a bite registration needs to be taken so that the devices can be custom fabricated for that particular patient. There is a dearth of information on how to obtain a proper jaw registration/working bite, which differs from a construction bite, for oral appliance therapy. A comprehensive discussion of the various techniques, some of which are arbitrary, used to capture the bite will not be argued here; suffice to say that the jaw registration/working bite represents the approximate finishing position of the mandible, and the starting position of treatment. This concept is based on the notion that changing the position of the mandible evokes a change in the pattern of gene expression (Fuentes *et al.*, 2003) as predicted by the spatial matrix hypothesis (Singh, 2004). But there are certain requirements for a successful jaw registration/working bite. First, the new position of the mandible should enhance the upper airway and not compromise it. This position is often achieved with biomimetic oral devices since these appliances invariably have occlusal coverage/pads built into their design as alluded to earlier in this chapter. In other words, a successful jaw registration/working bite position often provides sufficient space for occlusal coverage because of the curve of Spee (sometimes called the Christensen effect). This occlusal coverage increases the oral volume and, with the lips in light contact, the oral pressure will be reduced. The oral cavity communicates with the nasal cavity behind the soft palate. This anatomical arrangement means that the pressure is higher in the smaller (unchanged) nasal cavity, and the laws of physics ensure that air is sucked in through the nose to the region of lower pressure. In effect, a mouth-breather can quickly be converted into a nasal breather in most cases. Although the thickness of these occlusal pads will, to a certain extent, be determined by finding the jaw position noted above, in practice this thickness needs to be at least approx. 2–3mm in order to provide the dental technician with sufficient clearance to be able to construct a device that will not be too thin and liable to fracture if dropped or if a heavy bite is exerted, for example during bruxing, grinding, and/or clenching. In this case, the jaw registration/working bite position meets the criteria of the 'construction bite'. However, if the clearance is insufficient after the models have been mounted, the dental lab technician will adjust the clearance until there is sufficient space to fabricate a viable appliance. In these cases, the construction bite differs from the jaw registration/working bite position and clinical adjustments may become necessary at the time of device delivery.

Often, the above lab-based adjustment following mounting of the models on an articulator does not pose problems. However, in some cases a patient may complain that a device feels 'bulky'. In fact, this sensation is often caused by an appliance which had a poor jaw registration/working bite or has been poorly fabricated. In the first situation, if the jaw registration/working bite position does not enhance the upper airway there will be lack of functional space, and the patient may respond by saying the device feels 'bulky'. In this scenario, the jaw registration/working bite has to be corrected, and this will be discussed below. In the second situation, the device has not been well manufactured. For example, the fitting surface acrylic may be touching the palatal mucosa; the posterior border might not be beveled; the screw placement might interfere with tongue motion, or the occlusal pads might be too thick, encroaching on tongue space. In these instances, the device can either be sent back to the lab for refinement or it can be adjusted chairside, if feasible. For these reasons, it is best to have a cordial and professional working relationship with a reliable and skillful dental laboratory. Biomimetic oral appliances are precision-crafted devices that require great attention to detail.

In order to prevent any issues at the device delivery appointment, an appropriate jaw registration/working bite is essential. As noted above, there are many techniques to obtain the jaw registration/working bite; however, there are relatively few bite registration techniques for cases of OSA in the peer-reviewed literature. Frequently, an arbitrary degree of mandibular protrusion is attempted using a George gauge. There appears to be no evidence for this approach and the notion of 70–80% protrusion has not been corroborated. One technique that has been successfully deployed, however, is the neuromuscular jaw registration. Essentially, a neuromuscular bite registration is obtained in the upright-sitting position with a corrected jaw posture in the vertical axis specific for each subject. The protocol for capturing the physiological rest position of the mandible (Jankelson, 2005) starts with baseline data collection of the initial bite, jaw position, and posture, using 2D or 3D photography and 2D or 3D jaw-tracking hardware/software. The muscles of mastication are relaxed using ultra-low frequency, transcutaneous electrical neural stimulation (ULF-TENS) of cranial nerves V, VII, and XI for a minimum of 45 minutes (Fig. 77). These nerves are accessed through the coronoid notch and the

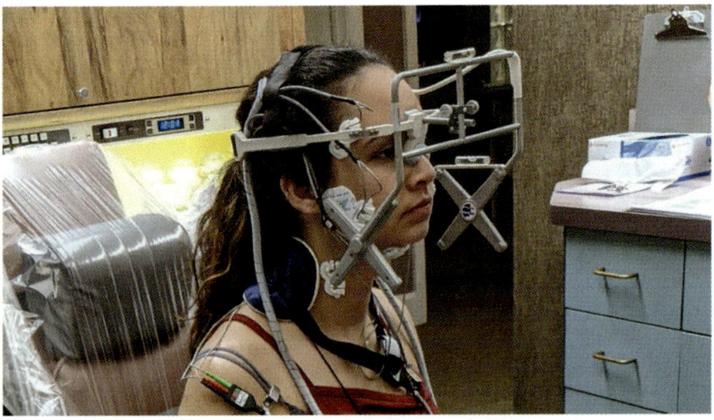

Figure 77: Patient with jaw-tracking system undergoing transcutaneous electrical neural stimulation. Courtesy: Dr Prabu Raman

upper portion of the middle one-third of the posterior cervical triangle, just posterior to the sternocleidomastoid muscle (SCM). Cranial nerve XI innervates SCM and trapezius, and if stimulated with ULF-TENS, these muscles and associated muscles can be relaxed simultaneously without risk of direct stimulation of the carotid sinus nerve (Raman, 2010). Following relaxation of the jaw and neck muscles, jaw-tracking data are used to find the most relaxed position of the mandible where the muscles coordinate together, documented at a single point in space. This physiological rest position is captured using a polyvinylsiloxane bite registration material when the electromyograph recordings are at their lowest. The bite position is then verified using jaw-tracking data. Thus, the physiological rest position is both measurable and repeatable (Heit *et al.*, 2015).

Patients with TMJ dysfunction (TMD) also require correction of the mandibular position, including anterior repositioning *inter alia*. However, determining the extent of the antero-posterior mandibular correction is essential in not increasing muscle tone, and inducing muscle spasm in some of these cases. Thus, an alternative method of obtaining the jaw registration can be used, not only for cases of TMD but also for cases of SDB that require mandibular repositioning. This procedure is colloquially referred to as the 'phonetic bite' or the sibilant phoneme registration (SPR) protocol more

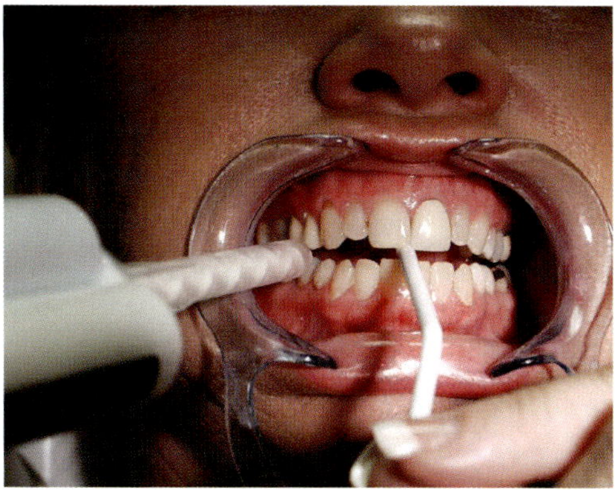

Figure 78: Capturing the 'phonetic bite' clinically using impression material while the patient rests the jaw on a suitable tip.

properly (Singh and Olmos, 2007) since it uses the 's' sound to determine the minimum speaking distance, which differs from the freeway space. In this technique, the patient is either sitting upright in a (dental) chair or standing against a wall. The patient is then instructed to count aloud between 60 and 70, repeatedly making an 's' sound. The clinician observes the jaw position showing the least speaking space (Fig. 78). In this position the tongue is likely sitting on the anterior part of the palate and the upper airway is opened. Studies have shown that when the baseline functional residual capacity (FRC) airway is measured and then compared to the (collapsed) residual volume (RV), a 25% reduction in the upper airway volume is typically demonstrable in patients with TMD. Using the SPR method or 'phonetic bite', however, when the RV airway was compared to the RV-SPR airway, a 15% increase in upper airway volume was found (Singh and Olmos, 2007). This jaw position would, therefore, prevent upper airway collapse during sleep if a device is made to that bite registration. Thus, the use of a SPR or 'phonetic bite' protocol may be useful in improving the upper airway in patients during treatment for TMD and/or SDB.

There are other methods that can also be used to obtain a jaw registration, including a 'biomimetic bite'. For example, it is known that the horizontal axis of rotation of the mandible passes through the first and second cervical vertebrae (C1/C2). However, if C1/C2 are misaligned (because of a forward head posture or subluxation) then it's unlikely that an optimal jaw registration can be achieved, simply because the mandible is compromised in its envelope of motion. In order to address this deficiency, professional collaboration with a chiropractor (specifically an atlas-orthogonal chiropractor) or, more generally speaking, an osteopath or other physical therapist that is professionally trained in cervical alignment, can be beneficial. Chiropractic adjustment can achieve improved cervical alignment, and the dentist can then record an optimized jaw registration with an enhanced upper airway space (Fig. 79). Although there is little data to support this claim currently, the principles of the kinetic chain apply. Put simply, it's wise to align the body, then align the jaws and finally align the teeth to enhance the upper airway. In one study, the effect of biomimetic oral appliance therapy combined with cervical adjustment was undertaken in adults (Chapman and Singh, 2013). Each subject was examined for malocclusion, and also for the presence of an atlas (C1) subluxation. The subjects were then asked to lie down horizontally on a chiropractic table and the leg lengths were measured: without the appliance; with the appliance in situ, and again after a transdermal atlas positioning procedure (TAPP) was performed by a chiropractor (atlas-orthogonist). It was found

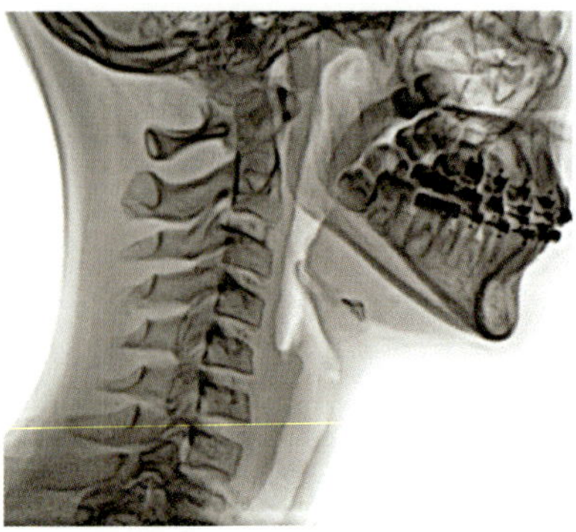

Figure 79a: Pre-treatment lateral radiograph showing cervical vertebrae, upper airway, and occlusion.
Courtesy: Dr Chris Chapman

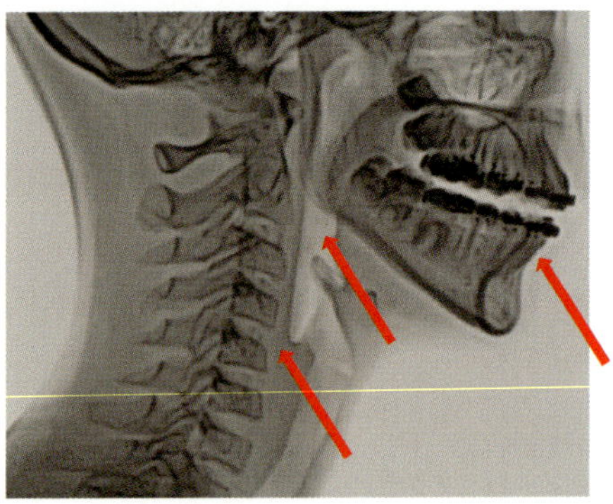

Figure 79b: 'Biomimetic bite' position showing improved cervical vertebrae, upper airway, and mandibular position (arrows).

that leg length discrepancy was about 12mm without the appliance in the mouth but was reduced to 6mm with the device in situ. In addition, the leg asymmetry was further reduced to about 2mm after the chiropractor TAPP procedure was completed. These data suggest that biomimetic oral appliance therapy in combination with chiropractor adjustment appears to significantly reduces leg length discrepancy in adults, in line with cranio-caudal gradient and kinetic chain concepts.

In fact, there are several chiropractic/osteopathic and other physical therapy techniques available to improve head and neck alignment, but none of these are typically combined with the PACE protocol. Therefore, another study investigated changes in head and neck alignment using combined chiropractic-TAPP and biomimetic oral appliance therapy in adults who had been evaluated for the presence of both malocclusion and C1 subluxation. Pre-treatment cranio-cervical relationships were assessed using frontal, horizontal, and axial radiography (T0). Each subject was treated for atlas subluxation by a chiropractor, and the radiographic procedure was repeated (T1). Next, the subject inserted the biomimetic device (DNA appliance®) and the radiographic procedure was repeated (T2). It was found that several parameters related to C1 and C2 showed improvements at both T1 and T2. After chiropractic adjustment (T1), the craniofacial alignment improved, but combining the chiropractic adjustment with the oral appliance (T2), the craniofacial alignment improved further, and the total postural decompensation was found to be about 70%. Thus, when biomimetic oral appliance therapy is used in combination with chiropractic adjustment, there appears to be a synergistic effect that improves craniofacial alignment in adults. Therefore, an optimized bite registration can be achieved and once this has been captured, the models can be mounted. Prior to doing so, however, it's important to check the study models for accuracy, especially if they have been hand-poured. Any bubbles or flaws need to be addressed since the study models need to accurately represent the patient's tissues. On the other hand, 3D intra-oral digital scans can be used, and the study models can be reproduced using a 3D printer. Once the study models have been produced, they can be mounted, preferably using the hamular notch/incisive papilla (HIP) technique, since the HIP plane is approximately parallel to the occlusal plane (Jayachandran *et al.*, 2008). Another advantage of this mounting (on an Acculiner articulator) is that the cranial base (represented by the hamular notches) is aligned with the maxilla (represented by the incisive papilla), to which the mandible is aligned after using cervical correction. Therefore, this procedure represents a biomimetic bite registration since the salient craniofacial components have been addressed to enhance the upper airway.

Professional co-operation and collaboration are essential for clinical excellence. An ongoing dialogue should exist between the dental office and the dental laboratory so that once the technician receives the laboratory prescription sheet there is no room for avoidable errors. The lab script should be clearly completed by the doctor's office, including diagrams for clarification, if needed. Prior to delivery, the doctor's office should first check the appliance for accuracy to ensure that it follows the script and that it has been well produced. The insert tray should be set-up with instruments most frequently used for delivery and adjustments, including pliers, articulating paper, etc. The most commonly used pliers in this respect are bird-beak pliers, sometimes called bird beak 139 or Angle 139 pliers. These pliers have one rounded beak and one flat beak. The actual beaks can be regular (short) in length or long bird beak pliers might be preferred to give additional access. Having said that, the preferred tool is the one that works best in the hands of the clinician since experience is the best teacher. Thus, some clinicians may choose to use Conlon lightwire pliers or Jarabak pliers or even hemostat pliers to attain a particular adjustment. Others might select Mathieu pliers or narrow forceps to adjust a component of the device. Yet another useful implement is the 3-prong pliers. These pliers can be used to adjust omega loops, clasps, and other wire components of the appliance. In this respect, Young's pliers are designed to help grasp wire since they have slots that prevent slippage. A comprehensive overview of actual device adjustments is provided in the next chapter.

References

Ansari S, Seagroves JT, Chen C, Shah K, Aghaloo T, Wu BM, Bencharit S, Moshaverinia A. Dental and orofacial mesenchymal stem cells in craniofacial regeneration: The prosthodontist's point of view. *J Prosthet Dent*. 2017;118(4):455–461.

Aytan S, Yukay F, Ciğler S, Enacar A, Aksoy A, Telli AE. Frankel III appliance. *Turk Ortodonti Derg*. 1989;2(2):338–345.

Banabilh SM, Suzina AH, Dinsuhaimi S, Samsudin AR, Singh GD. Dental arch morphology in south-east Asian adults with obstructive sleep apnoea: geometric morphometrics. *J Oral Rehabil*. 2009;36(3):184–192.

Basdra EK, Komposch G. Osteoblast-like properties of human periodontal ligament cells: an in vitro analysis. *Eur J Orthod*. 1997;19(6):615–621.

Becker MJ. Mandibular symphysis (medial suture) closure in modern Homo sapiens: preliminary evidence from archaeological populations. *Am J Phys Anthropol*. 1986;69(4):499–501.

Chapman DC, Singh GD. Combined effect of a biomimetic oral appliance and atlas orthogonist cervical adjustment on leg lengths in adults. *Annals Vert Sub Res*. 2013;46–50.

D'Attilio M, Filippi MR, Femminella B, Festa F, Tecco S. The influence of an experimentally-induced malocclusion on vertebral alignment in rats: A controlled pilot study. *Cranio*. 2005;23:119–129.

Di Ventura A, Lanteri V, Farronato G, Gaffuri F, Beretta M, Lanteri C, Cossellu G. Three-dimensional evaluation of rapid maxillary expansion anchored to primary molars: direct effects on maxillary arch and spontaneous mandibular response. *Eur J Paediatr Dent*. 2019;20(1):38–42.

El-Bialy T, El-Shamy I, Graber TM. Repair of orthodontically induced root resorption by ultrasound in humans. *Am J Orthod Dentofacial Orthop*. 2004;126(2):186–193.

Fuentes MA, Opperman LA, Buschang P, Bellinger LL, Carlson DS, Hinton RJ. Lateral functional shift of the mandible: Part II. Effects on gene expression in condylar cartilage. *Am J Orthod Dentofacial Orthop*. 2003;123(2):160–166.

Harris WG, Singh GD. Resolution of 'gummy smile' and anterior open bite using the DNA appliance™: Case Report. *J Amer Orthod Soc*. 2013;13(4):30–34.

Heit T, Derkson C, Bierkos J, Saqqur M. The effect of the physiological rest position of the mandible on cerebral blood flow and physical balance: an observational study. *Cranio*. 2015;33(3):195–205.

Jäger A, Polley J, Mausberg R. Effects of orthodontic expansion of the mandibular arch on the periodontal condition of the posterior teeth. *Dtsch Zahnarztl Z*. 1990;45(2):113–115.

Jankelson R. Neuromuscular dental diagnosis and treatment. Vol. 1. St Louis, MO: Ishiyaku EuroAmerica, 2005, pp. 87–96.

Jayachandran S, Ramachandran CR, Varghese R. Occlusal plane orientation: a statistical and clinical analysis in different clinical situations. *J Prosthodont.* 2008;17(7):572–575.

Jia B, Qiu X, Chen J, Sun X, Zheng X, Zhao J, Li Q, Wang Z. A feed-forward regulatory network lncPCAT1/miR-106a-5p/E2F5 regulates the osteogenic differentiation of periodontal ligament stem cells. *J Cell Physiol.* 2019;234(11):19523–19538.

Kopher RA, Nudera JA, Wang X, O'Grady K, Mao JJ. Expression of in vivo mechanical strain upon different wave forms of exogenous forces in rabbit craniofacial sutures. *Ann Biomed Eng.* 2003;31(9):1125–1131.

Lam B, Ip MS, Tench E, Ryan CF. Craniofacial profile in Asian and white subjects with obstructive sleep apnoea. *Thorax.* 2005;60(6):504–510.

Masset C. Age estimation on the basis of cranial sutures. In İşcan, MY (ed.): Age markers in the human skeleton. Springfield, IL: Charles C. Thomas, 1989, pp. 71–104.

Nicozisis JL, Nah-Cederquist HD, Tuncay OC. Relaxin affects the dentofacial sutural tissues. *Clin Orthod Res.* 2000;3(4):192–201.

Niinomi M, Nakai M, Hieda J. Development of new metallic alloys for biomedical applications. *Acta Biomater.* 2012;8(11):3888–3903.

O'Neal R, Wang HL, MacNeil RL, Somerman MJ. Cells and materials involved in guided tissue regeneration. *Curr Opin Periodontol.* 1994:141–156.

Proffit WR, Frazier-Bowers SA. Mechanism and control of tooth eruption: overview and clinical implications. *Orthod Craniofac Res.* 2009;12(2):59–6.

Raman P. Neurally mediated ULF-TENs to relax upper cervical and upper thoracic musculature as an aid to obtaining improved cervical posture and mandibular posture. In: The application of the principles of neuromuscular dentistry to clinical practice (Anthology Vol. IX). Seattle, WA: The International College of Cranio-Mandibular Orthopedics, 2010, pp. 77–85.

Roberts WE, Hartsfield JK Jr. Bone development and function: genetic and environmental mechanisms. *Semin Orthod.* 2004;10(2):100–122.

Singh GD, Abramson M. Effect of an intra-oral nasal dilation appliance on 3-D nasal airway morphology in adults. *Sleep Breath.* 2008;12(1):69–75.

Singh GD, Clark WJ. Localization of mandibular changes in patients with Class II division 1 malocclusions treated using Twin Block appliances: finite-element modeling. *Am J Orthod Dentofacial Orthop.* 2001;119(4):419–425.

Singh GD, Clark WJ. Soft tissue morphometry of subjects with Class II division 1 malocclusions treated using Twin Block appliances: finite-element scaling analysis. *Euro J Orthod*. 2003;25(3):225–230.

Singh GD, Cress SE. Craniofacial enhancement using a biomimetic oral appliance. *Dent Today*. 2013;329(12):92–94.

Singh GD, García AV, Hang WM. Evaluation of the posterior airway space following Biobloc therapy: Geometric morphometrics. *Cranio*. 2007;25(2):84–89.

Singh GD, Heit T, Preble D, Chandrashekhar R. Changes in 3D nasal cavity volume after biomimetic oral appliance therapy in adults. *Cranio*. 2016;34(1):6–12.

Singh GD, Heit T, Preble D. Changes in 3D midfacial parameters after biomimetic oral appliance therapy in adults. *J Ind Orthod Soc*. 2014;48(2):104–108.

Singh GD, Hodge MR. Bimaxillary morphometry of patients with class II division 1 malocclusion treated with twin block appliances. *Angle Orthod*. 2002;72(5):402–409.

Singh GD, Keropian B, Pillar G. Effects of the Full Breath Solution appliance for the treatment of obstructive sleep apnea: A preliminary study. *Cranio*. 2009;27(2):109–117.

Singh GD, Kim HN. Changes in nasal airway volume after biomimetic oral appliance therapy in Korean adults. *Am J Respir Crit Care Med*. 2020;201:A2442.

Singh GD, Kim KY. Facial enhancement using biomimetic oral appliance therapy in adults. *Dent Oral Craniofac Res*. 2016;2(4):313–317.

Singh GD, Krumholtz JA. Epigenetic orthodontics in adults. *Appliance Therapy Group*, USA, 2009.

Singh GD, Levy-Bercowski D, Santiago PE. 3-D effects of nasoalveolar molding in patients with orofacial clefts: geometric morphometrics. *Cleft Palate Craniofac J*. 2005;42(4):403–409.

Singh GD, Levy-Bercowski D, Yañez MA, Santiago PE. Three-dimensional facial morphology following surgical repair of unilateral cleft lip and palate in patients after nasoalveolar molding. *Orthod Craniofac Res*. 2007;10(3):161–166.

Singh GD, Maher GJ, Padilla RR. Customized mandibular orthotics in the prevention of concussion/mild traumatic brain injury in football players: a preliminary study. *Dent Traumatol*. 2009;25(5):515–521.

Singh GD, Olmos S. Use of a sibilant phoneme registration protocol to prevent upper airway collapse in patients with TMD. *Sleep Breath*. 2007;11(4):209–216.

Singh GD, Thind BS. Effects of the Headgear-Activator Teuscher Appliance in the treatment of Class II Division 1 malocclusion: a geometric morphometric study. *Orthod Craniofacial Res*. 2003;6:88–95.

Singh GD, Thind BS. Effects of the headgear-activator Teuscher appliance in the treatment of Class II Division 1 malocclusion: a geometric morphometric study. *Orthod Craniofac Res*. 2003;6(2):88–95.

Singh GD. On Growth and Treatment: The spatial matrix hypothesis. In: Ribbens KA and McNamara JA Jr (eds.) Growth and treatment: A meeting of the minds. Craniofacial Growth Series, Ann Arbor, USA,2004;41:197–239.

Trevizan M, Consolaro A. Premaxilla: an independent bone that can base therapeutics for middle third growth! *Dental Press J Orthod*. 2017;22(2):21–26.

Veis R, Christian J. Principles of appliance therapy for adults and children. Smile Foundation, Appliance Therapy Group, USA, 2004.

Vizzotto MB, de Araujo FB, da Silveira HE, Boza AA, Closs LQ. The quad helix appliance in the primary dentition — orthodontic and orthopedic measurements. *Clin Pediatr*. 2008;32(2):165–170.

Williams DE, Lynch JE, Doshi V, Singh GD, Hargens AR. Bruxism and temporal bone hypermobility in patients with multiple sclerosis. *Cranio*. 2011;29(3):178–186.

Williams MO, Murphy NC. Beyond the ligament: A whole-bone periodontal view of dentofacial orthopedics and falsification of universal alveolar immutability. *Semin Orthod*. 2008;14(4):246–259.

Zhao H, Feng J, Ho TV, Grimes W, Urata M, Chai Y. The suture provides a niche for mesenchymal stem cells of craniofacial bones. *Nat Cell Biol*. 2015;17(4):386–396.

Chapter 7

Biomimetic Oral Appliance Adjustments

Synopsis: This chapter describes biomimetic oral device adjustments. Retention and activation via clasps, screw mechanisms, and omega loops is noted. Equilibration of the occlusal pads/coverage and occlusal stops where present is discussed. Modification of the fitting surface, including wires extending from the omega loops is described. Adjustments of the 3D axial springs of the anterior six teeth are illustrated. Positioning of the labial bow is presented, and adjustment of the beaded, pharyngeal stent is reviewed.

Initial device adjustments

When inserting the appliance for the first time, it's a good idea to replicate the jaw-registration movements/positioning to ensure consistency. Muscle memory should permit duplication of the bite registration to within less than a couple of millimeters or so. On insertion, it's important to first check the fit for accuracy since the aim is that the device feels snug like a brand-new pair of shoes when first worn. Thus, step one is checking the retention and activation of the device. The job of the clasps is simply retention. This means that all things being equal, the clasps hold the device in place, so it doesn't feel loose or become dislodged on gentle pressure. There are different types of clasps that can be used for this purpose, depending on the degree of retention that is needed. For example, ball clasps (Fig. 74a) are often used to engage the undercuts of the teeth for retention without interfering with cheek tissues. On the other hand, some patients find it difficult to remove a device with this type of clasp and so Adams clasps (Fig. 74b) are a standard feature on many appliances. Sometimes, a more retentive clasp is needed, especially if the undercuts are shallow. In these cases, either delta clasps can be used or Crozat's clasps especially when extra retention is called for. Alternatively, the dentist may need to bond a composite ledge or button on the buccal aspects of the teeth for additional retention. This step is particularly useful in the case of 'C clasps' (Fig. 75b). C clasps are most often used in Wireframe or Hybrid appliances where they are soldered onto the framework and engage the undercuts in the same way as partial denture clasps. In this way, the clasps are passive and only provide retention of the device.

At the delivery appointment, it's unlikely that much adjustment will be required, especially if the device has been well fabricated. However, for any ball clasp adjustments, most clinicians use the round side of the bird-beak pliers on the inside of the clasp's loop (Fig. 80a) to bend the ball of the wire deeper into the undercut area. One or both loops may need to be adjusted on one or both sides. For Adams clasp adjustments, bird-beak pliers can also be used to grasp the delta portion of the clasp (Fig. 80b). This 'arrowhead' is then bent deeper into the undercut area, and the procedure is repeated for the other (mesial or distal) arrowhead, as well as on the other side of the appliance, if needed.

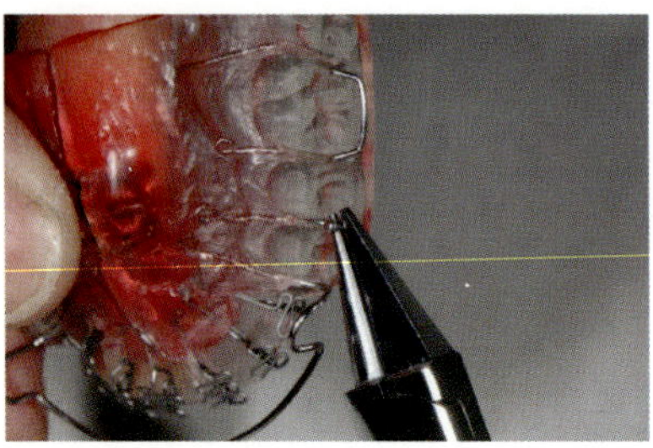

Figure 80a: The round side of the bird-beak pliers on the inside of the ball clasp, bending it deeper into the undercut.

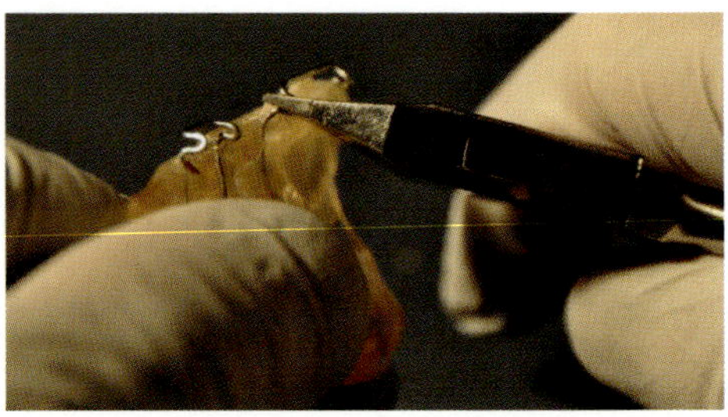

Figure 80b: Bird-beak pliers grasping delta of Adams clasp, bending it deeper into the undercut.

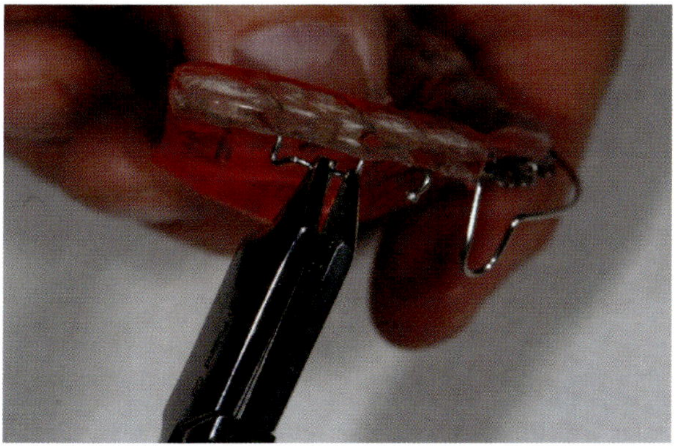

Figure 81: Single prong of 3-prong pliers placed on inside of Adams clasp. With light pressure both sides of the clasp bend inward.

Alternatively, it's also possible to use the 3-prong pliers for Adams clasp adjustments. In this case, the 1-pronged beak is simply placed on the inside (palatal/lingual) aspect of the device in the middle of the Adams clasp's 'bridge' and light pressure is applied (Fig. 81). In this procedure, both (mesial and distal) arrowheads are bent inward toward the tooth's undercut area in the interproximal regions. Sometimes, however, the source of the lack of retention is not the claps, which are gripping on to the teeth, but the dimensions of the device may be too small for it to be fully retentive. In these cases, the expansion screw or omega loop may need to be activated to add tension to the device.

The key or screwdriver is placed vertically into the screw (Fig. 82a) and following the direction of the arrow it is moved into an almost horizontal position (Fig. 82b). Moving from the original vertical position of the key to the new (horizontal) position represents 0.25mm (250μm) of activation in line with concept of sutural homeostasis. It is important to show the patient how to use the expansion key correctly and explain that the job of the screw is to keep up with tissues changes that will occur with prolonged wear — and not the other way around. In other words, the screw mechanism is not being used in the traditional way of other orthodontic expansion devices. It is only adjusted when the device feels loose. It is not

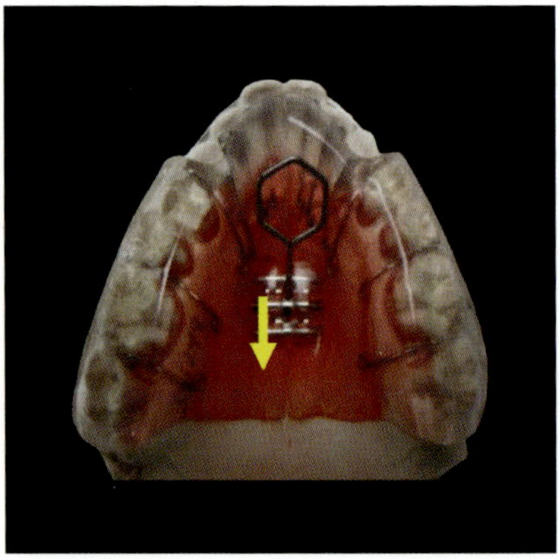

Figure 82a: Key in vertical position in screw mechanism. Note direction of yellow arrow.

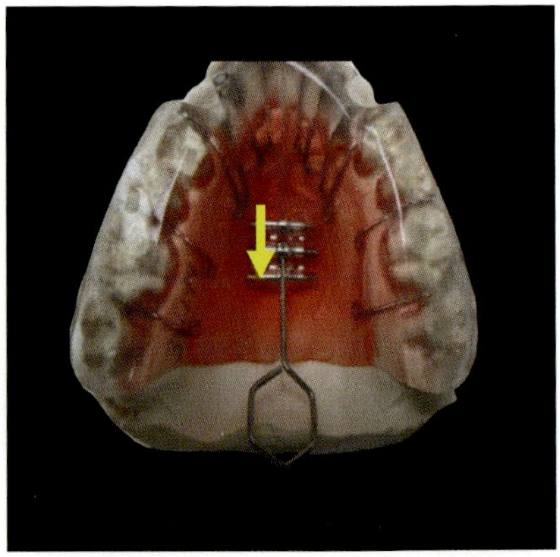

Figure 82b: Key in horizontal position in screw mechanism producing 0.25mm of activation.

used for 'rapid maxillary expansion', which can split the suture and evoke the healing process; instead, gentle sutural stretch results in new bone formation. Note that some devices may be acrylic-based with a 3-way screw mechanism. Thus, either the transverse and/or the sagittal screw can be used to gently add tension to the tissues. Mechanical, over-aggressive screw-turns must be avoided at all cost. If the device is used 'mechanically' there is a risk that tooth-tipping might occur, although in our experience this is unlikely. Neither tooth-tipping, dehiscence nor fenestration have been reported if the biomimetic protocol is followed. The reason for this finding is that over-expansion likely means that the device will not seat properly in the mouth, and the 3D axial springs will prevent excess forces being inappropriately applied. In any case, to gauge tissue response and remodeling, it is a good idea to record initial and progressive measurements with clinical photographs to help encourage patients visualize the progress being made, since the changes are sometimes subtle and difficult for a patient to assess by simply looking in the mirror.

Once the device is properly seated, it's important to check the occlusion with the device in situ. Generally speaking, the occlusal pads (if present) need to have a smooth and even surface with no occlusal

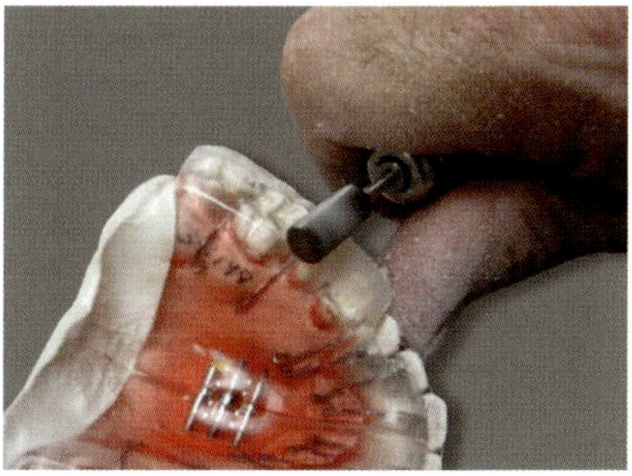

Figure 83a: A small amount of acrylic is removed on each visit, allowing the opposing teeth to supra-erupt.

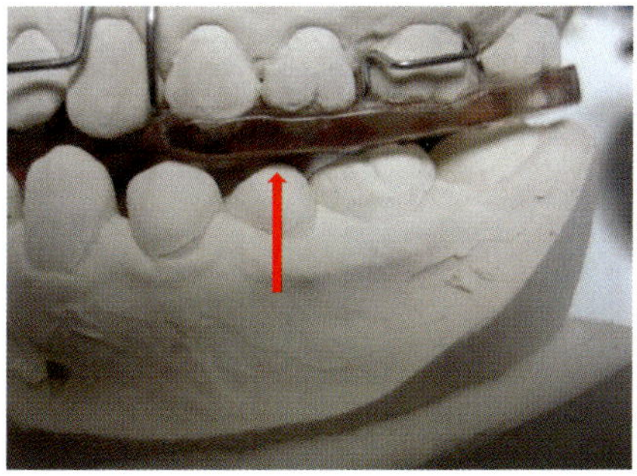

Figure 83b: Note the small space indicated (red arrow). This is repeated on each visit until the desired vertical dimension is obtained.

interference so that that midface is free to develop in 3D space while the mandible is free to move in 3D space. By using articulating paper, any high spots can be identified and ground out using an acrylic bur (Fig. 83a). Thus, using selective grinding, it's important to equilibrate the occlusal pads and gradually reduce/remove the occlusal acrylic to permit the lower teeth to track the subtle changes in occlusion (Fig. 83b). At the delivery appointment, it's unlikely that much occlusal grinding will be required, especially if the device has been fabricated following the bite registration provided. However, as treatment proceeds, this step may become increasingly important, as outlined below, and may lead to eventual perforation of the occlusal coverage.

Once the occlusion has been reviewed, it's important to check the labial bow. Since the device is not a retainer, the labial bow needs to be about 0.5mm away from the labial surfaces of the anterior teeth and not in contact with them. In this position, the labial bow is acting as a lip-bumper, keeping the soft tissues of the lip/cheek away from contacting the teeth. In effect, this is a new spatial matrix and provides sufficient space for minor tooth alignment even though this is not the primary purpose of the device. Again, if the appliance has been well-made, very little or no adjustment of the labial bow is needed at the delivery appointment. The clearance can be checked by passing floss between the teeth and the labial bow to gauge

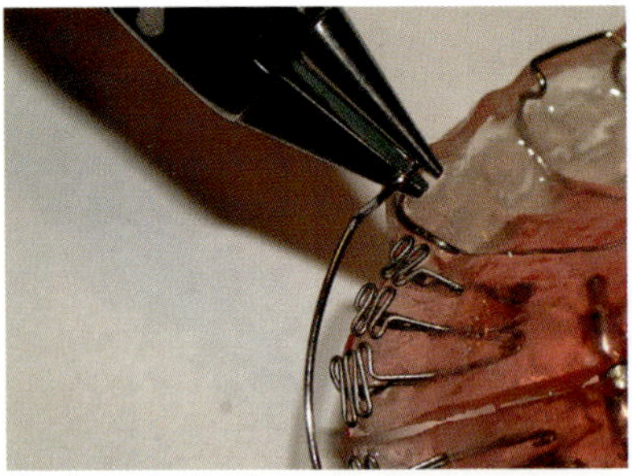

Figure 84a: Flat side of bird beak pliers on inside of U loop. Light pressure moves the bow away from the teeth.

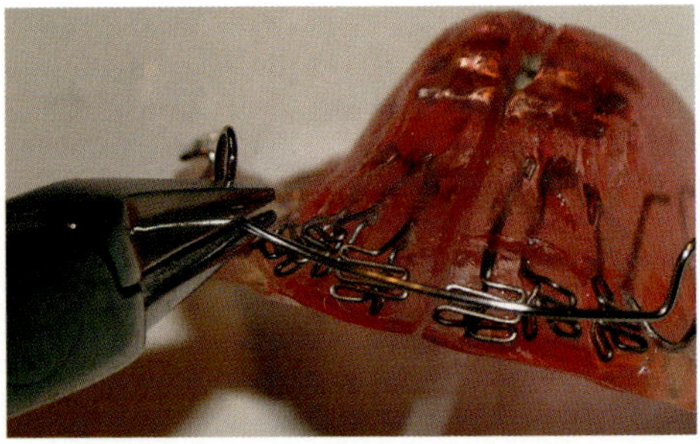

Figure 84b: Counter-bend to adjust labial bow back down to middle one-third of the anterior teeth.

the distance. If labial bow adjustment is needed, this can be easily achieved using bird-beak pliers. In this case, the flat side of the beak is positioned on the inside of the U loop of the labial bow (Fig. 84a), and light pressure is applied to move the wire away from the labial surfaces of the anterior teeth. This step moves the wire both upward and outward. Thus, the next step needs to reposition the wire downward so that it lies approximately in the middle-third of the labial aspect of the anterior teeth. For this counter-bend, the flat side of the beak is reversed and positioned on the inside at the base of the U loop (Fig. 84b). Light pressure is then applied to move the wire downward from its initial position. The U loops on one or both sides may need to be adjusted so that the labial bow comes to lie in middle-third of the labial surfaces of the anterior teeth.

At this initial visit, the dentist needs to check the palatal surface and posterior border of the device. Although it's unlikely, any sharp edges or flashes of acrylic that might irritate the oral mucosa need to be removed. Note that the fitting surface of the appliance should not contact the palatal mucosa. In a well-made device, the technician has already used a separating medium, so adjustments at this first appointment will probably be unnecessary. Conversely, it's important to ensure that the 3D axial springs are in light contact with the palatal aspect of the anterior six teeth. During device fabrication, the dental

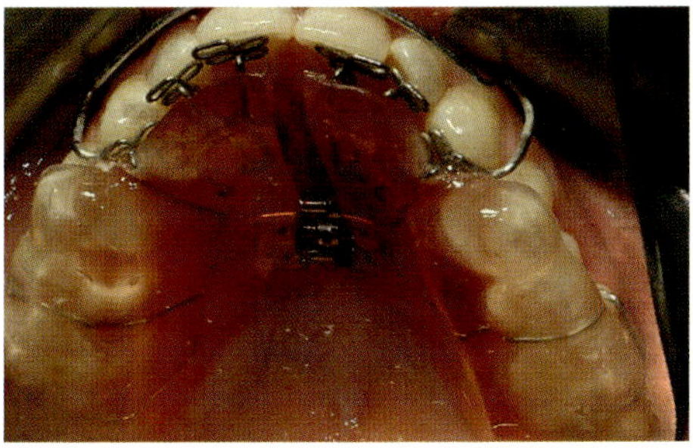

Figure 85a: Device showing lack of maximum area of contact between 3D axial springs and palatal surfaces of teeth.

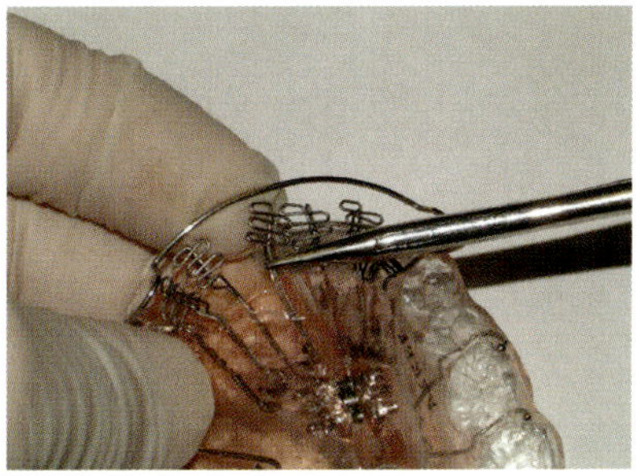

Figure 85b: Adjusting stems of 3D axial springs for 10 seconds since the memory wire will try to recover.

technician will ensure that the 3D axial springs are in intimate contact with the lingual surfaces of the anterior teeth, but this has to be checked clinically (Fig. 85a).

Finally, if a beaded, pharyngeal stent is present it needs to be thoroughly reviewed. This extension is used in cases of SDB, including OSA. As discussed previously, its role is to maintain a patent upper airway during sleep. For this reason, its placement is essential for success. Essentially, the extension is positioned halfway between the soft palate and the tongue (Fig. 73). It needs to be long enough to extend behind the posterior one-third of the tongue but not contact any soft tissues while the patient is sitting upright or standing, the so-called 'sweet spot'. The stent only becomes active on lying down when the relaxed tissues will cause collapse of the upper airway. In these circumstances, the tongue will roll upward and forward on to the anterior bite ramp/tongue-trainer, while the musculus uvulae muscle inside the soft palate will contract, preserving the patency of the upper airway. It is vital that the stent is long enough to extend past the circumvallate papillae of the posterior one-third of the tongue. If not, the glossopharyngeal nerve (IX) will be stimulated and the gag reflex might be evoked. Clinical experience suggests that patients can be sub-divided into two categories: those that have a desensitized gag reflex, and those that have a hypersensitive gag reflex. For the first group (who may have a history of CPAP use), the extension presents little or no problem and they are able to tolerate it well after about 24–72hrs of wear. In other cases, a topical anesthetic spray might be needed to dull the gag reflex when the device is first delivered, followed by a period of 48–72hrs of habituation. In the most severe category of patients with a hypersensitive gag reflex, other techniques will be called upon. For example, in some of these cases a cold (erbium or CO_2) laser may be beneficial. It is believed that the cold laser imparts energy to the tissues such that collagen cross-linking or neo-collagenesis is promoted. In this technique, the collagen fibrils contract, causing a shrinking of the oropharyngeal soft tissues, including the uvula and pillars of the fauces (Fig. 65). This increased space often permits most hypersensitive patients to adapt to the stent with a habituation period of approx. 24–72hrs.

After the device has been suitably installed for the first time, the patient is congratulated for their cooperation! The patient is then instructed on the proper removal and insertion of the appliance. With the device outside the patient's mouth, it's wise to go over the various components so that the patient understands their new appliance, including adjustments that will be done at home. It's important to educate the patient on how to turn the screw(s) in the direction of the arrow(s) but only when the appliance feels slightly loose. **Over-zealous screw turns must be avoided**. The device has an increased surface area intentionally, so it's advisable to use a sonic bath to clean the appliance and keep it exceptionally clean. The patient should be informed not to use a toothbrush to clean the device since the 3D axial springs may become distorted. Most patients will need to record their wear time and screw-turns, preferably in a journal, diary, or other suitable app, such as a calendar installed on a smart phone. Importantly, it is recommended that the appliance be protected like an investment or a diamond ring, by keeping the device in its case when it is not being worn. This simple step can prevent loss, breakage, or damage of the appliance,

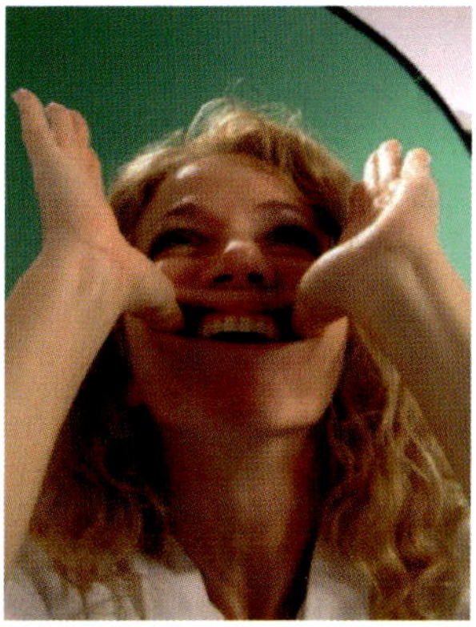

Figure 86: Zygoma or cheek bone lift exercise is done 3 times/day, 30 lifts each time, with thumbs inside or outside the mouth.

sometimes by the family's dog. In addition, when the device is not being worn, it is essential to follow the daytime-nighttime protocol by doing oral myofunctional exercises, as prescribed. For example, a patient may elect to do 'cheek bone lift' exercises (zygoma lift, Fig. 86a) three times per day with 30 lifts each time. When the appliance is first worn, the patient will experience increased salivation, which is a normal response that might actually help the patient because of an increased frequency of swallowing. While salivary adaptation will occur, the patient will likely also find it somewhat difficult to speak with the device in the mouth. To help with this transition, patients are encouraged to read aloud for 10mins three times per day until the speech sounds normal. A phonetic text that contains all the sounds of the English language can be used but, in some cases, especially children, normalization of speech occurs in a very short period of time. Finally, the patient is appointed for the next visit in approx. one week's time. However, some offices/practices will follow up with courtesy phone calls after 24–72hrs in case a patient needs further guidance, instruction, or assurance prior to the next appointment. In addition, an out-of-hours emergency phone number can also be supplied in the unlikely event that it may be needed in the interim.

One-week post insertion

At the one-week post insertion appointment, one of the first things to assess is patient compliance. In this biomimetic approach, elements of the circadian rhythm are invoked and without at least a minimum of 8hrs of wear, clinical changes may not be initiated. Ideally, prolonged wear of 12–16hrs is expected. In any case, this appointment's check list has six items. First, it's essential to re-check the retention and activation of the device. The dentist may simply ask the patient if the appliance feels a little loose. There will follow a subjective response, which may or may not reflect the clinical findings. If the device is loose after adjusting its retention, it's important to show the patient how to re-activate it, by gently turning the screw(s) in the direction of the arrow(s). Next, it's essential to re-check the occlusion with and without the appliance in situ. At this stage, the TM joints can also be palpated and assessed for comfort. Occlusal adjustments of the upper appliance are accomplished using articulating paper to find any high occlusal contacts (Fig. 87). In the generic protocol, an even number of uniformly spaced dots is typically the goal. In other cases, however, occlusal coverage adjustments are more proactively made to either reposition the mandible and/or encourage tooth eruption, for example to improve the vertical dimension of the occlusion. In this case, the general rule is to perform this step at each visit, starting from the anterior aspect (premolar region) to the more posterior molar region (Fig. 83a). The idea on each visit

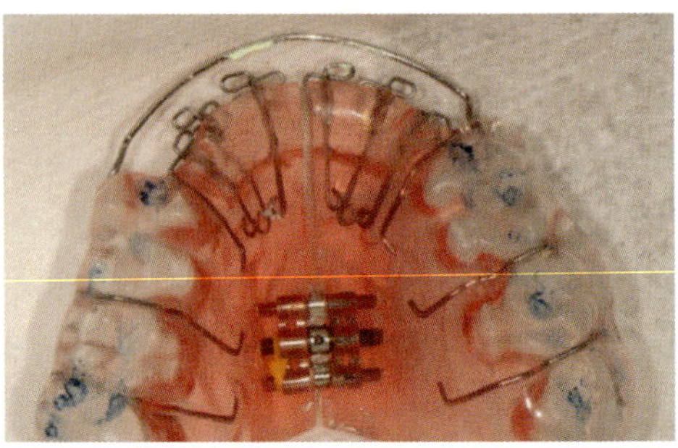

Figure 87a: Use of articulating paper to show occlusal contacts. Any heavy or premature contacts will need to be ground out.

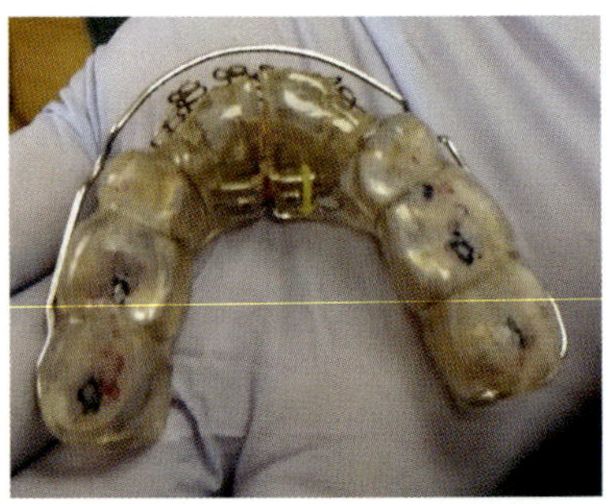

Figure 87b: Lower component of mRNA appliance showing heavy contacts that need to be ground out.

is to remove a very small amount of occlusal acrylic (say 0.25mm) from the bicuspid region using a flat acrylic bur until there is no occlusal contact with the opposing teeth. This spatial change will allow the opposing teeth to supra-erupt into that space (Fig. 83b) as predicted by the spatial matrix hypothesis. Thus, this procedure is repeated at each visit until the desired vertical height is obtained. Note that once the lower first premolar begins to supra-erupt, the selective grinding is extended to the second premolar, and sequentially onto the first molar, etc. until the proper vertical dimension has been sufficiently recaptured, for example, in a deep bite case. Note that this procedure might eventually lead to perforation of the occlusal coverage since the lower posterior teeth begin to supra-erupt, re-capturing the vertical dimension of the occlusion, as necessary. In other cases, a pattern of selective grinding is adopted that best suits the case. Take a 12yr-old patient with a deep bite as a clinical scenario. In this case, the second molars are undergoing active eruption. In these types of cases, the premolars and first molars could be covered with acrylic while the second molars 'over-erupt', recapturing the vertical dimension. Thereafter, the premolars/molars would be addressed as explained above. In yet another clinical situation, an adult may have an oral orthotic for the treatment of TMJ dysfunction. In these types of cases, it's probably best to correct the premolar region first before allowing the molar region to catch up with the occlusal changes achieved.

In the next step of this procedure, the fitting surface and posterior border of the device are checked. This is a significant component of the technique since, over a period of time, the palate will remodel inferiorly (Fig. 22). Subsequently, the posterior nasal spine will remodel downward, and the overlying mucosa will start to make contact with the appliance. In some cases where this feature occurs rapidly, a line can be seen extending across the palatal mucosa, demarcating the contact between the device and the tissues. If these clinical signs are not observable, then two further methods can be used to assess the fitting surface. The first of these is colloquially known as the 'slurp test'. If a separation exists between the palatal mucosa and the device, then this space will become filled with saliva.

As the patient swallows this saliva, a relative negative pressure is created and the patient 'sucks' on the device. This suction effect is well known in dental prosthetics when complete dentures are worn. The effect of this suction is that it pulls on the oral mucosa, which in turn gently stretches the mucoperiosteum including the midpalatal suture, thereby encouraging the remodeling process. Thus, to test for the presence of this gap, the patient is asked to suck air between the device and the mucosa, by making a slurping sound. The clinician then listens (or records) the sound. If the sound is moist, then saliva is passing through the space and the fluid flow suggests that there is sufficient clearance. On the other hand, if the sound is dry, then air is passing through the space but no fluids, which suggests that there is insufficient space between the palatal mucosa and the fitting surface of the appliance. Therefore, in this case the fitting surface needs to be adjusted to re-establish a space between the palate and the device. The second, more precise, method used to ascertain the goodness of fit is to use a pressure indicating paste. This paste can either be sprayed or painted onto the fitting surface (Fig. 88) and the device is then seated. When the appliance is carefully removed, high spots become evident since the pressure indicator paste has been displaced in areas of contact between the device and the mucosa, and these can be ground down using an acrylic

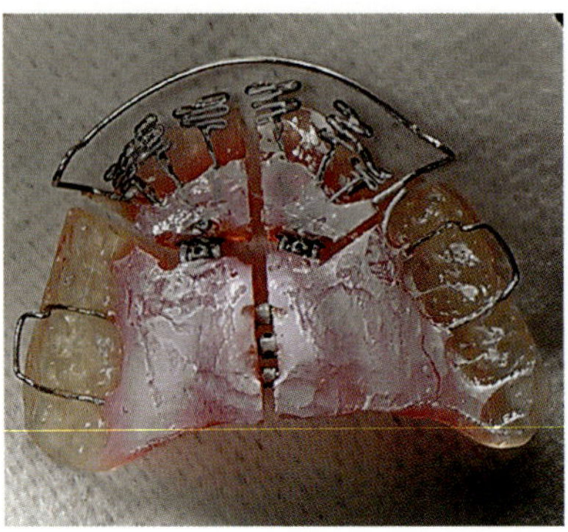

Figure 88a: Using pressure-indicating paste, the palatal surface and posterior border are checked.

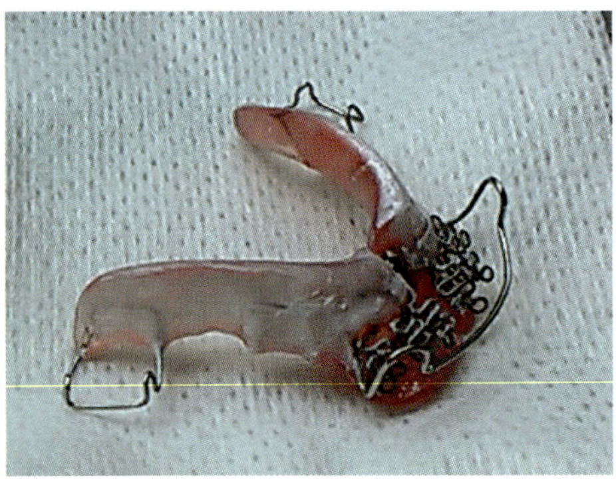

Figure 88b: On a lower device, it's important to check the disto-lingual flange using pressure-indicating paste.

bur. The device can then be re-seated, and the slurp test re-done, to see if sufficient clearance has been achieved, although some patients may need a sip of water if they have a dry mouth.

The above procedure can also be repeated on the lower device (Fig. 88b) to ensure that approx. 0.5mm of clearance is gained and the suction effect is maintained. Moreover, a variant of this step is required for the lower component of the mRNA appliance. In this specific design, the lower component of the mRNA appliance is adjusted on the bucco-occlusal aspect of the fitting surface (Fig. 89). The lower component of the mRNA appliance has occlusal coverage to embed the screw-fin mechanism for mandibular advancement, as well as making the device more robust and resistant to fracture due to bruxing, grinding, or clenching. However, clinical experience with the use of lower orthotics suggests that prolonged use can precipitate intrusion of the lower posterior segments, sometimes producing a posterior open bite. In order to avoid this possible sequela, the lower component of mRNA appliance is adjusted on the internal, bucco-occlusal aspect of the fitting surface, which helps the lower posterior segments to upright slightly. Continuing with this procedure throughout treatment might eventually lead to perforation of the occlusal coverage since the lower

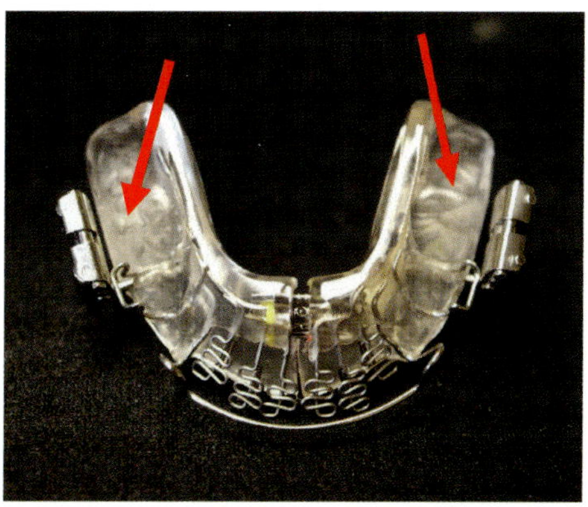

Figure 89: It is essential to adjust the lower component of the mRNA appliance on its bucco-occlusal aspect (indicated by arrows).

posterior teeth begin to supra-erupt, re-capturing the vertical dimension of the occlusion, as necessary. Nevertheless, it's imperative to make minor adjustments of the fitting surface as treatment proceeds.

If the device has a beaded pharyngeal stent for OSA, it needs to be re-checked at each visit. It's important to ensure that the extension is securely embedded in the device and that is has not become loose with wear or repeated bending. For the extension to be active, it can be bent to conform with the anatomy of the tissues. It can be elongated or shortened, and its position can be adjusted using bird-beak pliers to bend the extension as required. The extension has a 'C loop' design (Fig. 73), which can be used to either elongate the stent using the flat bird-beak pliers applied to the inside of the loop(s), or it can be shortened by using the single-prong of the 3-prong pliers applied to the inside of the loop(s). After this step, the same principles can be used to adjust the U loops of the labial bow to ensure that it is approx. 0.5mm away from the anterior teeth and not in contact with the labial surfaces, since the teeth may have moved in line with the remodeling process. Similarly, the dentist will check that the 3D axial springs continue to make contact with palatal/lingual aspects of the anterior teeth. First, it's worth noting whether the stem of the 3D axial spring is free of acrylic. If so, the stem can be grasped with long or short bird-beak pliers (Fig. 90) and bent toward the palatal/lingual aspects of

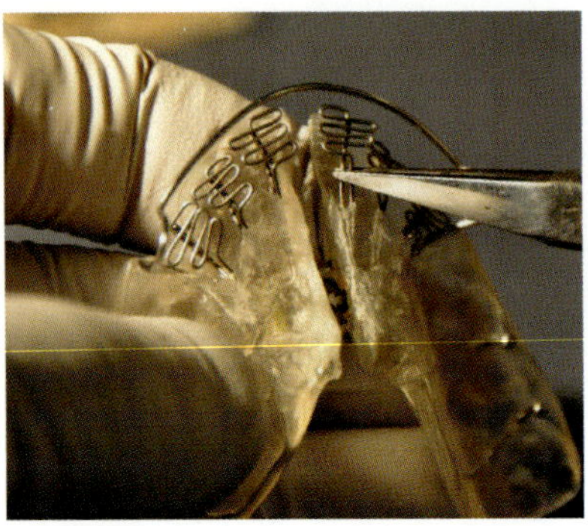

Figure 90a: Adjusting stem of 3D axial springs for maximum contact with palatal surface of tooth.

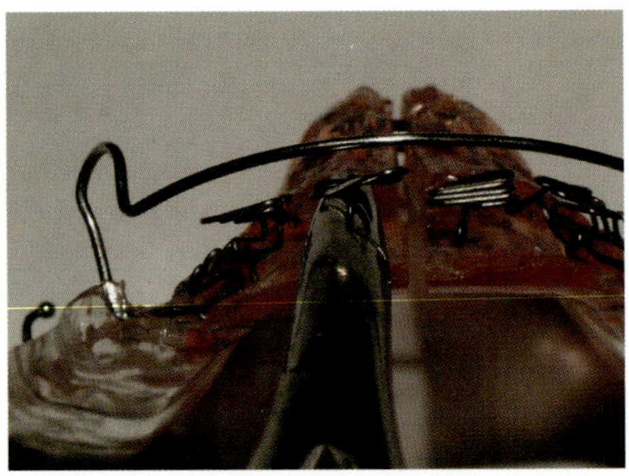

Figure 90b: Rotating stem of 3D axial springs for maximum area of contact with palatal surface of corresponding tooth.

the tooth. The 3D axial springs should not be repeatedly bent because they might become loosely embedded within the acrylic but, moreover, repeated bending can cause metal fatigue which could lead to fracture of a spring. Thus, it's better to grasp the stem of the spring, bend it as required, and then hold that position for about 10 seconds since the memory function of the wire will try to recover the spring back into its original position (Fig. 85b).

In addition, the 3D axial springs can be rotated to make maximum contact with the tooth surface. Fig. 90a shows the stem being grasped and rotated into place (Fig. 90b), by holding that position for approx. 10 seconds. In rare cases, it's sometimes necessary to add curvature to the head of the spring for it to make intimate contact with a palatal cingulum or lingual surface of a tooth. In this case, either bird-beak pliers can be used to bend the loops in the head of the spring or 3-prong pliers can be used to add a gentle curve by crimping the head of the spring (Fig. 91a). Sometimes, a C loop is added to the stem of 3D axial spring, especially when a tooth is palatally or lingually displaced/positioned with respect to the other teeth in the arch. In this case, the flat side of the bird-beak pliers is placed on the inside of the C loop (Fig. 91b) and gentle pressure will help elongate the stem of the spring, akin to an orthodontic adjustment to better align the tooth.

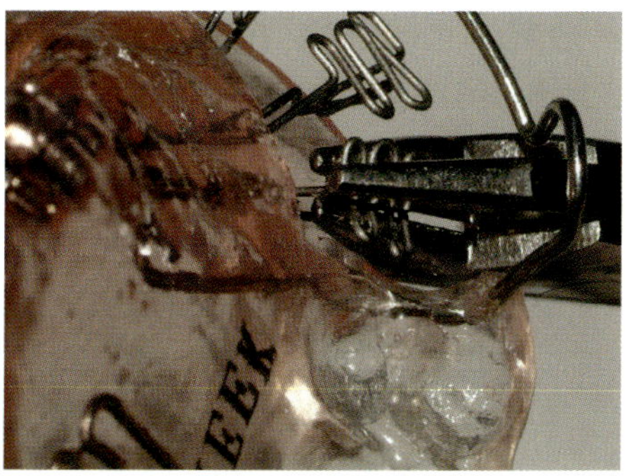

Figure 91a: Adjusting head of 3D axial spring for maximum contact with palatal surface of tooth.

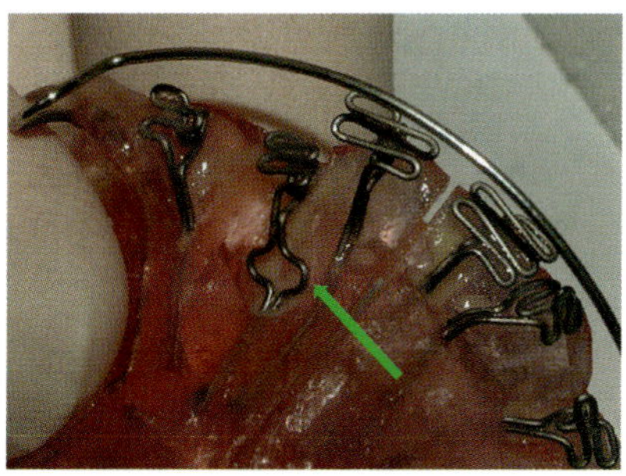

Figure 91b: C loop (arrow) in stem of 3D axial springs can be extended to improve orthodontic alignment of corresponding tooth.

The above six steps are slightly modified in the case of Wireframe or Hybrid appliances. In the first step (retention and activation), the retentiveness of the C clasps has to be established. Only minor adjustments should be necessary since a bonded button or ledge of composite can be used to provide a 'snap-on' fit. For activation of the device, the key is to not introduce any additional torque by keeping the minor and major omega loops flat in the same plane. Here, it's useful to review the omega loop principle. For practice purposes, an isolated omega loop can be fashioned from a piece of wire and laid flat on a piece of paper (Fig. 92a). Next, the width of the wire can be marked and measured (Fig. 92b) on graph paper or plain paper. The flat beak of the bird-beak pliers is placed on the inside of the omega loop at right angles to the axis of the wire. By applying a light pressure, the omega loop will spread and become wider; however, the ends of the wire will be displaced downward and the component becomes narrower (Fig. 93a). Therefore, counter-bends are needed. To achieve these counter-bends, the flat side of the beak is reversed and positioned on the inside of the base of the omega loops (Fig. 93b). By squeezing

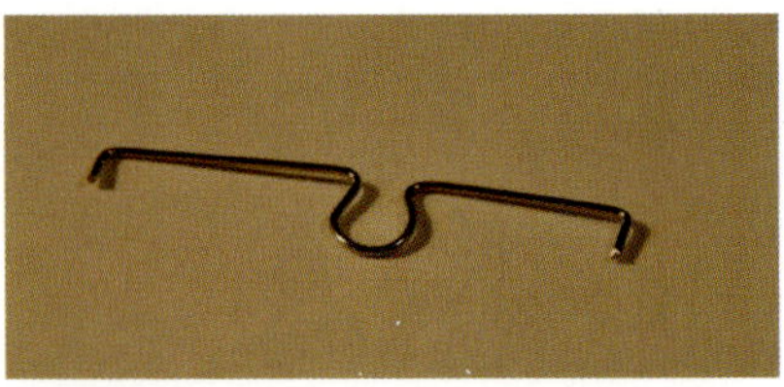

Figure 92a: Omega loop placed on paper on flat surface.

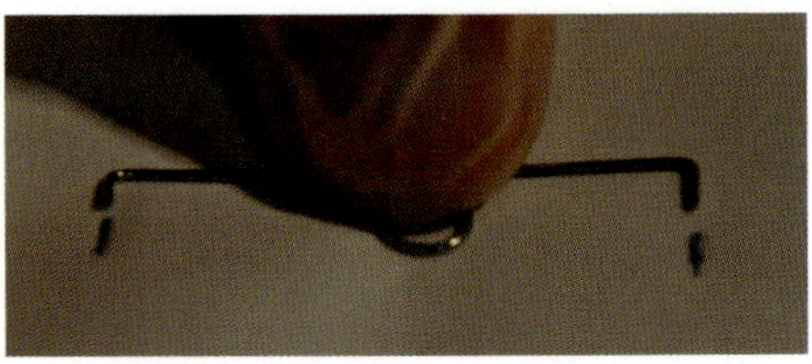

Figure 92b: Total width marked on paper.

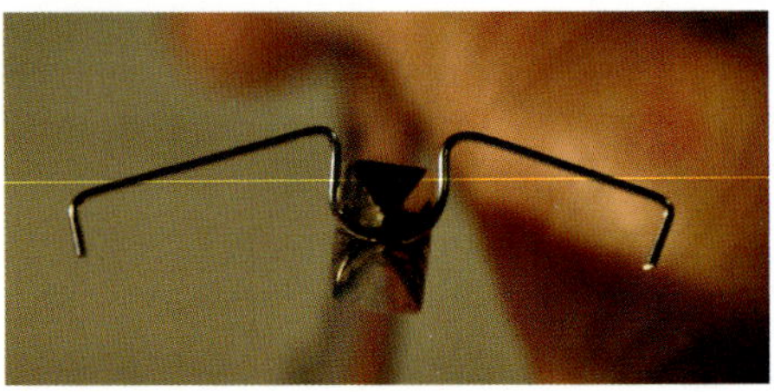

Figure 93a: Adjusting omega loop with flat side of pliers on inside of loop.

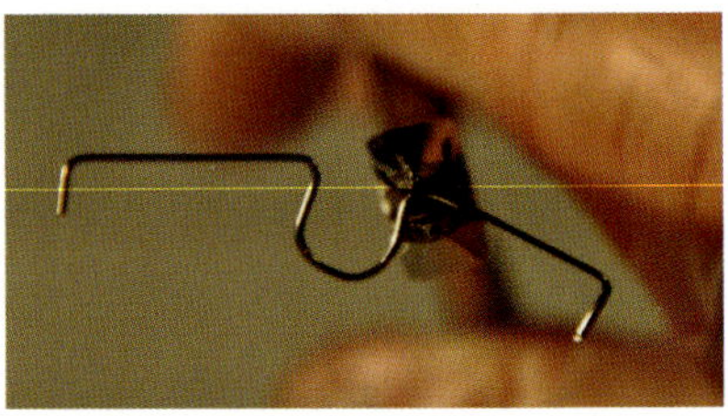

Figure 93b: Counter-bend on left of loop with pliers reversed.

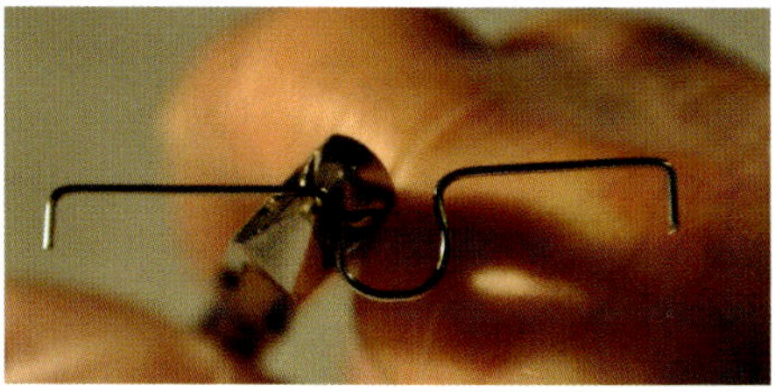

Figure 94a: Counter-bend on right side of loop with pliers reversed.

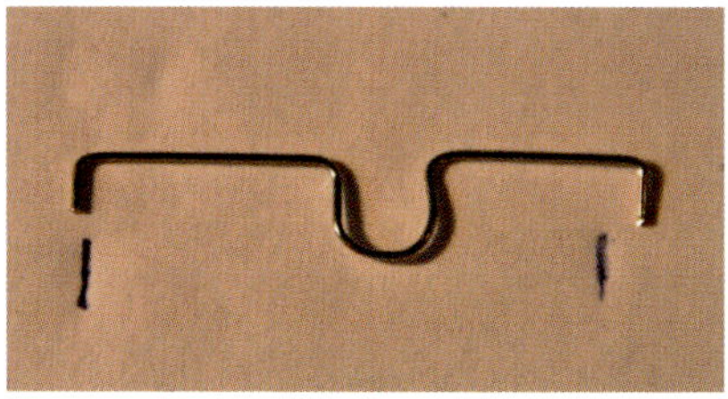

Figure 94b: Increased palatal width noted on paper.

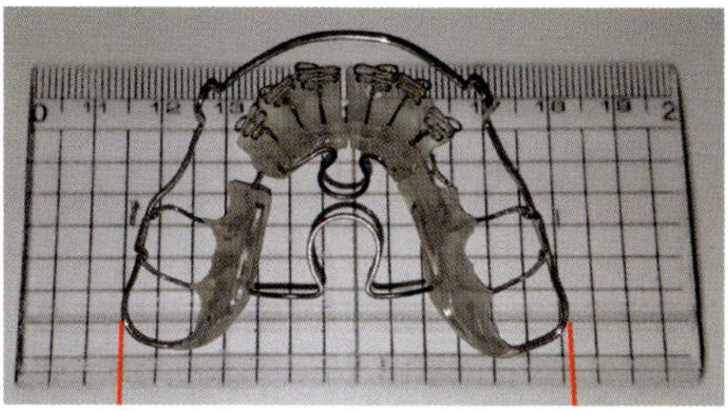

Figure 95a: Wireframe appliance on graph paper to measure width. Initial width measurement is 18 – 11.5 = 6.5cm.

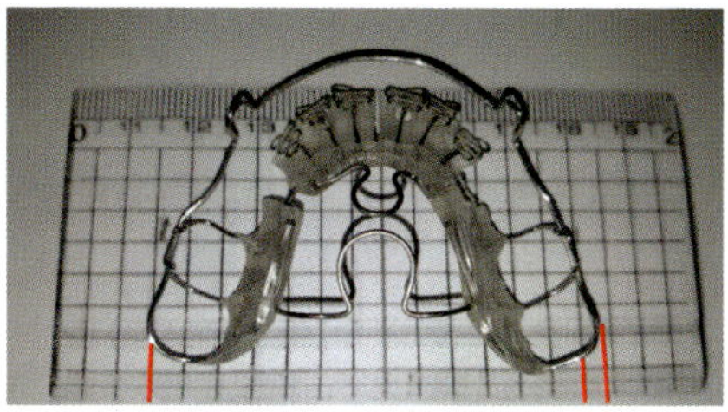

Figure 95b: Increased palatal width after adjustment is 18.5 – 11.5 = 7cm, providing 0.5cm of activation.

gently on both sides, the wire will become unbent while the omega loop itself becomes wider (Fig. 94a). These changes can be verified by placing the wire on a piece of paper and re-measuring its width (Fig. 94b). Note that the wire should lie flat on the paper if no torque has been introduced into the system.

The above principles can be applied in the clinical adjustment of a device following the assessment of retention. First, the width of the device can be marked and measured (Fig. 95a) on graph paper. For major (posterior) omega loop activation, the flat beak of the bird-beak pliers is placed on inside of the omega loop and squeezed gently to widen it by approx. 1mm. Next, a counter-bend is performed, by using the flat beak of the long bird-beak pliers on the inside of the base of the omega loop. These changes can be verified by placing the device back on the piece of paper and re-measuring its width (Fig. 95b). In addition, the wires extending from the major omega loop need to be moved away from the palatal mucosa, so they don't impinge on the tissues as the palate remodels inferiorly. This is achieved by using the single-pronged beak of the 3-prong pliers on the outside of device so that the wire is displaced away from the tissues by approx. 0.5mm when the pliers are gently squeezed. This degree of major omega loop activation should be sufficient for about 1 month until the next appointment, and it also parallels the approx. rate of screw turns (4 weeks × 0.25mm = 1mm). A similar procedure can be used for anterior (minor) omega loop activation also. Note that any acrylic obstructing the minor omega loop should be cleared using an acrylic bur prior to adjustment with, say, the long bird-beak pliers. It is also possible to measure the separation of the split in the acrylic components of the device (Fig. 96b), using a periodontal probe as ruler. With the device outside the mouth, the acrylic separation is measured. The appliance is then seated inside the mouth and the separation re-measured. Ideally, the acrylic separation should be 1mm narrower in situ compared to its width outside the mouth.

After the retention/activation and fitting surface of the device have been adjusted, the occlusal stops (in the case of a Wireframe device) or occlusal pads (in the case of a Hybrid device) are checked to ensure they are not interfering with the occlusion and have been equilibrated as noted above. The next three steps: adjustments of the 3D axial springs; positioning of the labial bow, and adjustment/extension of the beaded pharyngeal stent (if present) are identical to those described for the upper acrylic-based

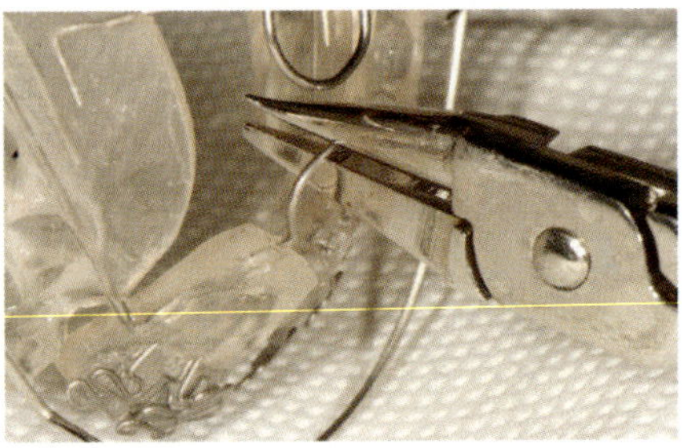

Figure 96a: Activation of the anterior omega loop of a Wireframe appliance with the flat beak on the inside of the omega loop.

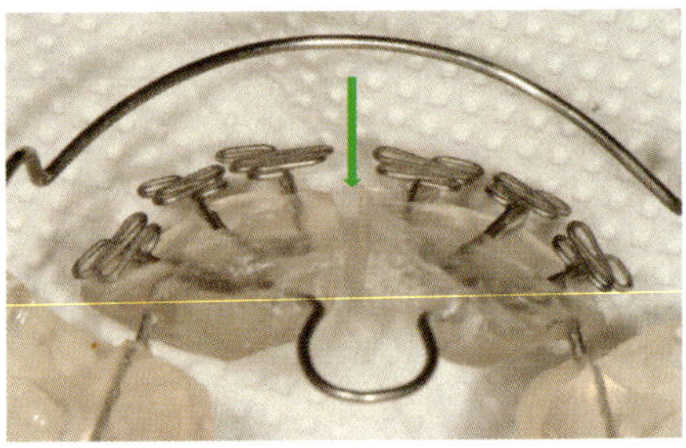

Figure 96b: Increased palatal width after adjustment with increased separation of the acrylic baseplate (arrowed).

appliance. Note that within approx. 1–3 months, a lower biomimetic device ought to be considered to help the lower arch gain its required alignment, especially if the lower arch is not keeping pace with changes in the upper arch. In some patients, the case can be finished following this empirical protocol. In other instances, however, it's necessary to plan final restorative reconstruction with crowns and bridges if there has been significant dental tissue loss through bruxism prior to treatment, or perhaps the provision of single-tooth implants if premolar spaces were recaptured during treatment. In other cases, a limited amount of orthodontic treatment using fixed appliances (Fig. 97) or clear trays may be indicated for orthodontic finishing. In the ideal setting, which is sometimes seen clinically, the holy grail is to provide sufficient functional space for the eruption of the third molars. In some cases, surgical exposure might be appropriate to permit these teeth to fully erupt and come into occlusion. Note that in approx. 30,000 years of human evolution, 32 teeth fully erupted and in occlusion was the norm; it is only within that last, say, 500 years or so that phenotypic variation from the norm has become more evident.

Appliance adjustments need to be done carefully and skillfully to avoid any breakages. The 3D axial springs are made of a nickel-free, super-elastic titanium alloy, which can fracture through metal fatigue if repeatedly bent. For this reason, 3D axial spring adjustments are done slowly, progressively, and deliberately, as required. On occasions, cold-cure acrylic can be used chairside for in-office 3D axial spring replacement.

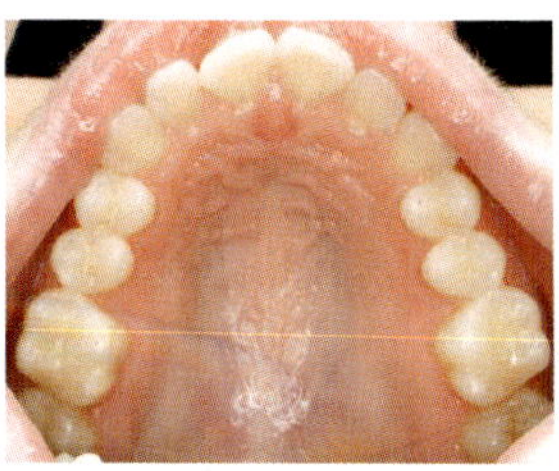

Figure 97a: Pre-treatment appearance of upper arch. Courtesy: Dr John Utama

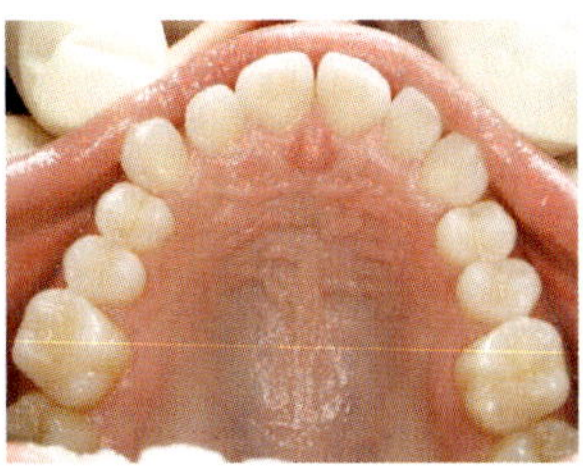

Figure 97b: Mid-treatment appearance after biomimetic oral appliance therapy.

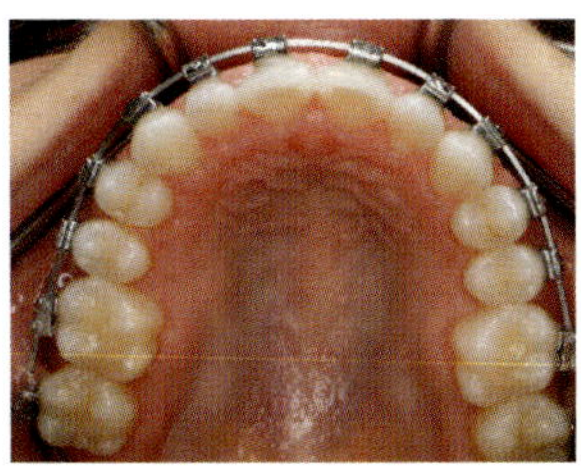

Figure 97c: Fixed orthodontic brackets for final finishing of the case.

Other components that can break include the C clasps. These clasps are soldered onto the wireframe and engage passively like partial denture clasps. While over-zealous adjustments of the claps can cause fractures, the use of a composite button/ledge bonded onto the buccal aspect of the tooth can provide additional retention and avoid frequent C clasp adjustments. Another feature that can sometimes facture due to thinning is the acrylic work. Patients should be advised that the acrylic will become thinner and perforated through continued equilibration and fitting surface adjustments as part of the protocol. However, sometimes dried acrylic will occasionally crack (especially if a patient is bruxing or grinding/clenching on the appliance) and will need to be repaired by relining or rebasing the device as needed. On the other hand, it is rare for either the omega loops or labial bow to break since they are fashioned from heavier gauge wire; however, they should be checked for looseness at each appointment to ensure they remain firmly embedded in the acrylic components. Similarly, while breakages of the pharyngeal stent/extension, including the roller bead are rare, they need to be re-checked carefully at each visit. The above breakages/occurrences do not represent a dental emergency *per se* and can be dealt with on the next business day or as appropriate.

Summary

The six appliance adjustments that are needed at each visit for these biomimetic devices are:

1. Retention and activation (clasps, screw mechanism, and omega loops)
2. Equilibration of the occlusal pads/coverage and/or occlusal stops
3. Modification of the fitting surface, including wires extending from the omega loops
4. Adjustments of the 3D axial springs to be in light contact with the palatal/lingual surfaces of the anterior six teeth
5. Positioning of the labial bow away from the labial surfaces of the teeth
6. Extension of the beaded pharyngeal stent (if present)

Each of these steps must be performed at each following visit, which are typically appointed every 4–6 weeks in adults and every 3–4 weeks in pediatric cases. But, perhaps the most important aspect of these appointments is encouragement of patients to continue with compliance, empowering them to reach a successful outcome. In addition, as treatment proceeds, the clinician is forward planning a finishing phase, if necessary. For example, some patients might require restorative reconstruction, especially in dentitions damaged by bruxism, etc. Other cases might require limited orthodontic finishing with either fixed appliances or clear tray aligners. In pediatric cases, there may be a need to monitor the case after an initial phase of biomimetic treatment, and pediatric craniofacial epigenetics is thoroughly discussed in the next chapter.

Chapter 8

Introduction to Pediatric Craniofacial Epigenetics

Synopsis: This chapter focuses on applying the concepts of pneumopedics and craniofacial epigenetics for the prevention and/or potential resolution of pediatric sleep disordered breathing (SDB), including upper airway resistance syndrome (UARS) and pediatric obstructive sleep apnea (pOSA). It is thought that a major risk factor for pediatric SDB is a deficiency in upper airway structure and function, often emanating from deficient craniofacial growth and development in non-syndromic children. This aberrant growth may be related to changes in child-rearing practices, ranging from sleep hygiene, changes in breasting-feeding and early nutritional behaviors, which might impact the child's developing microbiome. It should also be noted that poor food choices resulting in an inflammatory diet may precipitate nasal obstruction, which in turn can result in chronic mouth-breathing. In addition, a wide variety of systemic conditions, such as childhood obesity, enuresis, and attention-deficit hyperactivity disorder may be co-morbid with pediatric sleep disordered breathing.

In the previous chapters, I introduced the principles of pneumopedics and craniofacial epigenetics. These principles provide some knowledge and an appreciation of biomimetic oral appliance therapy, which can invoke epigenetic-orthopedic as well as epigenetic-orthodontic changes associated with non-surgical upper airway remodeling. In this chapter, I focus on applying these concepts for the prevention and/or potential resolution of pediatric sleep disordered breathing (SDB), including upper airway resistance syndrome (UARS) and obstructive sleep apnea (OSA) in a multi-disciplinary setting. The prevalence of SDB in children from 2–8yrs is estimated to be 2–3% (Chang and Chae 2010; Tsuda *et al.*, 2011; Gulotta *et al.*, 2019). It is thought that a major risk factor for pediatric SDB is a deficiency in upper airway structure and function, often emanating from deficient craniofacial growth and development in non-syndromic children. As early as the 20th century, Weeks (1913) and Green *et al.* (1917) discussed the relevance of perturbations of childhood facial growth and related these to disturbances in breathing associated with deficient structure and function of the upper airway. In addition, in most children, the tonsillar tissues become enlarged during upper airway infections, impairing physiologic functions, such as breathing during sleep. Kim and Guilleminault (2011) assessed craniofacial features in children and noted that a Mallampati score of 3 or 4 helped identify children with increased risk for SDB and a potentially inadequate response to adenotonsillectomy. Thus, when examining the upper airway of a child, attention should be given to both the soft tissues and the bony tissues surrounding the upper airway. Moreover, the interaction between craniofacial growth and muscle function starts early in development and continues throughout childhood. In this way, deviant tongue behaviors may perturb normal craniofacial growth and development. It should also be noted that poor dietary choices may precipitate nasal obstruction, which in turn can result in chronic mouth-breathing. This clinical sign is an important marker of orofacial muscle dysfunction, which is often associated with palatal dysmorphology, perpetuating the development of SDB.

In recent years, an increased awareness of the consequences of breathing disturbances during sleep in children has emerged. Evidence suggests that intermittent hypoxia, sleep fragmentation, obesity, and deterioration in daytime attentivity have accumulated in the pediatric population. In fact, further research has identified a link between pediatric sleep disorders and hyperactive behaviors, for example attention deficit hyperactivity disorder (ADHD). However, since there is considerable variation in the severity of these conditions, some suggest that both individual predisposition (genetic) and environmental (epigenetic) factors play a role in determining the extent of these morbidities, including: behavioral problems, cognitive function, loss of IQ, increased anxiety, attention deficit, and metabolic dysregulation in children due to fragmented sleep. As an alternative to prescription medications, such as methylphenidate (Ritalin) and dextroamphetamine (Adderall), etc., the prevention and treatment of pediatric SDB, including OSA, requires both the establishment and restoration of nasal breathing during wakefulness and during sleep. Preventive measures, such as the promotion of natural breast-feeding, allied with non-invasive interventions, in the form of oral myofunctional therapy, are thought to be important approaches to pediatric SDB and its sequelae. Indeed, if nasal breathing is not restored, despite short-term surgical improvements after tonsillo-adenoidectomy, continued mouth-breathing may be associated with abnormal upper airway growth, development, and function. Thus, screening during early childhood prior to the development of the mixed dentition is mandatory.

Typically, diagnostic pediatric features are often missed. This is not surprising since facial recognition and facial perception can obfuscate the casual observer. In fact, electroencephalography (EEG) recordings show a characteristic brain wave called N170, which is strongly associated with facial recognition (Schubert *et al.*, 2020). In other words, a child asleep with a pacifier in its mouth is regarded as normal behavior by most. However, in terms of temporo-spatial patterning, the pacifier represents an oral device, which is not biomimetic in its design. In this way, the pacifier can displace the tongue away from the palate and mold the primary alveolus and lips into a less than optimal form. The pliability of neonatal tissues is well documented. In one early study (Singh *et al.*, 2005), we evaluated 3D changes in nasal morphology in babies born with unilateral cleft lip and palate who were treated with a presurgical nasoalveolar molding

(NAM) appliance to correct the nasolabio-alveolar deformity. Note that human facial recognition draws attention to the facial deformity and our perception hinders our understanding of the dysfunction. In other words, these babies were unable to breathe through the nose on the cleft side, and that functional issue needs to be addressed primarily ahead of the perceived facial deformity. Thus, our treatment goal was to permit these babies to breathe through the nose and feed through the mouth. Using non-surgical NAM, nasal changes were captured using non-invasive, digital 3D stereo-photogrammetry. The results showed that using NAM, bilateral nasal symmetry in patients with unilateral cleft lip and palate was improved, which likely restored nasal breathing. Indeed, in a follow-up study, Singh *et al.* (2007) showed that the facial development in these children was virtually indistinguishable from a control group of non-cleft children. Thus, it's likely that the use of even a soft pacifier perturbs the spatial matrix and precipitates developmental compensation, precipitating a high-arched palate for example, that may in turn result in a mouth-breathing habit as the child grows. On the other hand, the biomimetic approach dictates that a baby or young child should exhibit physiologic behavior while asleep. Put simply, a child's sleep ought to be silent and friction-free. There should not be any labored breathing or stridor; nor should there be any sounds such as sleep bruxism in the primary or mixed dentitions. Therefore, one aspect of oral appliance design is to restore nasal function and enhance nasal symmetry, to improve the child's ability to breathe through the nose.

For the sake of simplicity, in this chapter, the phases of pediatric craniofacial development will be described as: the perinatal period, which encompasses the birthing process and the development of the biofilm; the early postnatal phase, which is dominated by breast-feeding; the deciduous dentition, which spans 3–6yrs of age; and the mixed dentition, which spans 6–12yrs of age. Note that for these four time periods, molecular compensations are occurring and, although epigenetic variations in the phenotype might be precipitated at much later stages in life (Khalyfa *et al.*, 2017), they may present earlier clinically, as discussed below. Childbirth represents the start of the perinatal period. Following natural vaginal

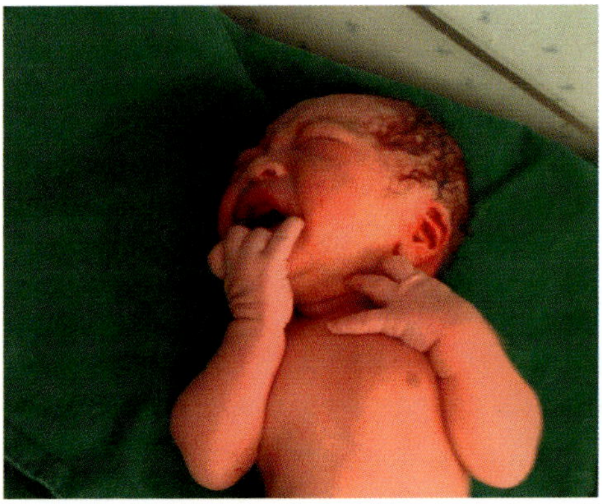

Figure 98: Newborn child at birth following natural vaginal delivery.

delivery (Fig. 98), four physiologic processes occur, which permit the fetus with placental oxygenation to become a baby with external respiration. There is closure of the: umbilical arteries, which becomes the (medial) umbilical ligaments; closure of the umbilical vein and ductus venosus in the liver, which become the ligamentum teres hepatis and ligamentum venosum, respectively; closure of the ductus arteriosus, which becomes the ligamentum arteriosum between the arch of the aorta and the pulmonary artery; and closure of the foramen ovale, which becomes the fossa ovalis between the two atria of the heart. These four physiologic changes produce separate arterial (oxygenated) and venous (de-oxygenated) blood circulations. In addition, during the birthing process, the fetus moves from a germ-free, sterile environment inside the placenta through the vaginal canal, picking up microflora from the mother's perineal fluids. In so doing the external biofilm is established *de novo* since the baby's skin becomes populated with microorganisms for the first time.

In fact, the mode of birth affects the formation of the microbiome. For example, establishment of the microbiota of the gut has been shown to differ between infants delivered vaginally and those delivered by Caesarian section; since their first contact is with the mother's skin and not with the vaginal mucosa (Penders *et al.*, 2006). Similarly, for the oral microbiota, Lif-Holgerson *et al.* (2011) reported that more diverse bacteria are detected in babies delivered vaginally compared with babies delivered by C-section. Thus, the microbiomes of C-section and vaginally delivered children form two distinct colonization patterns, which may impact later pediatric health. For example, by the age of 7yrs, children delivered vaginally showed higher numbers of clostridia compared with C-section born children (Salminen *et al.*, 2004). Moreover, children with a history of asthma had lower numbers of clostridia compared to healthy children. Thus, early colonization may influence the development of the microbiome, which may in turn predispose some children to specific diseases. In fact, babies born by C-section have higher rates of immune-related disorders later in life. To prevent this, when fecal transplants (microbiota from the mother's stool transferred to breast milk) were investigated, it was found that these babies developed gut microbiota that resembled those of vaginally born babies. In addition, the oral microbiome of the child is influenced by breast-feeding. In the maternal gastro-intestinal tract (GIT), gut bacteria pass through the GIT lining cells (entrocytes) and occupy the underlying connective tissues (lamina propria). From there, monocytes are thought to help microorganisms pass into the entero-mammary pathway by way of mesenteric lymph nodes and the lymphatic-venous blood circulation. This blood supply reaches the mammary glands in late pregnancy and its contents pass through the mammary gland epithelium to colonize the skin of the breast, forming the mammary microbiome. On breast-feeding, the colostrum/milk microbiota co-mingle with the breast-skin and populate the infant's oral microbiota. After swallowing, these microbiota will inhabit the infant's GIT. Thus, while human milk has been traditionally considered to be sterile, recent studies suggest that it may contain commensal, symbiotic, and probiotic bacteria. These bacterial populations, along with the secretory IgA molecules passed onto the suckling child, are helpful in many ways, including the ability to bind microorganisms to keep them away from the child's tissues, protecting the infant against infections, and contributing to the maturation of the child's immune system (Fernández *et al.*, 2013). Not surprisingly, in the absence of sufficient nursing, Hippocrates taught that 'all disease begins in the gut'. In fact, Greaves

(2018) considers that the child's developing immune system needs to be challenged by infection in the neonate's first year; otherwise there is a risk that it will not be primed. Recently, there has been a trend of parents using antiseptic wipes and disinfecting surfaces throughout the home, while breast-feeding of infants has become less common. These trends reduce a young child's exposure to microorganisms with a risk that the immune system may be unprimed; the so-called hygiene hypothesis (Bach, 2018). Consequently, it is thought that people in developed countries have a less diverse gut microbiome.

Originally, the early postnatal phase of human development was dominated by breast-feeding. Humans are, after all, mammals; and lactation by the mammary glands is the hallmark of mammalian evolution and behavior (Fig. 99). In the distant past, say 30,000 years ago, every human child that was born was either exclusively breast-fed or it didn't survive. Although child-rearing practices have changed dramatically, especially in more recent times, the 'caveman' genome persists along with human primitive reflexes. However, the mode, consistency, and contents of feeding have changed significantly since that time. For example, in the modern era, bottle-feeding is preferred by many women for a variety of reasons. This mode of feeding is, in fact, very different from nursing in many respects. As alluded to above, the teat of the milk-bottle represents a modified

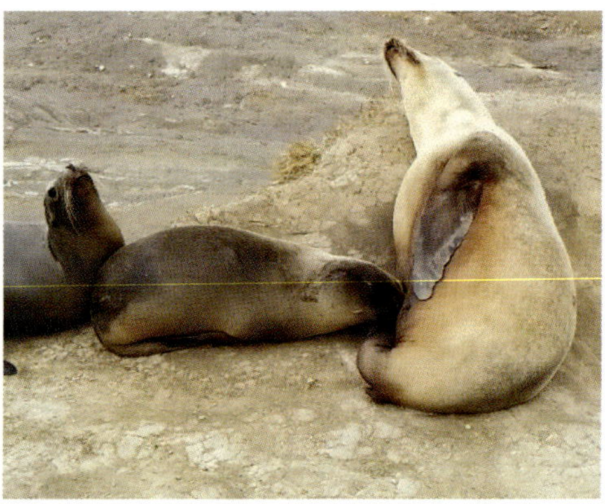

Figure 99: California sea-lion suckling newborn pup.

spatial matrix and, as such, initiates unintended epigenetic changes. In contrast, it is thought that suckling/breast-feeding promotes developmental mechanisms for midfacial morphogenesis. During nursing, jaw movements via the muscles of mastication provide gentle functional forces that stretch the craniofacial sutures, while the tongue shows peristaltic motion that is thought to mold the palate. In one study (López Del Valle *et al.*, 2006), we assessed the association of breast-feeding with the prevalence of malocclusion. The results of that study showed that about one-third of the mothers breast-fed their child for a period of about 3 months. Disturbingly, 90% of the children in that study showed some evidence of malocclusion by the age of about 3 years when the deciduous dentition was fully erupted and in occlusion.

On the other hand, another study investigated the plastic material of the milk bottle, benzyl butyl phthalate (BBP). The findings suggested that BBP exposure to mesenchymal stem cells enhances adipogenesis (fat cell formation) and lipid accumulation when compared to controls. Thus, it appeared that BBP tipped the epigenomic balance in the regulation of connective tissue stem cells toward adipogenesis. This epigenetic modification, associated with altered gene expression, might lead to excessive fat deposition and, eventually, childhood obesity (Sonkar *et al.*, 2016). However, obesity is a complex issue. Another study indicated that breast-feeding duration is related to methylation of the leptin gene, which plays a role in the risk of a child developing obesity during its lifetime (Obermann-Borst *et al.*, 2013). Thus, environmental factors in the early-life experience of the child, such as duration of breast-feeding, appear to be associated with variations in leptin methylation, which may be an epigenetic mechanism providing a protective effect against obesity. Despite the above contentions, some mothers and children find it difficult to breast-feed. On the one hand, lactation counselors can be usefully deployed to educate and support women of child-bearing age, including new and young mothers. On the other hand, a child may be unable to latch during lactation. For this reason, newly born babies ought to be screened after delivery or later at the dental office by a pediatric or general dentist. If tongue restriction or ankyloglossia/tongue-tie is diagnosed, a lingual frenectomy may be quickly performed, allowing the baby to latch immediately after the procedure to encourage nursing. It is thought that in the middle-ages, midwives did an oral sweep of the new-born child using the index finger, presumably to inoculate the oral flora of the mouth with the mother's perineal fluids and, using an elongated fingernail (pinky), released a tight or restrictive frenum (Obladen, 2010), prior to breast-feeding by the mother.

Note that malocclusions and maxillo-mandibular discrepancies have also been linked to dietary changes during evolution. Eyquem *et al.* (2017) suggest that epigenetic reductions in muscle mass and bite forces have resulted in reduced mechanical stimuli, leading to the development of smaller jaw bones. They investigated the relationship between masticatory function and facial morphology, using geometric morphometrics on 3D CBCT scans. They noted that people with a hunter-gatherer (HG) lifestyle had a more prognathic maxilla. The facial size of the HGs was also larger, while the maxilla of those with maxillo-mandibular discrepancies was smaller. In line with previous studies (Strand Viðarsdóttir *et al.*, 2002; von Cramon-Taubadel, 2011), it was suggested that the midface is influenced by the diet as well as by other factors, such as climate, population history, etc. and represents an adaptable, morphologic boundary between the cranial base above and the mandible below. Indeed, Yamamoto *et al.* (2020) studied morphologic correlation between craniofacial muscles and bones in mice. They noted that bone deformations were associated with a change in the shape of the corresponding muscles, suggesting epigenetic interactions that permit muscle and skeletal modifications to occur. Not surprisingly, it is currently thought that dentoskeletal abnormalities are associated with an increased risk of pediatric OSA. For example, Huynh *et al.* (2011) found that SDB in a pediatric cohort was associated with adeno-tonsillar hypertrophy, dolichocephaly, high mandibular plane (gonial) angle, narrow palate, and maxillo-mandibular crowding. The causative factors of these conditions likely relate to epigenetic/environmental parameters encountered during childhood development. Indeed, Eichenberger and Baumgartner (2014) consider that palatal expansion in children may play a role in improving nasal breathing, head position, OSA, nocturnal enuresis, and ear function, but Huynh *et al.* (2016) found little evidence for either maxillary expansion or mandibular advancement in addressing pediatric SDB. Similarly, Koretsi *et al.* (2018) found no prospective randomized clinical trials on the effectiveness of non-surgical or surgically assisted maxillary expansion in the treatment of pediatric OSA. On the other hand, Villa *et al.* (2011) and Camacho *et al.* (2017) suggest that palatal expansion is potentially curative in certain cases of pediatric OSA with normalization of the apnea-hypopnea index (Vale *et al.*, 2017). Similarly, Hoxha *et al.* (2018) reported that approx. 6 months of palatal expansion increased arch widths and pharyngeal airway size, while decreasing the AHI in children diagnosed with OSA.

Child-rearing practices have changed throughout the ages, and these changes include sleeping habits and feeding preferences. In recent times, there has been much discussion about sudden infant death syndrome (SIDS). In the neonate, the larynx is positioned considerably higher than in the adult so that the epiglottis and uvula can make contact, but later, descent of the larynx occurs. It is thought that this developmental change may be associated with SIDS. SIDS is characterized by the unexplained death of an otherwise healthy baby, typically less than one year old, usually during sleep. For these reasons, SIDS is sometimes referred to as crib death. In an investigation of etiologic factors (Li and Daling, 1991), it was found that maternal smoking was associated with SIDS in some but not all ethnic groups studied. Similarly, low birth weight was related to SIDS in Caucasian but not Asian families. In another study comparing Asian and European families, Balarajan *et al.* (1989) reported a lower incidence of SIDS in infants of Asian origin. This finding can likely be explained by sleeping habits, since it is known that Asian parents often prefer co-sleeping with the child in its formative years. For example, SIDS was not known amongst Thai mothers prior to their migration to Australia. Their family practices to prevent SIDS included breast-feeding, not leaving the baby alone at nighttime, placing the baby on its side or back to sleep, and bed-sharing. Thus, information derived from Asian child rearing practices may be useful in preventing SIDS

(Rice *et al.*, 1998). In any case, in order to prevent this tragic occurrence, the current pediatric advice is 'back to sleep', in other words putting the baby to sleep on its back with nothing else in the crib. This seemingly simple procedure has dramatically cut the incidence of SIDS. However, we suggested that more craniofacial research is required to elucidate the etiology of the condition (Mossey *et al.*, 1998).

While placing the baby on the back to sleep appears to beneficially impact the prevalence of SIDS, this practice does not necessarily reflect child-rearing skills in the past or those currently practiced in some non-westernized cultures (Fig. 100a). Consequently, in some cases, there has been an increased incidence of deformational plagiocephaly. Deformational plagiocephaly, also known as positional plagiocephaly, refers to an asymmetric or misshapen skull/head shape (Fig. 100b). This cranial deformity results from repetitive external pressure to an infant's skull, by the head being in one position for prolonged periods of time, e.g. in a baby crib or car seat. In Chapter 5 it was noted that a baby may have a bald patch on the occiput, which might be a clinical sign of early or developing deformational plagiocephaly. If left untreated, the child can develop ipsilateral frontal bossing, ipsilateral anterior ear displacement, ipsilateral occipital flattening, and contralateral occipital bossing, which gives rise to observable cranial asymmetry (Fig. 100b).

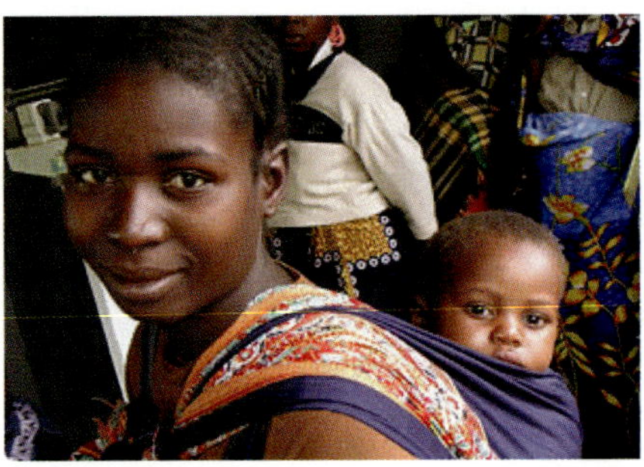

Figure 100a: African woman carrying child on her back.

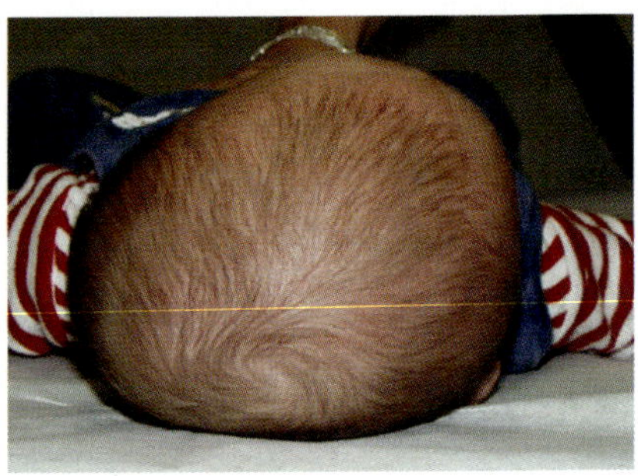

Figure 100b: Infant showing deformational plagiocephaly.

Deformational (positional) plagiocephaly can be regarded as an epigenetic phenomenon that represents (descending) cranial developmental compensation. The cranium and developing brain represent a spatial matrix. According to the spatial matric hypothesis (Singh, 2004), a spatial matrix is an arena/site in which development events unfold as (epigenetic) gene-environmental interactions proceed. In this case, the developmental event is brain development. Here, large amounts of hyaluronan are being produced, and this hydrophilic proteoglycan binds water. In effect, this macromolecule causes the brain to expand symmetrically, in line with temporo-spatial patterning. In other words, specific genes, such as HAR1, are being expressed at this time to permit neonatal brain development. This rapid, soft-tissue expansion gently stretches the cranial sutures, and the local stem cell populations (Zhao *et al.*, 2015) respond to this signal by differentiating into osteoblasts that lay down new (intramembranous) bone. However, this bony deposition is subject to remodeling by environmental pressure, mostly during sleep, which yields an asymmetric cranium associated with deformational plagiocephaly if the 'back to sleep' advice is followed exclusively.

It is believed that deformational plagiocephaly may be associated with developmental delay. One study (Collett *et al.*, 2013) found that preschool children with a history of deformational plagiocephaly received lower developmental scores when compared to controls. If a baby is diagnosed with deformational plagiocephaly, developmental delays in both motor and cognitive skills should be screened for, bearing in mind that babies develop at different times and rates. In addition, playing with babies to get them moving helps them to develop motor skills. Thus, rolling, crawling, pushing, reaching, pulling, holding, and grasping movements should be encouraged. To develop cognitive skills, it's important to play with the baby to get them babbling/talking and thinking. Similarly, other interactions with the environment including listening, looking, imitating, reading, singing, and talking can also be encouraged. In terms of SIDS prevention, it's wise to place babies to sleep on their backs. During the day when the baby is awake, active 'tummy time' can be encouraged by finding ways for the baby to play and move while lying on the tummy. In addition, parents can choose ways for the baby to be held, using a variety of different positions, such as on the parent's back, shoulders, or chest, etc. Car seats, strollers, infant seats, baby cribs, bassinets, and play pens can be used when necessary. However, prolonged head contact is best minimized since babies need frequent opportunities to move the head and not be limited to being in only stationary positions. Most cases of deformational plagiocephaly are diagnosed between 0–2yrs of age, but if the condition doesn't improve by age four months, active treatment might be needed. The treatment of deformational plagiocephaly can be divided into two main options: non-surgical and surgical. In the non-surgical approach, changes in the spatial matrix are effected by wearing a symmetrically shaped head orthotic (helmet) and pediatric physical therapy (Biggs, 2003), which molds the head — somewhat analogous to naso-alveolar molding. In other more complex cases, such as craniosynostosis where some of the cranial sutures are synostosed, a surgical approach, such as the floating cranium technique might be considered (Singh, 2004). If left untreated, some cases remain unresolved and the occipital asymmetry persists. In these cases, the squamous parts of the temporal bone become asymmetric, and its petrous part may also have some degree of asymmetry. In these cases, temporo-mandibular joint asymmetry leads to mandibular asymmetry, which may in turn precipitate maxillary asymmetry. Clinically therefore, features of untreated pediatric deformational plagiocephaly may first be observed intra-orally as a maxillary cant in an adult patient.

In general terms, the third phase of pediatric development can be considered during the deciduous dentition, which spans 3–6yrs of age. Quite often the general and/or pediatric dentist has likely already seen the child for dental check-ups, especially after the deciduous teeth first started to emerge. Thereafter, attention is usually focused on dental health and the prevention of dental diseases. However, tell-tale signs of upper airway compromise may be missed if not screened for, even at this early stage of life. As noted earlier, a child's sleep should be silent and friction-free. Some parents may notice grinding sounds as the child sleeps, and this may indicate a diagnosis of pediatric sleep bruxism (PSB). Sleep bruxism is a complex topic and here I will pose the question: Why would a child want to brux while asleep? Fonseca *et al.* (2011) and Vieira-Andrade *et al.* (2014) evaluated the prevalence of sleep bruxism in 3–5yr-olds and found it to be approx. 15% in Brazilian children. In addition, associations were found between sleep bruxism and dental crowding of the lower arch, as well as feeding-history, in these preschool children. On the other hand, PSB has been reported to occur in association with parasomnias. In fact, Weideman *et al.* (1996) reported that enuresis (bed-wetting), muscle cramps, and sleep talking (somniloquy) were significant findings in child-bruxers compared to non-bruxers, suggesting that a common sleep disturbance might underly parasomnias, such as PSB. Later, Serra-Negra *et al.* (2017) investigated associations between PSB and other sleep characteristics in children, using a pediatric sleep questionnaire (PSQ). They concluded that while sleep bruxism tends to be hereditary, pain, snoring, and mouth breathing are also associated with sleep bruxism in children. Earlier, this same research group (Serra-Negra *et al.*, 2014) had evaluated the association between environmental factors, sleep duration, and sleep bruxism in schoolchildren (aged about 8yrs old) using a PSQ. They concluded that children who slept for <8hrs per night are more likely to have PSB. In addition, both light and noise were two factors predisposing for PSB. Therefore, while sleep hygiene is imperative for children, the question of 'Why would a child want to brux while asleep?' appears to be unanswered.

In a study of PSB at the University of Miami and the Sleep Disorders Center (Marks, 1980), it was found that children with allergies showed a threefold increase in incidence of this parasomnia compared to controls. It was suggested that allergic edema of the mucosal membrane of the tympanic cavity might be causing intermittent blockage of the Eustachian tube. In an attempt to open the Eustachian tube, nocturnal bruxism may be initiated reflexively due to increased relative negative pressures in the tympanic cavities. However, the tympanic membrane and mucosa of the Eustachian tubes are very thin (approx. 3 cells in thickness), so intermittent allergic edema of these tissues is unlikely to cause significant blockage of the Eustachian tubes. On the other hand, hypertrophy of the tubal tonsils, which surround the openings of the auditory tubes, is a more likely candidate. Consider a child with allergic hypertrophy of the tubal tonsils. To open the Eustachian tubes, the child starts chewing movements due to the pressure differential. In fact, during upper airway collapse, pressure differentials are detected by mechanoreceptors in the pharyngeal walls (Marks, 1980). In PSB, upper airway obstruction during sleep may initiate chewing movements due to the pressure differential, and this learned behavior may present clinically as sleep bruxism in children with or without allergies. Thus, the hypothesis that a child learns bruxing behavior to open the Eustachian tube, and then uses this behavior reflexively as an adult when a pressure drop occurs in the upper airway in OSA, appears to be tenable. In addition, the pharyngo-tympanic tubes are more horizontally orientated in young children, and become more vertically disposed during growth and development. This means that infection is more likely to track to the middle ear from the throat in children, causing inflammation of the tympanic membrane and the mucosa of the Eustachian tubes.

Given that the embryologic, anatomic, and neurological relationships between the muscles of the middle ear, Eustachian tubes, and the mandible have a common evolutionary history, chronic middle ear blockage may promote a reflex action of the mandible by stimulating the trigeminal nuclei in the brainstem or Gasserian ganglion, and it's likely that abnormal pharyngo-tympanic tube function may be a significant etiologic factor for the development of PSB. For example, Schaller (2004) described the trigemino-cardiac reflex (TCR) as the rapid commencement of autonomic activities associated with stimulation of sensory branches of the trigeminal nerve, including parasympathetic dysrhythmia, sympathetic hypotension, apnea, and gastric hypermotility. Clinically, the TCR has been reported to occur during maxillofacial surgery, and it has been suggested that the

TCR represents a central neurogenic reflex leading to cerebrovascular vasodilatation from excitation of oxygen-sensitive neurons in the rostral ventrolateral medulla oblongata. Luco (2018) discusses the neural mechanism for sleep bruxism (SB) and the TCR. Stimulation of the maxillary (V2) and mandibular (V3) divisions of the trigeminal nerve, through the periodontal ligaments, the mental nerve, the masseter, and temporalis muscles during SB, initiates the stimulation of the TCR at the level of the Gasserion ganglion. Internuncial fibers in the reticular formation connect the trigeminal sensory nucleus to terminate at the dorsal motor nucleus and vagus nerve. Thus, V2 and V3 can stimulate an increase in heart rate, respiration and blood pressure. In fact, sleep studies demonstrate the effect of SB on the TCR. The heart rate and respiratory effort increase in response to major SB events, and these effects disappear when SB stops since the stimulation of the TCR is occurring at the level of the Gasserion ganglion. Thus, evidence suggests that adult and pediatric SB is centrally regulated, and the highest risk factor associated with sleep bruxism is OSA.

Current treatments for PSB include dental night-guards or occlusal splints, which are often provided without upper airway or sleep assessments. For the treatment of PSB, Bellerive *et al.* (2015) evaluated the effect of rapid palatal expansion (RPE). In 50% of patients, rhythmic masticatory muscle activity associated with PSB was decreased by more than 25% when compared to baseline recordings, while sleep and respiratory variables remained unchanged. In contrast, Liao and Singh (2015) used biomimetic oral appliance therapy to address SB by redeveloping the midface and repositioning the mandible in a 17yr-old female patient. This protocol resulted in the upper airway volume increasing from approx. 7.5cm^3 to 24cm^3, while the minimum upper airway cross-sectional area increased from approx. 120mm^2 to 275mm^2, which reduced the SB substantially. Therefore, it is possible that PSB may be either prevented and/or treated using a clinical technique that addresses the maxillo-mandibular features associated with PSB. However, other systemic and craniofacial conditions, such as bed-wetting (nocturnal secondary enuresis; natriuresis diuresis),

ADHD, childhood obesity, and malocclusion have also been linked with PSB. Therefore, a brief review of these disorders is warranted.

In this discussion, the fourth phase of pediatric development can be considered in the mixed dentition, which spans 6–12yrs of age. By this stage, although a fair amount of systemic health data is usually available, it may not be integrated into a typical dental treatment plan. In fact, many of these diseases may have overlapping causative agents, which sometimes go unnoticed. Mention has already been made of the importance of establishing a healthy GIT and oral microbiome. It is clear that foods shape the microbiota. For example, fermented foods and diets rich in fiber promote a diverse and robust microbiome. These foods have been a part of every human culture's culinary tradition, ranging from American dill pickle for hamburgers to Korean kimchi (a fermented, spicy cabbage dish), and many other items in between. It is now thought that a diet rich in fiber/foliage helps in the maintenance of a balanced GIT microbiota. Generally-speaking, fiber can be classified as soluble and non-soluble fiber. Non-soluble fiber, sometimes referred to as roughage, contains non-digestible cellulose that provides an environment for microflora to grow and flourish in the GIT. These microorganisms are referred to as prebiotics, which are the precursors of probiotics that are found in various foodstuffs, such as yogurts, etc. The probiotic colonies, once established, need to be nourished. This nourishment is achieved through soluble fiber, such as garlic, onions, etc. that provide a source of nutrition for the 'good' probiotic flora of the GIT. In addition, green vegetables provide a rich source of folate, which in turn helps donate methyl groups for biochemical methylation of various genes, such as the leptin gene. Folate supplementation is also recommended for women of child-bearing age since it has been shown to reduce neural tube defects, such as spina bifida in the developing fetus.

Fruit is another component of a healthy diet since it's rich in fiber and other nutrients, including vitamins and minerals. However, a major component of most fruits is fructose. Fructose is a simple (monosaccharide) sugar, which is absorbed directly into the bloodstream during digestion.

This process produces a glycemic index, increasing the blood-sugar level modestly, since fructose is often bonded to glucose to form the disaccharide, sucrose. However, fructose needs to be converted into glucose by the liver before it can be metabolized by the body. Prior to the mass production of refined sugar, humans rarely consumed fructose in large amounts, since the liver is the only organ that can metabolize it in significant amounts. Consequently, in a diet that is rich in fructose, the liver converts excess fructose into fat. In fact, at least historically, bears and other mammals that hibernate ate berries and other seasonal foods rich in fructose. By so doing the fat deposited throughout the body provided a source of energy during hibernation. Since the mammalian genome has a large degree of homology with the human genome, the liver converts fructose into fat in (obese) humans despite the fact that humans don't undergo prolonged periods of hibernation but, at least in some respects, sleep represents a microform of hibernation. Thus, in modern humans, high fructose consumption may be a key factor in many chronic diseases, including obesity, type II diabetes, heart disease, etc. In addition, high-fructose corn syrup (HFCS) is ubiquitous in the modern diet. The fructose in HFCS is not bound to glucose and, therefore, it goes directly to the liver for processing.

The importance of fish in a balanced diet has received much attention in recent times. Part of the reason lies in the fact that fish oils are rich in omega-3 fatty acids. The three main omega-3 fatty acids are α-linolenic acid (ALA), eicosa-pentaenoic acid (EPA), and docosa-hexaenoic acid (DHA). In humans, DHA levels are especially high in the retina of the eye, where it may help prevent macular degeneration, which can lead to blindness if left untreated. Omega-3 fatty acids are also crucial for brain development, especially during pregnancy — and later for brain health, being linked to higher intelligence and a lower risk of ADHD, hyperactivity, impulsiveness, and aggression in children. In adults, EPA seems to be effective at fighting depression, but ALA and DHA may also help prevent Alzheimer's disease and anxiety. Some studies suggest that omega-3 fatty acids, especially

DHA, may improve the length and quality of sleep in both children and adults. It is also known that omega-3 fatty acids are essential in preventing heart disease, since recent findings show omega-3 fatty acids may help to lower blood pressure in those diagnosed with hypertension, by reducing chronic, systemic inflammation. In addition, omega-6 fatty acids are a type of polyunsaturated fat found in vegetable oils, nuts, and seeds. Along with ALA, EPA, and DHA, omega-6 fatty acids when eaten in moderation play a crucial role in brain function, help stimulate skin and hair growth, maintain bone health, regulate metabolism, and maintain the reproductive system. A diet balanced in both omega-3 and omega-6 fatty acids is currently preferred.

As mentioned earlier, both fermented and flavored foods are highly beneficial for overall health. Fermented foods vary from wines and beers, which are found in almost all cultures of the world, to sauerkraut, which is made from shredded, fermented cabbage and salt, contains probiotics and fiber, and is high in antioxidants important for eye health. Subsequently, the advantages of these probiotic-rich foods include: GIT health/digestion, an improved immune response, and maintenance of a healthy weight/ body mass index (BMI). Fermented foods, like yogurt and kimchi, are rich in probiotics because beneficial bacteria, such as lactobacillus, grow during the fermentation process. Studies have shown that kimchi made from radishes may help reduce insulin resistance and blood cholesterol levels. On the other hand, probiotics in yogurt can help digest lactose (milk sugar). For example, kefir is a fermented dairy product that may improve lactose digestion, decrease tissue inflammation and boost bone health. Japanese tempeh, natto, and miso are made from fermented soybeans. Tempeh is high in probiotics and contains compounds that may act as antioxidants and improve heart health, while natto's high fiber content may promote digestion and prevent osteoporosis. It also produces enzymes that can help regulate blood pressure and thrombosis. On the other hand, miso is a seasoning that has been associated with a reduced risk of cancer and improved heart health. Similarly, kombucha is an effervescent, fermented tea. Initial studies suggest that it helps protect liver function, decreases blood sugar, and reduces the levels of cholesterol and triglycerides in the circulation. Apart from fermented foods, herbs and spices can be beneficial for human health. It has long been known that turmeric has several health benefits since its most active compound, curcumin, has the potential to prevent heart disease, Alzheimer's disease and even cancer. It has potent anti-inflammatory and antioxidant activities, and it may also help improve symptoms of depression and arthritis. Curcumin can suppress various molecules known to play major roles in chronic inflammation. Thus, its powerful antioxidant effects neutralize free radicals but also stimulate antioxidant enzyme synthesis, by improving endothelial function. This dietary approach contrasts with the current inflammatory diet of many children in the USA, which consists of processed, junk foods and fructose-enriched sodas. These refined foods, containing additives, preservatives, and stabilizers, etc. appear to be innocuous and biocompatible but, in some cases, can prove to be surprisingly harmful.

Childhood obesity occurs when a child consumes more energy than used for growth, development, and physical activities, etc. A child's BMI is based on age and is gender-specific because of changes associated with active growth and development. Ogden *et al.* (2006) studied the prevalence of obesity in American children and adolescents. They found that obesity among children and teenagers increased significantly from 14% to 18% during the period studied (1999–2004) and suggested that increases in BMI are a continuing trend in both children and adolescents. Later, Cockrell-Skinner and Skelton (2014) showed that the prevalence of obesity in 2–5yr-old American children increased from 5% to about 12% from the 1970s to 2013. In fact, this pattern can also be seen in other countries, including Australia, Chile, England/Scotland, Iceland, and Japan. Nevertheless, the causes and effects of childhood obesity are rather diverse. Some studies suggest that children of lower socio-economic status are at a higher risk of developing obesity, while Bonuck *et al.* (2015) noted that SDB increases the child's risk of being obese. However, other factors, such as the urban environment and its effect of a lack of physical activity, leading to a more sedentary lifestyle, has also been implicated. The modern, built environment may be also be associated with dietary habits and trends, including a diet rich in refined sugars, processed foods, food-like products (junk food), and foodstuffs containing stabilizers, additives, preservatives, artificial coloring, and flavoring, not to mention genetically modified organisms (GMO). In addition, fast foods may be inappropriately prepared with excess salt and saturated (hydrogenated) fats that can increase unhealthy high-density lipoprotein (LDL) cholesterol, while lowering healthy high-density lipoprotein (HDL) cholesterol, reflecting the notion of a 'super-sized' meal. In later life, the effects of these dietary habits can include conditions such as insulin-resistance and type II diabetes, hypertension/cardio-vascular diseases, asthma, obstructive sleep apnea, osteoarthritis, as well as psycho-social problems associated with obesity and body image. As alluded to above, fructose does not appropriately stimulate insulin, but stimulates the appetite and can lead to insulin resistance in the long term. In addition, fructose is converted into fat and deposited throughout the body, increasing the BMI. It is also thought that fructose metabolism elevates uric acid levels, which can in turn increase blood pressure, leading to hypertension. Some data suggest that adolescents spend an average of 7.5hrs per day engaged with cell phones, video games, computers, and watching television. If snacks such as popcorn and soda containing HFCS are consumed during these activities, it is easy to see how an epidemic of childhood obesity could be precipitated. However, childhood obesity is a preventable condition, especially if factors such as diet, lifestyle, and sleep are moderated.

Song and Jiang (2015) presented some preliminary findings on the association between sleep and dietary patterns in Chinese preschool children. Two major dietary patterns were identified: 'traditional' and 'western'. It was noted that a short sleep duration decreased the chances of children eating fruits and vegetables. Conversely, children who had an earlier bedtime were associated with higher traditional dietary pattern scores, lower western dietary pattern scores, a greater chance of eating more vegetables, less desserts, and less soft drinks, such as sodas containing HFCS. Similarly, Do (2015) investigated the effect of sleep duration on adolescent body weight in 10th and 11th graders since epidemiological studies have reported consistent associations between shorter sleep duration and increased BMI. The results of that pilot study showed that a 1-hour increase in sleep duration led to a $0.5kgm^{-2}$ reduction in BMI or a 4% decrease in the probability of obesity. While it was concluded that short sleep duration may be an important factor in overweight adolescents, the study also suggested that extra sleep can help address negative health consequences of a shorter sleep duration. Thus, the promotion of adequate sleep time can be proposed for the prevention of childhood obesity. In another preliminary study, Leblanc *et al.* (2015) considered associations between sleep characteristics and dietary intake patterns in 10yr-old Canadian children, since evidence suggests that short sleep duration is associated with increased food intake and childhood obesity. In this case, dietary intake was assessed using a food frequency questionnaire, which asked the participant how often they consumed 23 food items in a usual week. For assessment, two dietary scores were formulated: 'unhealthy diet' (e.g. hamburgers, soft drinks, fried food), and 'healthy diet' (e.g. vegetables and fruits, etc.). The initial results indicated that poor sleep efficiency was associated with a worse score for an unhealthy diet. In addition, a later bedtime was associated with a worse score for a healthy diet. Even after adjusting for age, sex, ethnicity, BMI, and level of physical activity, the relationships between sleep efficiency, unhealthy diets, later bedtimes, and healthy diets remained significant. Thus, it can be concluded that later bedtimes and poor sleep efficiency are associated with poor dietary patterns in children, which may result in increased childhood obesity.

Strategies for the prevention of childhood obesity can be formulated and implemented, starting as early as the neonatal period by avoiding the use of plastic (BPP) baby milk-bottles, as discussed above. In addition, as the child gets older, parents/guardians can help prevent childhood obesity by: educating the child on nutrition and developing awareness of healthy eating habits for a lifetime; providing healthy/organic meals, which provide nutrient-dense foodstuffs for growth and development; and by encouraging daily physical activity, which reduces the risk of obesity and helps with BMI management of the child. In addition, emerging data suggest that sleep hygiene is probably as important as the factors noted above. One aspect of sleep hygiene is to limit screen time for the child, especially at home. Blue light is thought to suppress melatonin release, which is a hormone that acts as a 'biomimetic alarm clock'. Typically, alarm clocks are used to wake a person up in the morning. A biomimetic alarm clock does the reverse; it signals the time to prepare to go to bed. In accord with the circadian rhythm, melatonin release from the pineal gland, starting in the early evening, marks the onset of the sleep drive in readiness for bedtime and sleep. That the sleep signal can be over-ridden is analogous to the snooze button being hit in the morning, due to insufficient quality or quantity of sleep. In any case, to promote sleep hygiene, the child's bedroom must be devoid of any blue screens such as cell phones, televisions, computers, etc. The room should be slightly less warm than the living room, as well as being very dark and quiet for restful, restorative sleep: a microform of hibernation.

Enuresis

In some children, bed-wetting (secondary nocturnal enuresis; natriuresis diuresis) can be problematic. At this juncture it's worth reviewing the physiologic process of micturition. As urine is produced, the volume of the bladder increases, leading to an expansion of its walls. This distention activates stretch receptors, which communicate with the spinal cord. Put simply, activation of the bladder-wall stretch receptors results in a decrease in sympathetic activity, which in turn leads to relaxation of the internal urethral sphincter. This decreased smooth muscle tone results in an opening of the internal urethral sphincter and permits micturition to proceed.

However, to eject the urine, there is an increase in parasympathetic activity at the level of the spinal cord. This neuromuscular process leads to contraction of the detrusor muscle in the bladder wall as well as opening of the internal urethral sphincter, which assists micturition. In addition, a decrease in somatic motor neuron activity leads to a relaxation of the external urethral sphincter. This action leads to opening of the external urethral sphincter, completing the process for micturition. As the bladder is emptied, the distention of the bladder walls is reduced, and the system returns to homeostasis.

Primary nocturnal enuresis is most often related to a developmental or neurologic abnormality of the uro-genital tract. However, in secondary or pediatric nocturnal enuresis, the etiologic factors are often external to a normally developed urogenital tract. For example, Carotenuto *et al.* (2011) noted that children with enuresis were predisposed to a dolicocephalic facial pattern and abnormal head posture when compared to controls. Sleep disordered breathing (SDB) is also a syndrome associated with an abnormality in both pediatric enuresis and arousal. The most common cause of SDB in childhood is adeno-tonsillar hypertrophy, which has a peak incidence in children aged 2–5yrs and has been discussed earlier. In contrast to pediatric enuresis, nocturnal polyuria has been reported in individuals with obstructive sleep apnea (OSA). In nocturnal polyuria, there is an increased amount of urine production, necessitating frequent bathroom visits at night. Studies suggest that a decrease in the nocturnal secretion of anti-diuretic hormone (ADH) and an increase in atrial natriuretic peptide (ANP) secretion are possible explanations for nocturnal polyuria. However, research reveals that nocturnal polyuria is found in some but not all children with enuresis. Thus, although nocturnal polyuria is important in the pathophysiology of enuresis, overproduction of urine *per se* cannot be the sole causal factor in enuresis. For example, nocturnal polyuria does not explain why children with enuresis do not wake up to the sensation of a full or contracting bladder at nighttime, using a mechanism that prevents accidents during the daytime. Thus, nocturnal polyuria in children with enuresis likely has multiple causes, including: increased fluid ingestion from the time a child arrives home from school through the afternoon and evening to bedtime; reduced fluid ingestion from the time a child wakes up through the school day; food consumption from the time a child arrives home from school through the afternoon and evening to bedtime; low nocturnal secretion of ADH; and an increased nocturnal solute excretion. Ingestion of fluids from the time a child arrives home from school through to bedtime is a common cause of nocturnal polyuria. Solid food ingestion is also a cause because excretion of solute by the kidneys is accompanied by an obligate amount of water. Many children with bed-wetting drink modest amounts of fluids at breakfast and throughout the school day. When they arrive home from school hungry and thirsty, most of their fluid intake often occurs in the few hours between arriving home and bedtime. This feeding/eating pattern favors nocturnal polyuria. Thus, production of urine is controlled by several factors, including ADH, which directly controls water absorption, atrial natriuretic peptide (ANP), and aldosterone, which controls solute and indirectly affects water excretion. Norgaard *et al.* (2007) first reported the absence of the expected nocturnal increase in ADH secretion in adults with enuresis. Subsequent reports suggested that low nocturnal secretions of ADH are present in some but not all children with enuresis.

Arousal to the sensation of a full or contracting bladder involves neurologic areas, including the cerebral cortex, the reticular activating system (RAS), the locus ceruleus (LC), the hypothalamus, the pontine micturition center (PMC), the spinal cord, and the bladder. The RAS controls the depth of sleep, the LC controls arousal, and the PMC initiates the command for detrusor contraction. Various neurotransmitters are also involved, including norepinephrine, serotonin, and ADH. Sleep studies reveal that children with enuresis do not wake up normally in response to an auditory signal; this finding confirms a problem in arousal. In pediatric enuresis, it is thought that the locus ceruleus (LC) does not produce arousal, but the pontine micturition center (PMC) initiates command for detrusor contraction, leading to bed-wetting. Zhenyun *et al.* (2015) conducted a study of arousals in children exhibiting primary snoring/OSA using electroencephalography (EEG). The values of various EEG arousal indices (e.g. total arousal index, respiratory arousal index, limb arousal index, and spontaneous arousal index) were compared in children considered to have primary snoring and/or OSA and a control group. The findings showed that there was no difference in total arousal index between children with primary snoring and those with OSA. However, in children with primary snoring, the limb arousal index was higher than in children with OSA and controls, especially during non-rapid eye movement (REM) sleep. The respiratory arousal index was notably higher in children with OSA than in the other two groups. Not surprisingly perhaps, significant differences in EEG arousal indices were apparent between children with SDB and controls, and these findings could impact children with nocturnal enuresis.

Atrial natriuretic hormone (ANP) is a cardiac hormone and its receptors are widely present in the body. ANP's main function is to lower blood pressure and to control electrolyte homeostasis (Evrard *et al.*, 1999). Its chief targets are the adrenal glands in the kidney and the cardiovascular system, but ANP interacts with many other hormones in order to regulate their secretion. Steroidogenesis, especially mineralocorticoid synthesis (e.g. aldosterone), is inhibited by ANP, but glucocorticoid production (e.g. cortisol) seems to be depressed also. On the other hand, ANP synthesis is enhanced by aldosterone and by thyroid hormone, suggesting it has a regulatory loop/positive feedback mechanism. The hypothalamus-pituitary-adrenal axis (HPA) is another important target. In this case, ANP inhibits adreno-corticotrophic hormone (ACTH) release while vasopressin enhances ANP synthesis, but growth hormone (GH) decreases it. As ANP synthesis is enhanced by vasopressin, this suggests another regulatory loop. Finally, the endocrine effects of ANP strengthen the cardiovascular and renal effects of the hormone, antagonizing salt and water retention due to aldosterone. Because of a local production, ANP may also act as a paracrine hormone that influences the function of many endocrine systems. Given this backdrop, the role of ANP in relation to nocturnal enuresis can now be considered. In children with SDB, upper airway obstruction, perhaps due to adeno-tonsillar hypertrophy, will increase upper airway resistance.

As the resistance increases, the diaphragm and chest wall work harder during respiration. As the chest wall expands, the volume of the thoracic cavity increases with a subsequent decrease in pressure. This means that the heart is beating against a decreased intra-thoracic pressure, which results in atrial distention. In addition, sympathetic stimulation increases the heart rate. As a result, ANP is produced. Its actions as noted above include decreased aldosterone biosynthesis as well as reduced amounts of angiotensin II and decreased renin release from the kidneys, resulting in urine formation. The net result of this process is natriuresis diuresis or bed-wetting. Once the bladder is vacated the event may not be repeated.

There is a relationship between sleep quality and regularity of sleep in children and adolescents. Kwon *et al.* (2015) found that as Korean children grow older, sleep duration consistently reduces between the ages of 10–19yrs. Sleep regularity also decreases from age 10–18yrs. In fact, from age 10–16yrs, sleep duration decreases by about 15 minutes on average, and drops significantly at age 17yrs. By age 15yrs, sleep quality is poor in these teenagers, but the lowest quality of sleep was observed at age 19yrs. Between age 16yrs and 17yrs, when Korean adolescents graduate from middle school and enter high school, the sleep duration drastically decreases and demonstrates a significant decrease in sleep quality. Therefore, the preliminary study of Kwon *et al.* (2015) concluded that as (Korean) adolescents get older, they sleep less, and the shortened sleep duration affects the quality and regularity of sleep negatively. Gaspar de Matos *et al.* (2015) also studied sleep deprivation in adolescents in an attempt to correlate it with academic achievement and quality of life. In their preliminary study, sleep duration was 7.5hrs during the week and 8.8hrs during the weekend. The total average amount of sleep was about 8hrs with 45% of pupils having a difference of >2hr between sleep during the week and during the weekend. It was also found that a perception of low achievement in school, disliking school, feeling pressured with schoolwork, and school truancy were correlated with extreme fatigue, total sleep duration, and difficulties in sleep initiation. Gaspar de Matos *et al.* (2015) concluded that poor sleep quality and insufficient sleep duration are important features during schooling, being associated with a perception of low achievement, and lack of well-being, but other features need to be considered. In that respect, Sekartini *et al.* (2015) investigated factors related to academic achievement in junior high school students with sleep disorders since it is thought that sleep disorders are prevalent in adolescents and may influence their academic achievement at school. This study, conducted in Indonesia, found that the prevalence of sleep disorders was 40% in junior high school; most of these students (70%) were having difficulty in initiating and maintaining sleep. Overall, approx. 50% of these students had an under-average academic achievement. It was concluded that the factors related to under-average academic achievement in junior high school students with sleep disorders in Indonesia were non-formal education, average IQ level, and male gender. Thus, sleep disorders have become an increasing health issue worldwide and its prevalence and consequences are viewed as a serious public health problem. For example, sleep disturbances in children with attention deficit hyperactivity disorder (ADHD) and learning disorders are also known to exist. In one study, Stokes-Brackett (2015) found a significant correlation between ADHD and learning disorders associated with lack of sleep hygiene, daytime sleepiness, and OSA.

ADHD is a complex condition. No single cause has been identified but it's most likely an epigenetic outcome of environmental factors and genetic predisposition. The symptoms of ADHD include: inattention, so the child does not appear to listen or is easily distracted; hyperactivity, so the child frequently talks too much or fidgets; and impulsivity, so the child acts and/or speaks without thinking, etc. On a positron emission tomography (PET) scan or EEG, children diagnosed with this condition may show high α-wave or θ-wave activity, allied with decreased cerebellar volume, and a hereditary dopamine deficiency (e.g. dopamine transporter and dopamine receptor-4 genes, and dopamine β-hydroxylase). Other parts of the brain can also be affected, including the frontal lobe, the posterior parietal lobe, the RAS, and the limbic system, which produce disturbed sleep patterns. Other co-morbidities with ADHD in children can include anxiety and/or depression, Asperger's syndrome, tics/Tourette's syndrome, dyslexia, and bipolar disorder, etc. In fact, environmental and/or lifestyle factors can exacerbate the symptoms, and these may include toxicity from lead and other heavy metals. In addition, there may be a nutritional deficiency of zinc, iron, and omega-3 fatty acids in the diet. The worldwide prevalence of ADHD in children varies from as high as 15–20% in places like the USA, Ukraine, and India to as low as 2–3% in countries like Ireland and the Netherlands (Faraone *et al.*, 2003; Biedermann and Faraone, 2005). Various pharmaceutical drugs have been prescribed for this condition, including dextroamphetamine (Adderall) and methylphenidate (Ritalin). Surprisingly, although the USA constitutes approx. 20% of the world population, it consumes 95% of the methylphenidate prescribed, which means that about 5% of American children are taking Ritalin. However, there may be an overlap of ADHD and SDB. For example, Yujing *et al.* (2015) studied EEG arousals in children with ADHD and children with SDB. They found that there were no significant differences in EEG arousal patterns among children with both ADHD/SDB and children with SDB alone. Therefore, healthcare professionals need to be aware of the various approaches to therapy. For example, about 25% of preschoolers diagnosed with ADHD are treated with medications alone, while 50% receive no behavioral therapy. However, a meta-analysis (Sedky *et al.*, 2014) found that ADHD symptoms are related to pediatric SDB. Therefore, they suggested that patients with ADHD should be screened for pediatric SDB and that treatment of SDB should be considered prior to medication for ADHD. In addition, it is thought that for children diagnosed with ADHD, the diet should be monitored to have a high protein content (such as meat, eggs, cheese, beans, and nuts); more complex carbohydrates (such as fruits and vegetables); more omega-3 fatty acids (such as fish, walnuts, and olive oil), and less simple carbohydrates (such as sugar and white bread).

On the other hand, an inflammatory diet may lead to allergies and/or allergic rhinitis that can precipitate mouth-breathing since a blocked nose can lead to oral respiration. In these children there may be local obstruction of the nares associated with allergic rhinitis, a deviated nasal septum, and/or a septal spur (Fig. 17a). Other features that may go undetected, unless screened for, include adeno-tonsillar hypertrophy (Fig. 25b), 'adenoid facies' or long face syndrome (Fig. 16), as well as snoring and/or SDB. For example, studies have indicated significant sleep fragmentation (reduced sleep time, reduced sleep quality, snoring, difficulty in maintaining sleep, and daytime sleepiness) in children with asthma. Thus, OSA may coexist with asthma since studies suggest that the prevalence of pediatric SDB and sleep fragmentation could be very high in children with asthma. It is also thought that non-well controlled asthma in children can produce a significant decrease in sleep efficiency, prolonged REM latency, and a reduction in percentage of REM sleep in children (Che and Lu, 2015). The effects of nitric oxide (NO) in asthma can be helpful since it promotes smooth muscle relaxation, vasodilatation, and tissue oxygenation (Zhang *et al.*, 2015) *inter alia*. Thus, NO is a reactive oxygen species that diffuses to the bronchi and lungs to produce bronchodilatory and vasodilatory effects. In fact, the critical role of the pneumocytes that line the paranasal air sinuses is to produce NO. In addition, NO is produced by healthy endothelial cells that line small blood vessels. NO synthase (NOS) is an enzyme that produces NO from L-arginine. In the smooth muscle cell, NO activates the enzyme guanylyl cyclase that, in turn, leads to the muscle relaxation and dilation of small blood vessels. Thus, a stimulus within the lumen, for example, airway collapse or hypertension, activates NOS, which promotes smooth muscle relaxation and vessel dilation to counteract the stimulus. Therefore, improved paranasal function might help asthmatic children sleep better.

In fact, it is now accepted that NO is one of the most important molecules produced by the endothelium, since it acts an essential regulator in a wide range of physiological functions, including blood pressure, immune response, and neural communication, depending on its level since it has a short half-life. Because of this vital role, healthy endothelial function is demonstrated by the ability to produce sufficient amounts of NO. Thus, in the respiratory tract, NO promotes lung tissue health and metabolism, including gas exchange. In the cardiovascular system, NO dilates small blood vessels and promotes nutrient exchange. In the cell cycle, NO reduces cell death/apoptosis and enhances angiogenesis. Perhaps one of the key roles of NO is that it regulates inflammation throughout the body and improves immunity. In the central nervous system, NO is involved in blood pressure regulation and the pain pathways, while it enhances metabolism and nutrient absorption in the GIT. Finally, NO's role in addressing sexual health, such as erectile dysfunction, has been well documented in the medical literature. Reactive oxygen species (ROS) also play a major role in NO-cell signaling. These ROS, such as superoxides, hydrogen peroxide, singlet oxygen, and hydroxyl radicals, can affect the bioavailability of NO either in terms of its production or post-production scavenging that can lead to numerous cardiovascular disorders since NO bioavailability is reduced in the presence of ROS (Pierini and Bryan, 2015). Lavie *et al.* (2001) found that patients with ischemic heart disease (IHD) and OSA had higher levels of homocysteine levels than patients with IHD alone, likely due to endothelial dysfunction combined with excess free-radical formation. Another factor to consider for health maintenance is that NO levels decline with age. Up to the age of about 30yrs, NO production is fairly constant, but then shows a steady deterioration. With declining levels of NO bioactivity, there is decreased vasodilation, vascular smooth muscle cell growth inhibition, and reduced antioxidant capacity. In response, there are increased levels of the enzyme NADPH oxidase, which: generates superoxides and increases the level of oxidative stress; increases the amounts of the hormone angiotensin II, which is a vasoconstrictor that regulates renal function, and, therefore, blood pressure; and enhances levels of endothelin-1, which is a potent vasoconstrictor that is encoded by vascular endothelial cells. The net result of these actions is the ageing mechanism. During ageing, typically there are increased levels of inflammation, fibrosis, and vasoconstriction, which can be associated with arterial stiffening and calcification. In addition, telomere shortening at the ends of the chromosomes is associated with premature ageing and damage of the DNA encoding the genes. These changes can lead to epigenetic modifications during the ageing process but also pathologic airway remodeling in conditions such as asthma, chronic obstructive pulmonary disease, bronchiectasis, emphysema, etc. Therefore, the consequences of endothelial dysfunction can include: hypertension, peripheral artery diseases, inflammatory diseases, atherosclerosis, immune deficiencies, hyperlipidemia, diabetes, heart failure, and coronary, as well as cerebral vasospasm *inter alia* (Rubanyi, 1993).

Individuals with NO deficiency associated with endothelial dysfunction may also develop asthma, skin allergies (e.g. eczema), 'leaky gut', Irritable Bowel Syndrome (IBS), Crohn's disease, etc. that dictate exclusion of gluten, dairy (lactose-sensitivity), and other foods (because of allergies, e.g. nuts) from the diet. In the craniofacial region, endothelial dysfunction associated with NO deficiency can lead to: inflammation of the respiratory mucosa, including allergies and/or infections; a blocked nose with discomfort and/or discharge or decreased mucus production; as well as mouth-breathing. To counteract the increasing levels of endothelial dysfunction with age, the diet can be supplemented with foods that are sources of NO such as: dark chocolate, tofu, pomegranate, meat, nuts (peanuts, Brazil nuts, almonds, hazelnuts, walnuts, pecans, and pistachios), spicy foods (cayenne peppers and jalapenos), watermelon, beans, beets, celery, spinach, fish (mackerel, salmon, and tuna), and certain soy products. Therefore, in the fourth phase of pediatric development (6–12yrs of age) while a developing malocclusion with crowding and unerupted/impacted third molars may be an obvious clinical sign, the framework for systemic health and longevity is developing concurrently and ought to be addressed clinically.

References

Bach JF. The hygiene hypothesis in autoimmunity: the role of pathogens and commensals. *Nat Rev Immunol.* 2018;18(2):105–120.

Balarajan R, Soni Raleigh V, Botting B. Sudden infant death syndrome and postneonatal mortality in immigrants in England and Wales. *BMJ.* 1989;298:716–720.

Bellerive A, Montpetit A, El-Khatib H, Carra MC, Remise C, Desplats E, Huynh N. The effect of rapid palatal expansion on sleep bruxism in children. *Sleep Breath.* 2015;19(4):1265–1271.

Biederman J, Faraone SV. Attention-deficit hyperactivity disorder. *Lancet.* 2005;366(9481):237–248.

Biggs WS. Diagnosis and management of positional head deformity. *Amer Family Phys*. 2003;67(9):1953–1956.

Bonuck K, Chervin RD, Howe LD. Sleep-disordered breathing, sleep duration, and childhood overweight: A longitudinal cohort study. *J Pediatr*. 2015;166(3):632–639.

Camacho M, Chang ET, Song SA, Abdullatif J, Zaghi S, Pirelli P, Certal V, Guilleminault C. Rapid maxillary expansion for pediatric obstructive sleep apnea: A systematic review and meta-analysis. *Laryngoscope*. 2017;127(7):1712–1719.

Carotenuto M, Esposito M, Pascotto A. Facial patterns and primary nocturnal enuresis in children. *Sleep Breath*. 2011;15(2):221–227.

Che D, Lu M. Sleep disorders in children with asthma. *Sleep Med*. 2015;16:S22-S23.

Cockrell-Skinner A, Skelton JA. Prevalence and trends in obesity and severe obesity among children in the United States, 1999–2012. *JAMA Pediatr*. 2014;168(6): 561–566.

Collett BR, Gray KE, Starr JR, Heike CL, Cunningham ML, Speltz ML. Development at age 36 months in children with deformational plagiocephaly. *Pediatrics*. 2013;131(1):e109-e115.

Do Y. Causal effect of sleep duration on adolescent body weight: Evidence from a natural experiment. *Sleep Med*. 2015;16:S90.

Eichenberger M, Baumgartner S. The impact of rapid palatal expansion on children's general health: A literature review. *Eur J Paediatr Dent*. 2014;15(1):67–71.

Evrard A, Hober C, Racadot A, Lefebvre J, Vantyghem MC. Atrial natriuretic hormone and endocrine functions. *Ann Biol Clin* (*Paris*). 1999;57(2):149–155.

Eyquem A, Aguilera J, Astudillo W, Toro-Ibacache V. Diet consistency, dental malocclusions and the shape of the human face. J Human Evol. 2017. In: Plavcan M, Alba DM, Elton S (eds.) *Proceedings of the European Society for the study of Human Evolution*. Vol. 6, page 63.

Faraone SV, Sergeant J, Gillberg C, Biederman J. The worldwide prevalence of ADHD: Is it an American condition? *World Psychiatry*. 2003;2(2):104–113.

Fernández L, Langa S, Martín V, Maldonado A, Jiménez E, Martín R, Rodríguez JM. The human milk microbiota: Origin and potential roles in health and disease. *Pharmacol Res*. 2013;69(1):1–10.

Fonseca CM, dos Santos MB, Consani RL, dos Santos JF, Marchini L. Incidence of sleep bruxism among children in Itanhandu, Brazil. *Sleep Breath*. 2011;15(2):215–220.

Gaspar de Matos M, Gaspar T, Tome G, Paiva T. Sleep deprivation in adolescents: Correlations with school achievement and health related quality of life. *Sleep Med*. 2015;16:S91.

Greaves M. A causal mechanism for childhood acute lymphoblastic leukaemia. *Nat Rev Cancer*. 2018;18(8):471–484.

Green RM, Smith GG, Burrage WL. Orthodontia in medicine. *Boston Med Surg J*. 1917;178(3):104.

Gulotta G, Iannella G, Vicini C, Polimeni A, Greco A, de Vincentiis M, Visconti IC, Meccariello G, Cammaroto G, De Vito A, Gobbi R, Bellini C, Firinu E, Pace A, Colizza A, Pelucchi S, Magliulo G. Risk factors for obstructive sleep apnea syndrome in children: State of the Art. *Int J Environ Res Public Health*. 2019;16(18):3235.

Hoxha S, Kaya-Sezginer E, Bakar-Ates F, Köktürk O, Toygar-Memikoğlu U. Effect of semi-rapid maxillary expansion in children with obstructive sleep apnea syndrome: 5-month follow-up study. *Sleep Breath*. 2018;22(4):1053–1061.

Huynh NT, Desplats E, Almeida FR. Orthodontics treatments for managing obstructive sleep apnea syndrome in children: A systematic review and meta-analysis. *Sleep Med Rev*. 2016;25:84–94.

Huynh NT, Morton PD, Rompré PH, Papadakis A, Remise C. Associations between sleep-disordered breathing symptoms and facial and dental morphometry, assessed with screening examinations. *Am J Orthod Dentofacial Orthop*. 2011;140(6): 762–770.

Khalyfa A, Cortese R, Qiao Z, Ye H, Bao R, Andrade J, Gozal D. Late gestational intermittent hypoxia induces metabolic and epigenetic changes in male adult offspring mice. *J Physiol*. 2017;595(8):2551–2568.

Kim JH, Guilleminault C. The nasomaxillary complex, the mandible, and sleep-disordered breathing. *Sleep Breath*. 2011;15(2):185–193.

Koretsi V, Eliades T, Papageorgiou SN. Oral interventions for obstructive sleep apnea. *Dtsch Arztebl Int*. 2018;115(12):200–207.

Korpela K, Helve O, Kolho KL, Saisto T, Skogberg K, Dikareva E, Stefanovic V, Salonen A, *et al*. Maternal fecal microbiota transplantation in Cesarean-born infants rapidly restores normal gut microbial development: A proof-of-concept study. *Cell*. 2020 Sep 18:S0092-8674(20)31089-8. doi: 10.1016/j.cell.2020.08.047. Epub ahead of print.

Kwon Y, Oh S, Hong J. The relationship between quality and regularity of sleep based on Korean adolescents' sleep duration by age. *Sleep Med*. 2015;16:S60.

Lavie L, Perelman A, Lavie P. Plasma homocysteine levels in obstructive sleep apnea: association with cardiovascular morbidity. *Chest*. 2001;120(3):900–908.

Leblanc A, Tremblay M, Boyer C, Borghese M, Leduc G, Chaput J. Associations between sleep characteristics and dietary intake patterns in 10-year old Canadian children. *Sleep Med*. 2015;16:S113.

Li DK, Daling JR. Maternal smoking, low birth weight, and ethnicity in relation to sudden infant death syndrome. *Am J Epidemiol*. 1991;134(9):958–964.

Liao F, Singh GD. Resolution of sleep bruxism using biomimetic oral appliance therapy: A case report. *J Sleep Disord Ther*. 2015;4:204–208.

Lif-Holgerson P, Harnevik L, Hernell O, Tanner AC, Johansson I. Mode of birth delivery affects oral microbiota in infants. *J Dent Res*. 2011;90(10):1183–1188.

López Del Valle LM, Singh GD, Feliciano N, Machuca Mdel C. Associations between a history of breast feeding, malocclusion and parafunctional habits in Puerto Rican children. *PR Health Sci J*. 2006;25(1):31–34.

Luco K. The relationship of the trigemino-cardiac reflex to sleep bruxism. *On J Neur Br Disord*. 2018;1(2).

Marks MB. Bruxism in allergic children. *Am J Orthod*. 1980;77(1):48–59.

Mossey P, Singh GD, Smith ME. More extensive analysis is needed when assessing facial structure in SIDS. *BMJ*. 1999;318:396–397.

Nørgaard JP, Hashim H, Malmberg L, Robinson D. Antidiuresis therapy: Mechanism of action and clinical implications. *Neurourol Urodyn*. 2007;26(7):1008–1113.

Obermann-Borst SA, Eilers PH, Tobi EW, de Jong FH, Slagboom PE, Heijmans BT, Steegers-Theunissen RP. Duration of breastfeeding and gender are associated with methylation of the leptin gene in very young children. *Pediatric Res*. 2013;74(3):344–349.

Obladen M. Much ado about nothing: Two millenia of controversy on tongue-tie. *Neonatology* 2010;97(2):83–89.

Ogden CL, Carroll MD, Curtin LR, McDowell MA, Tabak CJ, Flegal KM. Prevalence of overweight and obesity in the United States, 1999–2004. *JAMA*. 2006;295(13): 1549–1555.

Penders J, Thijs C, Vink C, Stelma FF, Snijders B, Kummeling I, *et al*. Factors influencing the composition of the intestinal microbiota in early infancy. *Pediatrics*. 2006;118:511–521.

Pierini D, Bryan NS. Nitric oxide availability as a marker of oxidative stress. *Methods Mol Biol*. 2015;1208:63–71.

Rice PL, Naksook C. Child rearing and cultural beliefs and practices amongst Thai mothers in Victoria, Australia: Implications for the sudden infant death syndrome. *J Paediatr Child Health*. 1998;34(4):320–324.

Rubanyi GM. The role of endothelium in cardiovascular homeostasis and diseases. *J Cardiovasc Pharmacol*. 1993;22(Suppl 4):S1-S14.

Salminen S, Gibson GR, McCartney AL, Isolauri E. Influence of mode of delivery on gut microbiota composition in seven year old children. *Gut*. 2004;53(9):1388–1389.

Schaller B. Trigeminocardiac reflex. A clinical phenomenon or a new physiological entity? *J Neurol.* 2004;251(6):658–665.

Schubert TM, Rothlein D, Brothers T, Coderre EL, Ledoux K, Gordon B, McCloskey M. Lack of awareness despite complex visual processing: Evidence from event-related potentials in a case of selective metamorphopsia. *Proc Natl Acad Sci.* 2020; 117(27): 16055–16064.

Sedky K, Bennett DS, Carvalho KS. Attention deficit hyperactivity disorder and sleep disordered breathing in pediatric populations: A meta-analysis. *Sleep Med Rev.* 2014;18(4):349–356.

Sekartini R, Auliyanti F, Mangunatmadja I. Factors related to academic achievement in junior high school students in Jakarta with sleep disorders. *Sleep Med.* 2015;16:S97.

Serra-Negra JM, Paiva SM, Fulgêncio LB, Chavez BA, Lage CF, Pordeus IA. Environmental factors, sleep duration, and sleep bruxism in Brazilian schoolchildren: A case-control study. *Sleep Med.* 2014;15(2):236–239.

Serra-Negra JM, Ribeiro MB, Prado IM, Paiva SM, Pordeus IA. Association between possible sleep bruxism and sleep characteristics in children. *Cranio.* 2017;35(5): 315–320.

Singh GD, Levy-Bercowski D, Santiago PE. Three-dimensional nasal changes following nasoalveolar molding in patients with unilateral cleft lip and palate: Geometric morphometrics. *Cleft Palate Craniofac J.* 2005;42(4):403–409.

Singh GD, Levy-Bercowski D, Yáñez MA, Santiago PE. Three-dimensional facial morphology following surgical repair of unilateral cleft lip and palate in patients after nasoalveolar molding. *Orthod Craniofac Res.* 2007;10(3):161–166.

Singh GD. On Growth and Treatment: The spatial matrix hypothesis. In: McNamara JA Jr (ed.) Growth and treatment: A meeting of the minds. Vol 41, Craniofacial Growth Series, Ann Arbor, USA, 2004, pp. 197–239.

Singh GD. Report on a Symposium "Advances in the modeling of form: Clinical and computational interfaces". *Amer J Orthod Dentofac Orthop.* 2004;125(1):124–125.

SJ Chang, KY Chae. Obstructive sleep apnea syndrome in children: Epidemiology, pathophysiology, diagnosis and sequelae. *Korean J Pediatr.* 2010;53(10):863–871.

Song Y, Jiang F. Association between sleep and dietary patterns in preschool children. *Sleep Med.* 2015;16:S22.

Sonkar R, Powell CA, Choudhury M. Benzyl butyl phthalate induces epigenetic stress to enhance adipogenesis in mesenchymal stem cells. *Mol Cell Endocrinol.* 2016;431:109–122.

Stokes-Brackett AC. Sleep disturbances in children with attention-deficit/hyperactivity disorder and learning disorders. *Sleep Med.* 2015;16:S69.

Strand Viðarsdóttir U, O'Higgins P, Stringer C. A geometric morphometric study of regional differences in the ontogeny of the modern human facial skeleton. *J Anat.* 2002;201:211–229.

Tsuda H, Fastlicht S, Almeida FR, Lowe AA. The correlation between craniofacial morphology and sleep-disordered breathing in children in an undergraduate orthodontic clinic. *Sleep Breath.* 2011;15(2):163–171.

Vale F, Albergaria M, Carrilho E, Francisco I, Guimarães A, Caramelo F, Maló L. Efficacy of rapid maxillary expansion in the treatment of obstructive sleep apnea syndrome: A systematic review with meta-analysis. *J Evid Based Dent Pract.* 2017;17(3):159–168.

Vieira-Andrade RG, Drumond CL, Martins-Júnior PA, Corrêa-Faria P, Gonzaga GC, Marques LS, Ramos-Jorge ML. Prevalence of sleep bruxism and associated factors in preschool children. *Pediatr Dent.* 2014;36(1):46–50.

Villa MP, Rizzoli A, Miano S, Malagola C. Efficacy of rapid maxillary expansion in children with obstructive sleep apnea syndrome: 36 months of follow-up. *Sleep Breath.* 2011;15(2):179–184.

von Cramon-Taubadel N. The relative efficacy of functional and developmental cranial modules for reconstructing global human population history. *Am J Phys Anthropol.* 2011;146:83–93.

Weeks SM. Relation between abnormal breathing and malocclusion. *Arch Ped.* 1913;30:46–51.

Weideman CL, Bush DL, Yan-Go FL, Clark GT, Gornbein JA. The incidence of parasomnias in child bruxers versus nonbruxers. *Pediatr Dent.* 1996;18(7):456–460.

Yamamoto M, Takada H, Ishizuka S, Kitamura K, Jeong J, Sato M, Hinata N, Abe S. Morphological association between the muscles and bones in the craniofacial region. *PLoS One.* 2020;15(1):e0227301.

Yujing Y, Dabo L, Zhenyun H, Jianwen Z. EEG arousals in attention-deficit/hyperactivity disorder (ADHD) children with sleep-disordered breathing (SDB). *Sleep Med.* 2015;16:S87.

Zhang R, Hess DT, Qian Z, Hausladen A, Fonseca F, Chaube R, Reynolds JD, Stamler JS. Hemoglobin βCys93 is essential for cardiovascular function and integrated response to hypoxia. *Proc Natl Acad Sci USA.* 2015;112(20):6425–6430.

Zhao H, Feng J, Ho TV, Grimes W, Urata M, Chai Y. The suture provides a niche for mesenchymal stem cells of craniofacial bones. *Nat Cell Biol.* 2015;17(4):386–396.

Zhenyun H, Yujing Y, Dabo L, Jianwen Z, Shuyao Q, Jiajian X, Jing Z, Xinhua Y, Shaofeng L. EEG arousals in children exhibiting primary snoring. *Sleep Med.* 2015;16:S88.

Chapter 9

Introduction to Craniofacial Sleep Medicine

Synopsis: This chapter provides a brief overview of the speciality of sleep medicine as well as a review of normal sleep physiology. The purpose of natural sleep is discussed and the consequences of a lack of quality sleep are noted. It should be noted that sleep disordered breathing (SDB), including upper airway resistance syndrome (UARS) and obstructive sleep apnea (OSA) in adults varies significantly from its pediatric counterpart although a deficiency in upper airway structure and function, often emanating from deficient craniofacial growth and development, is common in both adults and children. This chapter also briefly examines current therapies for sleep-related breathing disorders and contrasts them with biomimetic oral appliance therapy, which aims to eliminate sleep-related breathing disorders by the provision of therapeutic devices predicated on evidence-based preventive and curative principles.

Sleep medicine is a diverse medical speciality, and the international classification of sleep disorders (ICSD) has defined at least 64 known sleep disorders (Sateia, 2014). Before discussing any of these disorders, it's worth briefly reviewing normal sleep physiology. Sleep is a natural physiologic state in most mammals, characterized by reduced consciousness, sensory activity, and voluntary muscle activity. One question that can be posed is: What is the value of sleeping for part of the 24hr cycle? The reasons most often advocated are that sleep is a restorative phase that decreases fatigue, while improving the immune system and neurologic functions (such as memory consolidation), as well as showing increased anabolic activity (growth and development), along with a safe discharge of emotions through dreams and rapid eye movement (REM) sleep. However, Schmidt (2014) hypothesized that sleep evolved for the conservation of energy and optimal allocation of energy. For example, we use metabolic energy for different purposes, which can be classified into two main groups: activities directed toward environmental exploitation (e.g. mobility, foraging, reproduction, avoidance of predators, etc.), and biological activities of the internal environment of the body (e.g. repair/healing; neuronal plasticity; cellular processing; immune function, growth and maintenance of organs, etc.). Most recently, Cao *et al.* (2020) used mathematical modeling to predict how sleep varies during both evolution and ontogeny. Their approach shows a sudden change in sleep function during early childhood (< 2–3 yrs. of age) associated with neural reorganization and learning; whereas sleep after 2–3 yrs of age is primarily concerned with repair, especially during REM sleep. In this way, it's likely that REM sleep evolved to support energy availability for somatic and neurophysiologic processes at the expense of muscle tone. Furthermore, the alternating non-REM and REM stages of sleep help conserve energy by decreasing the need for a constant core body temperature. Thus, healthy sleep is associated with longevity, while sleep disorders, such as fatal familial insomnia, are associated with a shortened lifespan, while others can be life-threating (Medori *et al.*, 1992).

In order to transition from wakefulness to sleep, melatonin is synthesized by the pineal gland and its rhythm of secretion is regulated by the suprachiasmatic nuclei in normal light/dark conditions. In other words, exposure to light coordinates melatonin production. The overall function of melatonin is to communicate the light-dark cycle information to the body, which is used to produce functional changes (photoperiodism/circadian rhythm), including lowering the core body temperature while asleep. But there are many situations where melatonin secretion can be perturbed (Claustrat and Leston, 2015). For example, the suprachiasmatic nucleus also coordinates the circadian rhythm of the hypothalamo-pituitary-adrenal (HPA) axis. Specifically, cortisol acts as a messenger between the suprachiasmatic nucleus and the body tissues. In night-shift workers, alterations of the HPA axis can result in metabolic disturbances, leading to health issues, including jetlag, depression, anorexia nervosa, etc. (Liyanarachchi *et al.*, 2017). Since OSA is associated with increased cortisol secretion, it is not uncommon for these patients to gain weight as cortisol acts as an anabolic steroid precipitating an inappropriate increase in the BMI. On the other hand, slow-wave sleep (SWS) is associated with growth hormone (GH) secretion, which is dependent on the production of growth hormone-releasing hormone (GHRH); since GHRH has been shown to decrease wakefulness and increase SWS (Van Cauter and Plat, 1996). Thus, sleep-related GH output in adults likely plays a major role in maintaining decreased amounts of body fat. In contrast, ghrelin is a GIT hormone that acts as a ligand of the GH secretagogue receptor and is known to stimulate the appetite. It is involved in systemic energy metabolism as well as sleep rhythm, taste sensation and glucose metabolism (Müller *et al.*, 2015), acting as an antagonist to leptin.

It is thought that most adults need about 8hrs of sleep per night on average (Watson *et al.*, 2015), although the actual time lying in bed at night might exceed this. For example, the amount of time it takes to fall asleep is referred to as sleep latency, and this can normally last for about 10–20mins. Thereafter, the normal sleep architecture is typically: 5% Stage 1 sleep, 50% Stage 2 sleep, 15–25% Stage 3 slow wave sleep, and about 25% REM sleep. On the other hand, a newborn infant may require up to 16hrs of sleep per 24hr cycle. Paruthi *et al.* (2016) recommended that infants aged 4–12mths should sleep 12–16hrs per day (including naps). Children aged 1–2yrs should sleep 11–14hrs per day (including naps). Children aged 3–5yrs should sleep 10–13hrs per day (including naps), while those aged 6–12yrs should sleep 9–12hrs per day on a regular basis. For teenagers (13–19yrs of age), 8–10hrs of sleep per day on a regular basis is thought to promote optimal health. In addition, some data suggest that not only do teenagers require approx. 9hrs of sleep, but they prefer to go to bed later (and wake up later the next morning). Some studies suggest that permitting adolescents to start school later often helps in improving educational grade scores (Marx *et al.*, 2017), while it is thought that older adults prefer to go to sleep earlier and wake up earlier, perhaps accompanied by a mid-afternoon siesta or nap. Thus, sleep requirements appear to be an age-related phenomenon.

In all cases, sleep starts from the stage of wakefulness, which is characterized by α-waves on an electro-encephalograph (EEG). Whilst awake, responses to external stimuli are maintained partly by arousals. Arousal mechanisms are governed by the reticular formation in the brainstem, referred to as the reticular activating system (RAS). The RAS communicates with the cerebral cortex through the thalamus: sensory input from the cerebral cortex can activate the RAS and cause arousal. During sleep, fewer stimuli arise from the cortex because of a feedback loop to the cortex from the RAS. Specifically, in the brainstem, the dorsal raphe nucleus and the locus ceruleus are active both while awake and during non-REM sleep. These two nuclei suppress the pedunculo-pontine tegmental (PPT) nucleus which, when not suppressed, sends output to both the lower brainstem and to the thalamus (Simmons, 2012). While awake, a person maintains a focused attention by the RAS-thalamic ability to filter out stimuli. If that process fatigues, failure to filter out stimuli results in attention deficit. During non-REM sleep, the cortex is being inhibited by the reticular thalamic nucleus, which wraps around the thalamus, so there is little cortical processing. To remain awake when sleep deprived, a person can try to use increased stimulation, which is often achieved in children with ADHD by changes in behavior, including fidgeting, being distracted, getting up, etc. Thus, the child becomes hyperactive as a compensation to the enhanced sleep drive of the reticular thalamic nucleus. During non-REM sleep in adults, the RAS/thalamus attenuates incoming sensory stimuli to achieve sufficient filtration of sensory input necessary to fall asleep. In other words, the brain utilizes a filtering mechanism within the reticular thalamic nucleus to block the sensory input coming from the body from reaching the cerebral cortex at the thalamic level (Simmons, 2012). REM sleep occurs when the locus ceruleus and the dorsal raphe nucleus stop their inhibitory activity over the PPT nucleus. In effect, this results in activation of the pathways of the PPT nucleus. The first of these pathways ascends into the thalamus as part of the ascending reticular activating system, having an activating effect on the cortex, creating hallucinatory phenomena during REM sleep. The second pathway descends to the medulla ending at the reticulo-spinal track nucleus, which consists of neurons that descend into the spinal cord. Here, neurotransmitter (glycine) release causes inhibition of the motor neurons that leave the spinal cord, resulting in paralysis of the body during REM sleep. Therefore, during REM sleep the body becomes paralyzed while the cortex is very actively dreaming. This muscle paralysis prevents the body from acting out on the impulses generated from the brain's cortex during REM sleep (Simmons, 2012).

The actual stages of sleep are classified as Non-REM and REM sleep. NREM sleep has three stages. In stage 1 (N1) sleep, the eyelids start to droop (ptosis), accompanied by slow, rolling eye movements, and the heart rate begins to slow. This stage of sleep lasts about 1–7mins, and during that time a subject can wake up easily since it's a transitional stage between wakefulness and deep sleep. In fact, a common sign of disrupted sleep is an increase in the percentage amount of stage N1 sleep for the whole night (α-wave intrusion). These α-waves were the first waves discovered on an EEG since they are predominant in relaxed wakefulness, having a frequency of 8–13Hz. In stage N1 sleep, there is increased drowsiness, and the EEG rhythms slow to mixed δ- and θ-waves. The θ-waves have a frequency of 12–14Hz and dominate stage N1 sleep, which is associated with reduced muscle activity, decreased minute ventilation, and increased partial pressure of carbon dioxide in arterial blood ($PaCO_2$). At this time, the heart rate and cardiac output decrease from an increase in parasympathetic tone. In stage 2 (N2) sleep, conscious awareness of the surroundings is gradually lost. The duration of stage N2 sleep is about 10–25mins per cycle, and it normally represents about 50% of the total sleep time. The EEG is characterized by sleep spindles and K-complexes, which occur in a setting of variable, low-frequency waves.

After stage N2, stages 3 and 4 are now combined into N3, which represents deep sleep or slow, δ-wave sleep. In stage N3 sleep: brain metabolism is slowed; there is a lower respiratory rate; the heart rate and blood pressure are lowered; and there is a lower core body temperature. By stage N3, it's difficult to awaken a sleeping subject, any if they are awoken, they may awake feeling confused. Stage N3 sleep is also associated with parasomnias, such as sleepwalking (somnambulism), which is a sleep disorder that results in walking or performing other behaviors while asleep. It is more common in children than adults and is more likely to occur if a person is sleep-deprived. In stage N3 sleep, slow, δ-waves dominate the EEG with a frequency of between 0.5 and 2Hz. There is elevated electromyographic (EMG) activity and growth hormone levels peak during this stage of sleep. The respiratory rate is the most regular in this phase, which represents approx. 13–23% of the total sleep time in adults. This stage is mostly associated with restful, restorative sleep, and requires the highest intensity stimuli for arousal. If a subject is woken from stage N3 sleep, they appear groggy on awakening. Parasomnia behaviors may also occur during this stage of deep sleep. On the other hand, the stage of sleep during which dreaming can occur is REM sleep. It is characterized by rapid eye movements, rapid low voltage electroencephalography (EEG), and vivid dreams. There is muscle atonia since skeletal muscle tone is decreased. Notably, upper airway muscle tone is also decreased. On the other hand, memories of skills are consolidated, and erections can occur in males. The EEG shows mixed frequencies with α-waves. There are sometimes surges in autonomic activity that can destabilize the heart rate. Conversely, while the respiratory rate can increase, airflow can be decreased, and the hypoxic ventilatory response is depressed. Thus, REM sleep is 'paradoxical' sleep with rapid eye movements, a highly active brain, and active muscles of the eyes/diaphragm, accompanied by vivid dreams, while the body remains in a state of paralysis. REM sleep represents 50% of infant sleep, about 20%

of adult sleep, and approx. 15% of elderly sleep. In contrast, NREM is 'slow wave' or quiet sleep that lasts most of the night. Non-REM represents about 50% of infant sleep, 80% of adult sleep and approx. 85% of elderly sleep. Non-REM (stage 1, 2, and 3 sleep) and REM sleep cycles last approx. 90–110 minutes in normal sleep, and there are typically 4–6 cycles per night.

In sleep medicine, sleep latency (or sleep onset latency, SOL) is the amount of time it takes to transition from wakefulness to sleep (stage N1), or in other words, to fall asleep. An ideal sleep latency of around, say, 15–20mins also lays the foundation for a good night's sleep. The time it takes to fall asleep after the lights are turned off is also related to an individual's sleep debt and sleep efficiency. Sleep efficiency is the actual amount of time (%) spent sleeping compared to the total time spent in bed, since awakenings can occur during sleep. On the other hand, sleep debt is the accumulated amount of sleep loss from a deficiency of sleep. It most often occurs when insufficient sleep was obtained to meet an individual's requirements. For example, a sleep debt may occur due to sleep deprivation, in which insufficient hours are spent sleeping. Thus, if an individual needs 8hrs of sleep but only obtains 6hrs, there will be a 2hr sleep debt for that night. This sleep deficiency may have important consequences, especially if the debt builds up. Sleep debt may lead to increased daytime sleepiness, poor concentration or short-term memory, and mood problems such as anxiety, depression, and irritability. Pain perception is also worsened by poor sleep since it is thought that pain thresholds decrease with fatigue. In addition to the quantity of sleep, the quality of sleep is also important. For example, if the oxygen saturation of the blood hemoglobin (SaO_2) is <90% for significant amounts of time, then the quality of sleep is less than adequate for restorative purposes and likely represents one symptom of a possible sleep disorder.

Introduction to OSA

Along with insomnia, obstructive sleep apnea (OSA) is one of the most prevalent sleep disorders with a variable pathophysiology that includes upper airway dysmorphology, genioglossus dysfunction, changes in arousal threshold, and instability of the respiratory center *inter alia* (Subramani *et al.*, 2017). OSA is characterized by intermittent cessation of airflow through the nose and/or mouth during sleep. Apnea means 'absence of breath' and an apneic event has been defined to last at least 10 sec in duration. Thus, absence of breathing for 9sec is not recorded, but in most cases the apneas last between 20 and 30sec and can last as long as 2–3mins or more. In fact, apneic events of long duration are associated with postoperative complications in patients undergoing surgical procedures (Suen *et al.*, 2019). In addition, these recurrent bouts of asphyxiation and subsequent arousal from sleep lead to clinical complications, including cardiorespiratory disturbances, such as cyclical bradycardia during apnea and tachycardia during ventilation, which may precipitate sudden death during sleep (Gami *et al.*, 2013). For example, the neuropeptide somatostatin is involved in the control of respiration and modulation of respiratory rhythm, and can induce irreversible apnea (Llona and Eugenín, 2005). It is also thought that sympathetic disturbances occurring as a result of the respiratory dysregulation play a role in increasing the risk of sudden death, since OSA is associated with nocturnal arrhythmias, myocardial ischemia/infarction, stroke, and heart failure (Mansukhani *et al.*, 2015). More typically, the systemic blood pressure fails to decrease during sleep in patients with OSA (the so-called 'non-dippers'). Instead, the blood pressure increases at the termination of each apnea due to sympathetic nerve activation and reflex vasoconstriction. Not surprisingly, therefore, approx. half of all patients with OSA have systemic hypertension, while a diagnosis of OSA is an independent risk factor for the development of systemic hypertension. In patients with a chronic history, OSA may precipitate myocardial ischaemia, especially in those with coronary artery disease; and OSA in patients with congestive heart failure may acutely or chronically depress left ventricular function. In fact, Zhang *et al.* (2013) reviewed unexpected sudden death in people with OSA. The causes of demise included cardiomyopathy with and without ventricular hypertrophy. In addition, it is suspected that OSA is common in patients undergoing surgery, and has been associated with adverse events post-operatively, including neurologic injury and death (Fouladpour *et al.*,

2016; Feng *et al.*, 2019). Interestingly, Anandam *et al.* (2013) reported that oral appliance therapy may reduce cardiovascular mortality in patients with severe OSA that are intolerant to CPAP. In fact, Rotenberg *et al.* (2016) noted that CPAP compliance remains low and cannot be considered the best option in some cases. But in addition to the cardiovascular system, the central nervous system may also be affected. Thus, OSA is associated with cognitive and behavioral disturbances, excessive daytime sleepiness, intellectual impairment, memory loss and personality changes. Other physiologic processes are also perturbed, including erectile dysfunction in adult males, and an increased overall risk of developing cancer. For example, in an epidemiologic study, Brenner *et al.* (2019) reported that patients aged <45yrs with severe OSA have a higher incidence of prostate, hematologic, colorectal, and breast cancer compared to the general population. Thus, screening young patients suspected of having OSA is recommended.

The prevalence of OSA was thought to be 2% in middle-aged women and 4% in middle-aged men (Young *et al.*, 1993) but a more recent systematic review (Senaratna *et al.*, 2017) reported that for an apnea-hypopnea index (AHI) of >5 events/hr, the overall prevalence ranged from 9%–38%. The prevalence is higher in men and increases with age and body-mass index. At an AHI of >15 events/hr, the prevalence of OSA in adults ranges from 6%–17%, and in patients with a history of orthodontic treatment, the prevalence of OSA was found to be approx. 10% (Larsen *et al.*, 2015). OSA differs from central sleep apnea (CSA) where the neural drive to the respiratory muscles (via C3–C5) is abolished. In OSA, airflow ceases despite continuing respiratory effort because of a closure of the upper airway. Overall, Osman *et al.* (2018) consider that there are about four phenotypes associated with the pathogenesis of OSA including: a small or crowded upper airway, low/collapsible pharyngeal muscle tone, a low arousal threshold, and loop gain, which is unstable control of breathing. Thus, the patho-etiology of OSA includes collapse of the upper airway, leading to progressive asphyxia until there is a brief arousal from sleep so that upper airway patency is restored and airflow resumes. The subject then returns to sleep and the process is repeated numerous times during the night so that the sleep architecture becomes perturbed and fragmented. The main factor leading to collapse of the upper airway is generation of a sub-atmospheric pressure during inspiration, which exceeds the ability of pharyngeal muscles, etc. to maintain airway patency. Thus, a measure of upper airway collapsibility during sleep is the pharyngeal critical closing pressure (Pcrit), which is the estimated nasal pressure at which the 'passive' upper airway collapses and airflow ceases (Smith *et al.*, 1988). Pcrit progressively decreases (i.e. the airway becomes more collapsible) in those who snore and in patients with OSA, compared with healthy individuals. However, this collapsing pressure is not reached during wakefulness since the higher upper airway muscle tone is able to compensate for airway narrowing and upper airway resistance.

In children, upper airway resistance may not result in hypoxia but may still produce fragmented sleep. In these cases, the AHI may be ≤3 events/hr but abnormal breathing patterns, flow limitation and mouth-breathing can often be observed. In addition, the respiratory disturbance index (RDI) may be increased to about 5 events/hr. The RDI includes respiratory effort-related arousals (RERAs) and may help confirm the typical symptoms of pediatric OSA (Fig. 101). All of these respiratory sleep disorders (RSD)

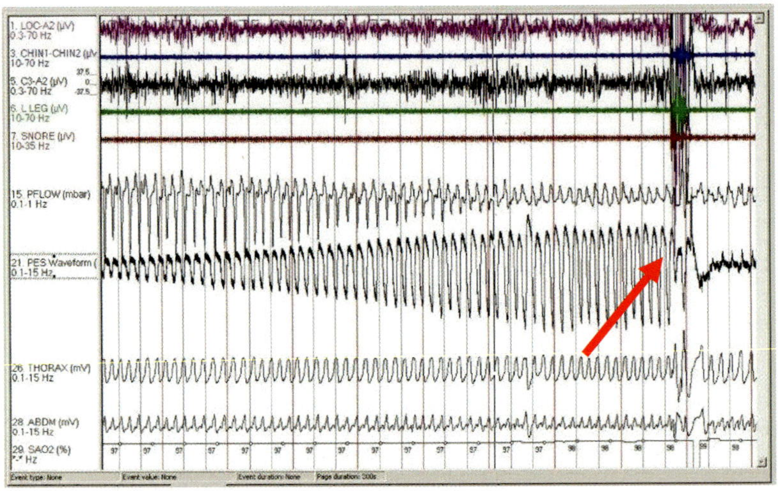

Figure 101: Classic respiratory effort-related arousal (RERA, arrowed) seen on EEG. The arousal precedes the bruxing event. Courtesy: Dr Ravindra Chandrashekhar.

are associated with EEG disturbances in these cases of 'non-hypoxic' SDB (Guilleminault *et al.*, 2019). Thus, RSDs include primary snoring and upper airway resistance syndrome (UARS). In children aged 2–8yrs, UARS is typically correlated to the size of the adenoidal tissues of the upper airway (Gulotta *et al.*, 2019). These tissue abnormalities produce variable obstruction of the upper airway and an alteration of gas exchange during sleep (Schechter, 2002; Gozal and Kheirandish-Gozal, 2009). The clinical consequences of these disturbances are not only sleep fragmentation, but daytime sleepiness, cognitive and behavioral disorders, with consequent poor school performance. These neurocognitive, behavioral and metabolic conditions form a neurobehavioral syndrome which, in turn, has social implications (Paglia, 2019). In adults, Arnold and Guilleminault (2019) consider that a diagnosis of UARS is aimed at preventing the development of features associated with SDB. For example, on the one hand, when comparing inspiratory sleep airflow parameters and sleep fragmentation, Gold *et al.* (2013) found virtually no differences when comparing adults diagnosed with UARS and controls. On the other hand, Broderick *et al.* (2014) noted that UARS is an indicator of chronic stress and that patients with UARS show increased levels of somatic arousal. In Asian patients with UARS, Tay and Pang (2018) also noted high arousal indices but a low AHI (<5 event/hr), while the RDI was much higher (19 events/hr). Unlike patients with OSA, however, hypertension was rare, but depression was more commonly found in these cases. Also, as expected, many had a history of chronic pain such as headaches, neck aches, muscle myalgia, as well as sleep bruxism (SB) and temporo-mandibular joint disorders (TMD). In fact, Shapira (2013) opines that resolution of sleep disorders is a key principle in the successful management of TMD. Moreover, Lynn and Curry (2011) hypothesized that arousals are associated with mechanisms of SpO_2 cycling that may contribute to a fall in upper airway tone/collapse leading to paroxysmal cluster patterns of desaturations.

In addition, structural abnormalities of upper airway morphology may also predispose to nocturnal collapse. There is a range of structural compromises, including a reduction in post-oral airway size, which can be

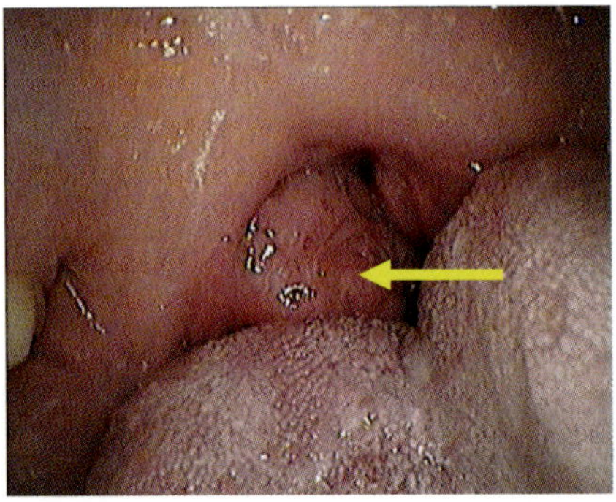

Figure 102a: Intra-oral photograph showing 'crowding' of post-oral airway by enlarged tonsils (arrowed). Courtesy: Dr Tammarie Heit.

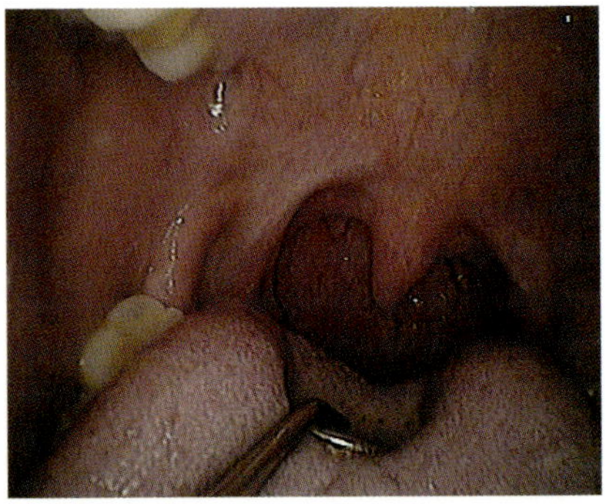

Figure 102b: Intra-oral photograph of same patient showing post-surgical aperture of post-oral airway.

described as 'crowding' (Fig. 102a). The Mallampati score is a qualitative method of describing the degree of oropharyngeal airway crowding, where a Mallampati Class I score means that the tip of the uvula and the base of the tongue are visibly separated. A Mallampati Class II score means that the tip of the uvula and the base of the tongue are visibly in contact. A Mallampati Class III score means that the base of the tongue lies approx. halfway across the uvula, and a Mallampati Class IV score means the base of the tongue and the soft palate are in contact. These classifications are made at rest. In the Pneumopedics protocol, I first suggested that the oropharyngeal airway be assessed during function. In this case, the patient is asked to make the 'Aaaah' sound aloud for about 5–10sec. During this time, it's possible to observe the behavior of the post-oral airway, and this may indicate the functional requirement of the upper airway during sleep since the upper airway may have high compliance with a 'flaccid' muscle tone that may be prone to collapse. In addition, obesity may contribute to a reduction in upper airway size, by increasing fat deposition in the salpingopharyngeal fold in the lateral pharyngeal wall of the pharynx (Agrawal, 2015) or by compressing the pharynx by superficial fat masses in the neck. However, Sforza *et al.* (2019) found that 3D facial measurements were not associated with an increased risk of metabolic syndrome.

In children, adeno-tonsillar hypertrophy may impede airflow and, along with other craniofacial features such as bimaxillary retrognathia and macroglossia (secondary to obesity), may predispose an individual to sleep disordered breathing. Witzel and Posnick (1989) studied velopharyngeal behavior in children with cleft palate. They discovered that the predominant pattern of upper airway closure (68%) was in the coronal plane, followed by a concentric pattern of closure (28%), with only 4% showing a sagittal pattern of velopharyngeal closure. The significance of this study is that the pattern of upper airway opening and closing appears to be diverse and may have implications in the treatment of SDB.

Watanabe *et al.* (2002) studied craniofacial characteristics in patients with sleep disordered breathing. The types of pharyngeal closure were determined by endoscopic evaluations of the pharynx in paralyzed and anesthetized patients with SDB. Compared with lateral cephalometric radiographs of normal subjects, patients with SDB demonstrated retrognathic mandibles and longer faces with downward mandibular development. Patients with SDB also demonstrated smaller maxillae and mandibles. These findings were corroborated by Banabilh *et al.* (2009) who demonstrated that the upper arch in patients with OSA was 7–11% narrower in the transverse plane while the lower arch was 10–11% shorter in the antero-posterior plane when compared with the control configurations. Similarly, using cephalometric radiographs in both obese and non-obese Chinese patients diagnosed with OSA, Chang and Shiao (2008) reported finding a narrower upper airway in patients with non-positional OSA compared to those with positional OSA. Neelapu *et al.* (2017) also consider that craniofacial disharmony is a critical risk factor for the development of OSA in individuals of a particular ethnic group. Using a meta-analysis, they also reported that a reduced pharyngeal airway space *inter alia* was a cephalometric feature characteristic of patients with OSA compared to controls. Furthermore, comparing Chinese and Caucasians patients with the same OSA severity, Lee *et al.* (2010) noted that Chinese patients with OSA showed more craniofacial disharmony while Caucasian patients with OSA had a higher BMI.

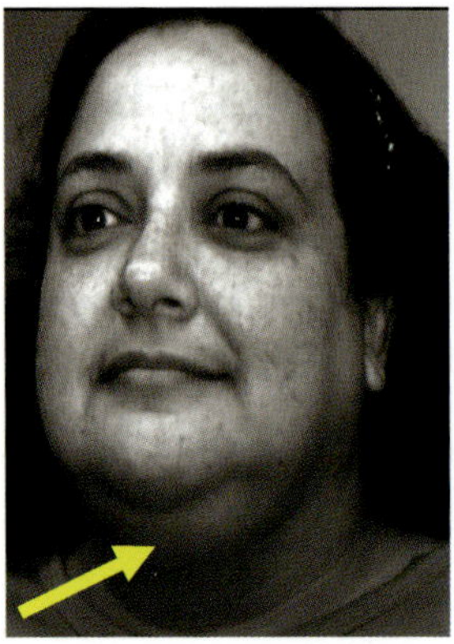

Figure 103a: 3D photograph showing submandibular pannus or 'double chin' (arrowed).

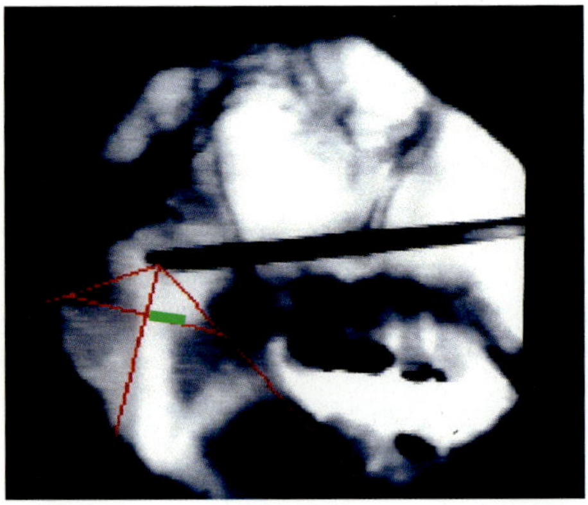

Figure 103b: Video-nasofluoroscopy showing velopharyngeal isthmus (green line) viewed from above.

Earlier, Watanabe *et al.* (2002) had suggested that obesity and craniofacial abnormalities may contribute to the pathogenesis of obstructive sleep apnea. These findings were also supported by Banabilh *et al.* (2009) who reported that craniofacial obesity is associated with OSA, and a submandibular pannus (Fig. 103a) may be a valuable screening sign in the identification of patients with undiagnosed OSA. Indeed, Watson (2016) noted in two white papers commissioned by the American Academy of Sleep Medicine that in the USA approx. 80% of potential patients remain undiagnosed. Craniofacial obesity may contribute to reduction in upper airway size by increasing fat deposition in the soft tissues of the pharynx and tongue or by tissue pressure compressing the pharynx by superficial fat masses in the neck. Furthermore, nasoendoscopy can be used for a retropalatal examination of the upper airway where the velopharyngeal isthmus (the narrowest point between the soft palate and posterior pharyngeal wall) can be viewed from above (Fig. 103b).

In order to improve the oropharyngeal airway, mandibular advancement devices (MADs) are often used. However, based on the pattern of velopharyngeal opening, one study found that 80% of patients had a smaller cross-sectional airway area with excessive mandibular protrusion, while 18% showed no difference in cross-sectional area, the so-called 'non-responders'. Sutherland and Cistulli (2011) compared upper airway responses to MADs in 'responders' and 'non-responders'. In responders, there was an increase in the lateral width and cross-sectional area of the velopharynx. Conversely, in non-responders, no increases in upper airway dimensions were evident. Morrison *et al.* (1993) studied sites of upper airway obstruction. They reported that the nasopharynx was a site of primary narrowing in 80% of patients, but two or more sites of narrowing were also commonly observed (82%). This study suggests that the site and severity of the upper airway obstruction needs to be addressed, but the precise localization of the site(s) of obstruction cannot be detected using PSGs or HSATs alone (Neelapu *et al.*, 2017). Thus, thorough craniofacial diagnosis may be the key to successful therapeutic interventions.

Apart from craniofacial features, there are other clinical findings that are associated with a suspected diagnosis of sleep disordered breathing. In adults, these systemic conditions include obesity, hypertension, cardio-pulmonary diseases, diabetes (Reutrakul and Mokhlesi, 2017), etc. Although snoring may predate a diagnosis of OSA by several years, primary snoring in the absence of other symptoms, may not warrant investigation for OSA, but counseling for weight/BMI management and/or alcohol use may be required. The stereotypical presentation of OSA is often thought of in terms of a middle-aged male with obesity/submandibular pannus, who snores and has daytime sleepiness. In addition, there may be witnessed apneas during sleep, nocturnal choking and/or gasping, with a history of hypertension. In contrast, women suspected of having OSA may be post-menopausal with less frequent snoring, but daytime fatigue accompanied by chronic pain, which may be a presenting symptom perhaps overlapping with chronic fatigue syndrome or fibromyalgia. However, it is important to note that a much larger and broader spectrum of individuals may have SDB, ranging from upper airway resistance syndrome and sleep bruxism to mild/moderate and even severe OSA. Because of this diverse range of presentations, thorough history-taking is mandatory when a report of snoring is first encountered. Other signs and symptoms may include: morning headaches, nocturnal urinary frequency/nocturnal enuresis, nasal congestion, etc. History-taking can include general questions such as past medical history and family history; and sleep-related questions can then be introduced, such as sleep hygiene, sleep position, and the quality and quantity of dreams, since relative changes in dreaming (dreaming more often, remembering dreams, and dreaming in color) are sometimes reported during or post-treatment. However, to assess the sleep quality a sleep questionnaire (such as the Epworth Sleepiness Scale, STOP-Bang Questionnaire, or Pediatric Sleep Questionnaire; Appendix) is often deployed clinically.

Following comprehensive history-taking, a physical examination can be performed. Craniofacial features need to be assessed including: nasal morphology and function as well as the retropalatal, retroglossal, and hypopharyngeal regions, which may require special investigations, such as nasendoscopy or 3D cone-beam CT scans. In addition, the oral cavity needs to examined, including: the dentition and occlusion, the Mallampati score, the oropharyngeal size and shape, the presence of adenoids and/or tonsils, tongue features (such as scalloping and lingual frenum), the palatal vault height/width assessment, as well as the length of the uvula. After reviewing the findings of the head and neck exam, which includes cone-beam CT scan findings as discussed previously, diagnostic tests for OSA may be indicated. Currently, the preferred diagnostic procedure for sleep disorders is polysomnography (PSG), which is a detailed overnight sleep study with various channels being recorded using:

- Electrocardiography (ECG: to identify any arrythmias and cardiovascular behavior)
- Electroencephalography (EEG: to assess brain waves, indicating the stages of sleep)
- Electro-oculography (EOG: to detect eye movements, especially during REM sleep)

- Electromyography (EMG: to detect muscle tone/bruxism, especially during REM sleep)
- Plethysmography (to assess ventilation via movements of the chest and abdominal walls)
- Pulse oximetry (to assess arterial oxygen saturation, using finger, ear, or toe sensors)
- Heart rate monitoring (if an ECG channel is not available)
- Actigraphy (using a device worn on the wrist to record movements that can be used to estimate sleep parameters, using algorithms in software programs.)
- Nasal/oral airflow sensors (used to measure the breathing rate in a patient while asleep)

While PSGs are the standard of care, especially for sleep physicians, not all patients are willing to undergo a sleep study in a laboratory or sleep clinic since some find it difficult to sleep in an unfamiliar environment. As an alternative, an array of home sleep apnea tests (HSAT) have become available. Accordingly, there are different types of sleep studies. For example, a Level 1 sleep study is most often an attended laboratory-based sleep study (PSG). A Level 2 sleep study uses the same Level 1 testing equipment, but is performed without a respiratory technician in attendance. In contrast, a Level 3 sleep test is most often a portable sleep apnea study, which is performed in the patient's home. This test is used to diagnose mild/moderate OSA but is not able to diagnose other sleep disorders. Finally, a Level 4 sleep study refers to OSA screening using pulse oximetry, which measures blood oxygen levels. This test also includes measuring the heart rate, and Level 4 studies are usually used to screen for pediatric OSA. However, if a pediatric sleep questionnaire identifies a child at high risk of OSA but a subsequent Level 3 or 4 sleep apnea study returns a negative result, the sleep study needs to be repeated using PSG to confirm the initial findings. Children require thorough sleep testing since an AHI >1 represents a diagnosis of pediatric OSA. Thus, portable sleep tests for children should feature: oximetry for SpO_2, thoracic and abdomen belts, audio signal for snoring, airflow signal through a nasal cannula, and signals for pulse and body position.

Once a representative sleep study has been performed, the data requires interpretation to reach a working diagnosis. For example, episodes of airflow cessation or reduction at the nose and mouth despite continuing respiratory effort (chest wall movement) are diagnostic of OSA. During an apneic event, abnormal nasal and oral airflow may be followed by EMG activity, representing bruxism and/or clenching. However, a PSG is both expensive and time consuming. Thus, if an HSAT can confirm a suspicion of OSA based on episodes of arterial O_2 desaturation, etc. then this option can decrease the need for a PSG. However, increased upper airway resistance during sleep may be associated with arousals in the absence of apneas or hypopneas, and can still result in clinically important sleep-related syndromes, such as UARS, but this data might not be picked up with an HSAT. In addition, it is thought that some HSATs tend to underestimate the severity of OSA. In any case, some modern portable HSAT units now include: analysis and reporting software, simplified patient attachments, fast data download with rapid study results, and multi-night recordings, which can be extended for pediatric patients. Despite these advantages, it is important to remember that when an HSAT result is negative, a PSG may be indicated, especially where there are clinical signs and symptoms.

Management of OSA

The body's circadian rhythm includes sleep. In the late evening various hormones (such as melatonin) are released from the brain that lead to the individual feeling sleepy. However, just like an alarm clock, the 'go to sleep' signal can be overridden, which can disturb the circadian rhythm to a certain extent. Getting ready for a good night's sleep is called sleep hygiene. Classically, exposure to blue light needs to be minimized, which means devices like cell phones, TV screens, computers, etc. need to be put away since they can delay or suppress melatonin release. For children and adults, there should be no device use in the bedroom, which should be slightly cooler than the living room. Ideally, the bedroom should be very dark (some people use blackout blinds or eye shades) and quiet. Sleep is, in some respects, a microform of hibernation, so the bed should be snug to allow the body to reduce its core temperature, lower the heart rate and blood pressure, with regular nasal breathing. One of the first things to address in adults diagnosed with OSA is sleep hygiene. Thus, preparing for a good night's sleep starts with no exposure to blue screens within 1–2hrs of bedtime. It's best not to eat a heavy meal, including alcohol, within 3–4hrs of bedtime. Some people prefer relaxation/breathing techniques to help get ready for bedtime, while others may use various techniques to optimize nasal breathing, sometimes by using lip-tape. Sleep and head position also contribute to the quality and quantity of sleep. Some people have a preferred sleeping-side and others use pillows, etc. to find the best sleeping position, especially those with positional OSA.

Individuals who are tired during the day may be suffering from a condition known as excessive daytime sleepiness (EDS). This type of EDS is a classic symptom of OSA. In OSA, breathing stops intermittently during sleep, which leads to transient awakenings/arousals during the night that are associated with poor quality sleep. The individual wakes up the next morning without feeling refreshed from a good night's sleep, and this leads to excessive tiredness during the day. One of the first things that can be done to address this issue is to fill out a sleep questionnaire (such as an Epworth Sleepiness Scale; Appendix). This questionnaire helps identify individuals that may be at a higher risk of having OSA. If the questionnaire suggests an increased risk of OSA, a physician may then suggest an overnight sleep study, which can verify a diagnosis of OSA and indicate the degree of its severity. Once diagnosed, various forms of sleep therapy can be considered to help restore normal, restful sleep. Treatment options for OSA include: assessment of sleep position, especially in those with positional OSA; weight management, particularly in those with an increased BMI; continuous positive airway pressure (CPAP) ventilation;

oral appliances, especially for those patients that are unable to comply with CPAP; and various surgical procedures in selected/complex adult cases. In children, it's important to rule out co-morbidities such as ADHD, in which 25–50% of children suffer from sleep-breathing problems. These children are hyperactive during the day, although there may be exceptions. In one study, about 30% of children scheduled for tonsillectomy and adenoidectomy had a differential diagnosis of ADHD. Post-operatively, 50% of these children no longer had ADHD, thus there appears to be an overlap of symptoms in ADHD and pediatric OSA. Therefore, treatment in children might at first be conservative with attention being paid to diet, lifestyle, behavioral issues, allergies, etc. In principle, airway obstruction can be avoided by increasing or maintaining upper airway muscle tone during sleep. Thus, in adult cases of mild OSA, alcohol and sedatives may need to be avoided prior to going to sleep. Similarly, upper airway obstruction can be avoided by increasing or maintaining its lumen size. If the upper airway lumen caliber is decreased in adults diagnosed with mild to moderate OSA, then empirical measures, such as weight/BMI reduction and avoidance of the supine position while asleep might help to keep the airway patent. Thus, the range of treatments option for SDB is diverse. For example, in mild cases of upper airway resistance syndrome, improved nasal patency may be sufficient to address the issue. In severe cases of adult OSA, nasal CPAP with adaptive servo-regulation (ventilatory support that is adjusted based on the detection of apneas or pauses in breathing during sleep) might be preferred by sleep physicians. In fact, Ito *et al.* (2014) consider that for successful nasal CPAP, craniofacial parameters, such as tongue and maxillo-mandibular size, may need to be taken into account.

In addition to these options, dental professionals are often called upon in the management of mild to moderate OSA. The vast majority of oral appliances are based on the principle that mandibular advancement leads to an increased aperture of the oropharyngeal airway. Thus, mandibular advancement devices are designed to protrude the mandible. However, complications and side effects can arise with long-term use. In rats, long-term mandibular protrusion leads to increased mandibular growth and, it appears that a similar phenomenon also occurs in some patients, in that some MAD procedures have an effect on the facial profile. In fact, unwanted tooth movement following MAD treatment of OSA has been reported (Almeida *et al.*, 2006) and Korngut (2010) reported inappropriate mandibular prognathism in a patient treated with long-term MAD therapy for OSA. It is thought that these craniofacial outcomes might not be acceptable to some patients and by orthodontists that have been trained to correct Class III malocclusions in adults and children. In children, symptoms of OSA can be quite different from adults. Thus, behavioral problems, learning issues, lack of attentiveness, and hyperactivity can characterize sleep disordered breathing more than classic signs of fatigue in children. In one study, Singh *et al.* (2007) studied the effect of palatal expansion on the pediatric airway and found that midfacial development using a palatal expander was associated with an enhanced upper airway space in children. In another study, Singh and Krumholtz (2009) found that the upper airway changes in non-growing adults were similar to those of actively growing children undergoing midfacial development therapy. These novel findings suggested that genetically encoded developmental mechanisms may be modulated by biomimetic oral appliances to enhance the upper airway in adults as well as children and help in the management of patients diagnosed with OSA using a Pneumopedic effect. In summary, regardless of whatever method is chosen to address OSA, a comprehensive patient history and diagnosis is mandatory. Once a diagnosis has been achieved, it's important to treat the patient, not the numbers, by carefully observing clinical responses and outcomes. Although it's important to provide evidence-based medicine, it's also important to practice what you preach, and remain cognizant of the triad of airway, breathing and sleep.

References

Agrawal V. Role of salpingopharyngeal fold in lateral pharyngeal wall collapse causing obstructive sleep apnea. *Sleep Med.* 2015;16:S199.

Almeida FR, Lowe AA, Otsuka R, Fastlicht S, Farbood M, Tsuiki S. Long-term sequellae of oral appliance therapy in obstructive sleep apnea patients: Part 2. Study-model analysis. *Am J Orthod Dentofacial Orthop*. 2006;129(2):205–213.

Anandam A, Patil M, Akinnusi M, Jaoude P, El-Solh AA. Cardiovascular mortality in obstructive sleep apnoea treated with continuous positive airway pressure or oral appliance: an observational study. *Respirology*. 2013;18(8):1184–1190.

Arnold WC, Guilleminault C. Upper airway resistance syndrome 2018: non-hypoxic sleep-disordered breathing. *Expert Rev Respir Med*. 2019;13(4):317–326.

Banabilh SM, Suzina AH, Dinsuhaimi S, Samsudin AR, Singh GD. Craniofacial obesity in patients with obstructive sleep apnea. *Sleep Breath*. 2009;13(1):19–24.

Banabilh SM, Suzina AH, Dinsuhaimi S, Samsudin AR, Singh GD. Dental arch morphology in south-east Asian adults with obstructive sleep apnoea: geometric morphometrics. *J Oral Rehabil*. 2009;36(3):184–192.

Brenner R, Kivity S, Peker M, Reinhorn D, Keinan-Boker L, Silverman B, Liphsitz I, Kolitz T, Levy C, Shlomi D, Pillar G, Peled N. Increased risk for cancer in young patients with severe obstructive sleep apnea. *Respiration*. 2019;97(1):15–23.

Broderick JE, Gold MS, Amin MM, Gold AR. The association of somatic arousal with the symptoms of upper airway resistance syndrome. *Sleep Med*. 2014;15(4):436–443.

Cao J, Herman AB, West GB, Poe G, Savage VM. Unraveling why we sleep: Quantitative analysis reveals abrupt transition from neural reorganization to repair in early development. *Science Adv*. 2020;6(38):eaba0398.

Chang ET, Shiao GM. Craniofacial abnormalities in Chinese patients with obstructive and positional sleep apnea. *Sleep Med*. 2008;9(4):403–410.

Claustrat B, Leston J. Melatonin: Physiological effects in humans. *Neurochirurgie*. 2015;61(2–3):77–84.

Feng TR, White RS, Ma X, Askin G, Pryor KO. The effect of obstructive sleep apnea on readmissions and atrial fibrillation after cardiac surgery. *J Clin Anesth*. 2019;56:17–23.

Fouladpour N, Jesudoss R, Bolden N, Shaman Z, Auckley D. Perioperative complications in obstructive sleep apnea patients undergoing surgery: A review of the legal literature. *Anesth Analg*. 2016;122(1):145–151.

Gami AS, Olson EJ, Shen WK, Wright RS, Ballman KV, Hodge DO, Herges RM, Howard DE, Somers VK. Obstructive sleep apnea and the risk of sudden cardiac death: a longitudinal study of 10,701 adults. *J Am Coll Cardiol*. 2013;62(7):610–616.

Gold AR, Broderick JE, Gold MS, Amin MM. A comparison of inspiratory airflow dynamics during sleep between upper airway resistance syndrome patients and healthy controls. *Sleep Breath*. 2013;17(4):1169–1178.

Gozal D, Kheirandish-Gozal L. Obesity and excessive daytime sleepiness in prepubertal children with obstructive sleep apnea. *Pediatrics*. 2009;123:13–18.

Guilleminault C, Huang YS, Chin WC, Okorie C. The nocturnal-polysomnogram and "non-hypoxic sleep-disordered-breathing" in children. *Sleep Med*. 2019;60:31–4.

Gulotta G, Iannella G, Vicini C, Polimeni A, Greco A, de Vincentiis M, Visconti IC, Meccariello G, Cammaroto G, De Vito A, Gobbi R, Bellini C, Firinu E, Pace A, Colizza A, Pelucchi S, Magliulo G. Risk factors for obstructive sleep apnea syndrome in children: State of the art. *Int J Environ Res Public Health*. 2019;16(18):E3235.

Ito E, Tsuiki S, Namba K, Takise Y, Inoue Y. Upper airway anatomical balance contributes to optimal continuous positive airway pressure for Japanese patients with obstructive sleep apnea syndrome. *J Clin Sleep Med*. 2014;10(2):137–142.

Korngut R. Case study: A persistent positive outcome treating OSA with a MAD following the treatment protocol. *Dialogue*. 2010;1:26–27.

Larsen AJ, Rindal DB, Hatch JP, Kane S, Asche SE, Carvalho C, Rugh J. Evidence supports no relationship between obstructive sleep apnea and premolar extraction: An electronic health records review. *J Clin Sleep Med*. 2015;11(12):1443–1448.

Lee RW, Vasudavan S, Hui DS, Prvan T, Petocz P, Darendeliler MA, Cistulli PA. Differences in craniofacial structures and obesity in Caucasian and Chinese patients with obstructive sleep apnea. *Sleep*. 2010;33(8):1075–1080.

Liyanarachchi K, Ross R, Debono M. Human studies on hypothalamo-pituitary-adrenal (HPA) axis. *Best Pract Res Clin Endocrinol Metab*. 2017;31(5):459–473.

Llona I, Eugenín J. Central actions of somatostatin in the generation and control of breathing. *Biol Res*. 2005;38(4):347–352.

Lynn LA, Curry JP. Patterns of unexpected in-hospital deaths: a root cause analysis. *Patient Saf Surg*. 2011;5(1):3.

Mansukhani MP, Wang S, Somers VK. Sleep, death, and the heart. *Am J Physiol Heart Circ Physiol*. 2015;309(5):H739–H749.

Marx R, Tanner-Smith EE, Davison CM, Ufholz LA, Freeman J, Shankar R, Newton L, Brown RS, Parpia AS, Cozma I, Hendrikx S. Later school start times for supporting the education, health, and well-being of high school students. *Cochrane Database Syst Rev*. 2017;7:CD009467.

Medori R, Tritschler HJ, LeBlanc A, Villare F, Manetto V, Chen HY, Xue R, Leal S, Montagna P, Cortelli P, *et al.* Fatal familial insomnia, a prion disease with a mutation at codon 178 of the prion protein gene. *N Engl J Med*. 1992;326(7):444–449.

Morrison DL, Launois SH, Isono S, Feroah TR, Whitelaw WA, Remmers JE. Pharyngeal narrowing and closing pressures in patients with obstructive sleep apnea. *Am Rev Respir Dis*. 1993;148(3):606–611.

Müller TD, Nogueiras R, Andermann ML, *et al.* Ghrelin. *Mol Metab.* 2015;4(6):437–460.

Neelapu BC, Kharbanda OP, Sardana HK, Balachandran R, Sardana V, Kapoor P, Gupta A, Vasamsetti S. Craniofacial and upper airway morphology in adult obstructive sleep apnea patients: A systematic review and meta-analysis of cephalometric studies. *Sleep Med Rev.* 2017;31:79–90.

Osman AM, Carter SG, Carberry JC, Eckert DJ. Obstructive sleep apnea: Current perspectives. *Nat Sci Sleep.* 2018;10:21–34.

Paglia L. Respiratory sleep disorders in children and role of the paediatric dentist. *Eur J Paediatr Dent.* 2019;20(1):5.

Paruthi S, Brooks LJ, D'Ambrosio C, Hall WA, Kotagal S, Lloyd RM, Malow BA, Maski K, Nichols C, Quan SF, Rosen CL, Troester MM, Wise MS. Recommended amount of sleep for pediatric populations: A consensus statement of the American Academy of Sleep Medicine. *J Clin Sleep Med.* 2016;12(6):785–786.

Reutrakul S, Mokhlesi B. Obstructive sleep apnea and diabetes: A state of the art review. *Chest.* 2017;152(5):1070–1086.

Rotenberg BW, Murariu D, Pang KP. Trends in CPAP adherence over twenty years of data collection: a flattened curve. *J Otol Head Neck Surg.* 2016;45:43–52.

Sateia MJ. International classification of sleep disorders — third edition: highlights and modifications. *Chest.* 2014;146(5):1387–1394.

Schechter MS. Technical report: Diagnosis and management of childhood obstructive sleep apnea syndrome. *Pediatrics.* 2002;109(4):e69.

Schmidt MH. The energy allocation of sleep: A unifying theory of sleep, torpor, and continuous wakefulness. *Neurosci and Biobehav Rev.* 2014;47:122–153.

Senaratna CV, Perret JL, Lodge CJ, Lowe AJ, Campbell BE, Matheson MC, Hamilton GS, Dharmage SC. Prevalence of obstructive sleep apnea in the general population: A systematic review. *Sleep Med Rev.* 2017;34:70–81.

Sforza C, Bertoli S, Leone A, Rosati R, Menezes M, Battezzati A. Three-dimensional soft-tissue facial morphometry in Caucasian obese adults. *Pesqui Bras Odontopediatria Clín Integr.* 2019;19:e4550.

Shapira IL. TMJ alias, the Great Imposter, has a co-conspirator: poor sleep. *Cranio.* 2013;31(1):1–2.

Simmons JH. Neurology of sleep and sleep-related breathing disorders and their relationships to sleep bruxism. *J Calif Dent Assoc.* 2012;40(2):159–167.

Singh GD, Garcia-Motta AV, Hang WM. Evaluation of the posterior airway space following Biobloc therapy: geometric morphometrics. *Cranio.* 2007;25(2):84–89.

Singh GD, Krumholtz J. Epigenetic Orthodontics in Adults. *Appliance Therapy Group*, USA, 2009.

Smith PL, Wise RA, Gold AR, Schwartz AR, Permutt S. Upper airway pressure-flow relationships in obstructive sleep apnea. *J Appl Physiol*. 1988;64(2):789–795.

Subramani Y, Singh M, Wong J, Kushida CA, Malhotra A, Chung F. Understanding phenotypes of obstructive sleep apnea: Applications in anesthesia, surgery, and perioperative medicine. *Anesth Analg*. 2017;124(1):179–191.

Suen C, Ryan CM, Mubashir T, Ayas NT, Abrahamyan L, Wong J, Mokhlesi B, Chung F. Sleep study and oximetry parameters for predicting postoperative complications in patients with OSA. *Chest*. 2019;155(4):855–867.

Sutherland K, Cistulli P. Mandibular advancement splints for the treatment of sleep apnea syndrome. *Swiss Med Wkly*. 2011;141:w13276.

Tay DKL, Pang KP. Clinical phenotype of South-East Asian temporomandibular disorder patients with upper airway resistance syndrome. *J Oral Rehabil*. 2018;45(1):25–3.

Van Cauter E, Plat L. Physiology of growth hormone secretion during sleep. *J Pediatr*. 1996;128(5):S32–S37.

Watanabe T, Isono S, Tanaka A, Tanzawa H, Nishino T. Contribution of body habitus and craniofacial characteristics to segmental closing pressures of the passive pharynx in patients with sleep-disordered breathing. *Am J Respir Crit Care Med*. 2002;165(2):260–265.

Watson NF, Badr MS, Belenky G, Bliwise DL, Buxton OM, Buysse D, Dinges DF, Gangwisch J, Grandner MA, Kushida C, Malhotra RK, Martin JL, Patel SR, Quan SF, Tasali E. Recommended amount of sleep for a healthy adult: A joint consensus statement of the American Academy of Sleep Medicine and Sleep Research Society. *Sleep*. 2015;38(6):843–844.

Watson NF. Health care savings: the economic value of diagnostic and therapeutic care for obstructive sleep apnea. *J Clin Sleep Med*. 2016;12(8):1075–1077.

Witzel MA, Posnick JC. Patterns and location of velopharyngeal valving problems: atypical findings on video-nasopharyngoscopy. *Cleft Palate J*. 1989;26(1):63–67.

Young T, Palta M, Dempsey J, Skatrud J, Weber S, Badr S. The occurrence of sleep-disordered breathing among middle-aged adults. *N Engl J Med*. 1993;328(17):1230–1235.

Zhang M, Li L, Fowler D, Zhao Z, Wei D, Zhang Y, Burke A. Causes of sudden death in patients with obstructive sleep apnea. *J Forensic Sci*. 2013;58(5):1171–1174.

Chapter 10

Biomimetic Correction: Pneumopedics and Craniofacial Epigenetics

Synopsis: This chapter focuses on the outcomes of biomimetic oral appliance therapy. Using a quantitative approach, various parameters used to measure the quality and quantity of sleep are presented. Different structural and functional techniques, ranging from 3D CBCT scans, study models, intra-oral and facial photographs, as well as data such as the apnea-hypopnea index, oxygen saturation of the blood and the amount of REM sleep from overnight sleep studies are used to assess the degree of clinical success. Significantly, the post-treatment sleep evaluations are based on data captured with no device in the patient's mouth while sleeping to determine whether physiologic sleep can be restored and long-term device use avoided, using the principles of pneumopedics and craniofacial epigenetics.

In the latter part of the 20th century, the idea of biomimetic dentistry was introduced (Magne and Douglas, 1999), acknowledging that biomimetics is an interdisciplinary field in which scientific principles from engineering, chemistry and biology, etc. are applied to the development of materials, systems or machines that mimic biological processes. In the context of this discussion, *biomimetic oral devices rely on the natural human* model (32 teeth, bilateral symmetry, cephalization, and klinorhynchy, etc.) in an attempt to resolve a complex human problem, sleep disordered breathing (SDB). Using my pneumopedics and craniofacial epigenetics (PACE) protocol, we have deployed devices to deliver biomimetic oral appliance therapy, which is based on the novel idea of pneumopedics or non-surgical upper airway remodeling. During this clinical procedure, epigenetic orthopedics in evoked and tangible skeletal changes in both children and adults are discernible and quantifiable, as presented below. Simultaneously, epigenetic orthodontics is harnessed to improve the occlusion, although this is not the specific issue of concern. Nevertheless, unlike other approaches that might precipitate unwanted bite changes, the biomimetic approach attempts to harness anticipated tooth movements to benefit the patient. In fact, the position paper of the American Association of Orthodontists (2019) suggests that long-term oral appliance therapy results in progressive occlusal changes, and these unwanted tooth movements occur in conjunction with skeletal adaptations. Thus, the pneumopedic procedure differs radically from conventional thinking as it aims to deploy these adaptive mechanisms for biomimetic correction. While the upper airway changes evoked through this protocol are likely associated with the mechanism of craniofacial pneumatization, the dentoskeletal changes rely on sutural homeostasis, so that an enhanced level of craniofacial homeostasis is achieved. In the same way that blood pressure, body temperature, etc. are subject to homeostatic regulation, the craniofacial region is no different; the system will regress to homeostasis, given the clinical conditions to do so. Examples of this phenomenon include orthodontic relapse. Clinically therefore, a foundational correction is often required of the skeleto-dental tissues, as well as a functional correction of the soft tissues (mostly muscles) and functional spaces to secure stability of the outcome. This equilibrium is achieved by building retention into the system as a proactive component of biomimetic correction, and not as an after-thought, as exemplified by orthodontic retainers.

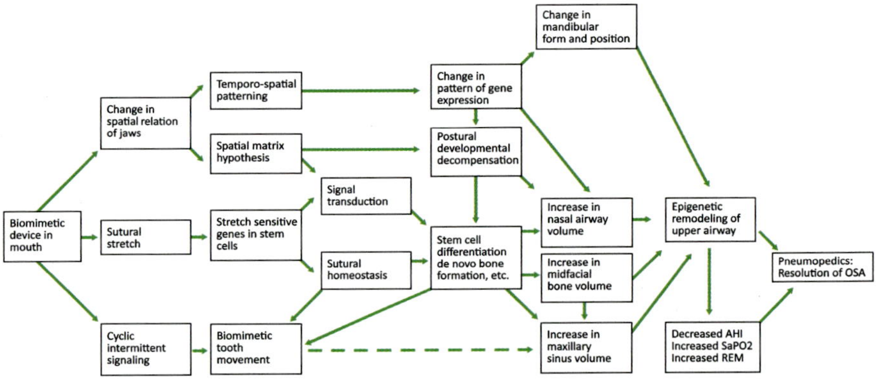

Figure 104: Summary of pathways thought to be involved in craniofacial correction using pneumopedics and craniofacial epigenetics delivered through biomimetic oral appliance therapy.

How does it work?

The above question has been posed to me over the past ten years or so. Fig. 104 above summarizes the response. Craniofacial correction is initiated when a biomimetic oral appliance is inserted into a patient's mouth. The design, materials and protocols of these devices have been discussed in previous chapters, and it's sufficient to say here that intra-oral placement of the device results in a change in spatial relations of the jaws and teeth (Fig. 105). The spatial matrix hypothesis is an attempt to encompass the clinical behavior of the craniofacial system during its growth and development, and during its clinical therapeutic manipulation. According to the spatial matrix hypothesis, this change in spatial positioning is detected by mechanoreceptors on the cell surfaces of the periodontal and periosteal cells, and this process evokes a change in the pattern of gene expression, according to temporo-spatial patterning. In turn, due to signal transduction, a cascade of events is initiated, resulting in gene transcription and mRNA biosynthesis, as demonstrated by Fuentes *et al.* (2003). Clinically, postural decompensation is observable since the mandible changes its position, and it is well known that mandibular

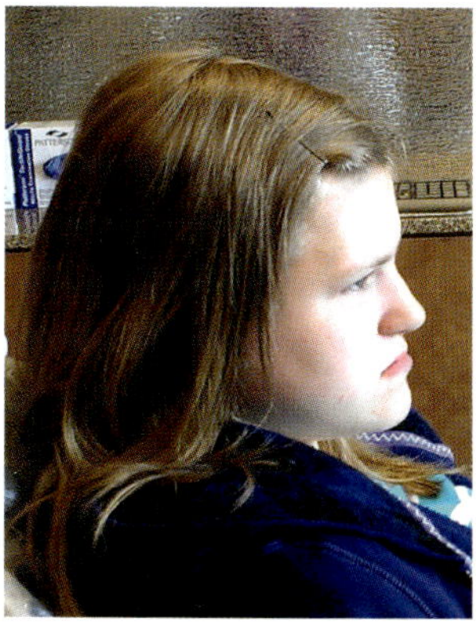

Figure 105a: Pre-treatment lateral photograph with no device in patient's mouth. Courtesy: Dr Dennis Klemp.

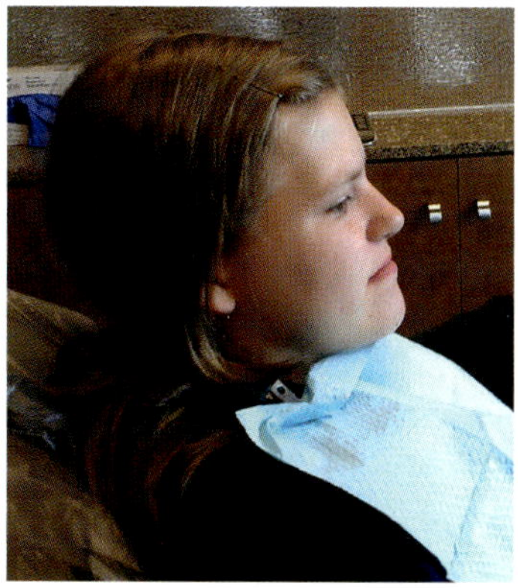

Figure 105b: Note change in facial profile immediately upon delivery of biomimetic oral appliance.

repositioning can enhance the lower pharyngeal part of the upper airway.

In addition to spatial signaling, biomimetic oral devices also impart tensile stress. This gentle stretch is targeted at local sutural sites that are found in the midfacial region, specifically. It is now known that craniofacial sutures provide a niche for mesenchymal stem cells (Zhao *et al.*, 2015), and that mechano-responsive genes (Wu *et al.*, 2017) can undergo signal transduction, for example by differentiating into osteoblasts that lay down new woven bone is response to tensile stress. Because of sutural homeostasis, physical bone parameters, such as bone width and volume can increase, while the width of the suture returns to it normal limits and thus appears to be unchanged (Vizzotto *et al.*, 2008). Interestingly, some are of the opinion that the periodontal ligament is, in fact, more akin to a modified suture. In this way, Coura *et al.* (2008) consider that the human periodontal ligament represents a niche of neural-crest-derived stem cells. Moreover, by changing the signal to these stem cells from a static stretch to one that invokes cyclic, intermittent signaling, the connective tissue effects can be enhanced (Schmidt *et al.*, 2016). Consequently, biomimetic tooth movement can be achieved clinically, while obeying the physiologic principles of sutural homeostasis. The clinical effects of the above mechanisms and pathways are significant. Studies in adults have shown non-surgical, non-pharmaceutical: increases in midfacial bone volume (Singh *et al.*, 2014); improved nasal airway volume; increased maxillary sinus volume (Singh and Kim, 2020); and enhanced mandibular form and position in adults (Singh and Kim, 2016). In turn, these structural changes have been associated with functional improvements, such as: decreased AHI in patients with mild/moderate OSA (Singh *et al.*, 2014; Singh and Cress, 2017); decreased AHI in patients with severe OSA (Singh *et al.*, 2016; Heit *et al.*, 2016); increased $SaPO_2$ (Singh and Callister, 2013); and increased amounts of REM sleep (Singh *et al.*, 2019). These preliminary findings support the notion of epigenetic remodeling of the upper airway or pneumopedics for the potential resolution of OSA.

Epigenetic-pneumopedic protocol

The developmental dynamics of the biomimetic approach, in accord with the cranio-caudal gradient of human development, are captured in the Pneumopedic® and Craniofacial Epigenetic (PACE) protocol (Appendix). The epigenetic-pneumopedic protocol begins at birth as the child abruptly changes from placental to external oxygenation *inter alia*. Generally speaking, this physiologic event is probably best handled by midwives unless other concerns require medical attendance. Historically, midwives used to perform an oral sweep of a young baby soon after birth to inoculate the oral flora with the mother's internal microbiome from her perineal/vaginal fluids after giving birth. In fact, it is now accepted that development of the intestinal microbiome begins immediately following birth. Next, breast-feeding would be encouraged, which would also transfer the mother's external microbiome from her skin to the neonate. It is now understood that further evolution of the infant's microbiome is defined by contact with the mother, since colonizing bacteria rapidly adapt to breast milk and epithelial mucins as sources of nutrients. These steps are thought to assure enhanced immunogenicity for the newborn child. However, some babies are delivered through Caesarian section. Recent studies (Salminen *et al.*, 2004) suggest that Caesarean-born babies are deprived of contact with the maternal/vaginal microbiome and have a more slowly diversifying microbiota. Thus, the microbiome of Caesarian-delivered infants is less robust due to sterile operating theater conditions, which may in the long-term be less beneficial. But, regardless of the birthing procedure, some infants are unable to suckle adequately at birth and, more recently, dentists have taken a renewed interest in this process. Thus, an oral examination of a young baby soon after birth by a general dentist or pediatrician is strongly suggested. If tongue restriction, ankylosis, or tongue-tie is diagnosed, lingual frenectomy may be provided by a dentist or an oral surgeon, and breast-feeding is encouraged immediately thereafter so that the baby learns how to latch onto the breast and nurse more effectively.

The natural birthing process also necessitates passage through the birth canal. Some suggest that vaginal compression of the baby during birth extracts excess hyaluronan and other hydrophilic glycosaminoglycans, which are abundant in the neonate and give the neonatal skin its increased resilience. However, these pressures also act on the cranium, which distorts due to the patent cranial sutures. Thus, cranial examination of a young baby soon after birth can be performed either by a (cranial) osteopath, a chiropractor, or a naturopath, but most commonly the parents take the child to a pediatrician. In any case, if cranial asymmetry/deformational plagiocephaly is diagnosed, appropriate cranial therapy may be provided as indicated. In older babies, a review of sleep hygiene might also be required. For example, parents might notice a bald patch on the back of the baby's head. This occipital hair-loss likely represents the fact that the baby is spending prolonged periods of time lying on its back. This behavior may precipitate positional or deformational plagiocephaly. For correction, it might simply be sufficient to change the baby's position; for example, 'tummy time', changing sides and varying the positions in which the baby is held. If these simple measures don't rectify the asymmetry, then helmets might be used to mold the cranium back toward symmetry, as discussed in Chapter 8.

Children start to erupt teeth at about 6–12mths of age, and their oral behaviors start to change. Thus, in the epigenetic-pneumopedic protocol, an oral examination by an oral myofunctional therapist, by the age of three years is highly recommended. If oral habits, such as digit-sucking, lip-sucking, etc. are diagnosed, oral myofunctional therapy (OMT) may be provided. In fact, OMT is a central part of the PACE protocol; put simply, in most cases OMT is required prior to, during, and after biomimetic oral appliance therapy. As a child grows, further habits and behaviors start to change and develop. Parents might note that nocturnal bruxism is developing or diagnosed, possibly in association with nocturnal enuresis. If so, a pediatric sleep questionnaire and/or pediatric sleep study may be provided and a TMJ examination by a dentist or neuromuscular dentist might be indicated, especially if the child has a history of middle-ear issues, such as otitis media. In addition, there may be a need for an orthodontic examination by an orthodontist or general dentist, before the age of five to six years. If a malocclusion is developing or diagnosed, epigenetic-orthodontic therapy may be provided; however, note that the specialist orthodontists are largely undecided on the merits of 'early treatment'. Nevertheless, the philosophy adopted here is simply: **align the body; align the jaws, and then align the teeth** — in that sequence. Therefore, prior to any orthodontic intervention, the PACE protocol recommends a cervical examination by a chiropractor, osteopath, etc., by or before the age of nine years or so because by that age the first permanent molars should be fully erupted and in occlusion with complete root formation. If cervical subluxation is diagnosed, chiropractic adjustment or some other appropriate physical therapy may be provided, as clinically indicated. Note that the horizontal axis of rotation of the mandible is a plane passing through the first cervical vertebra (C1), which articulates with C2 at the intervertebral disk. Thus, if C1/C2 are misaligned, the mandible is not free to move into its optimal functional space, and as a result either a malocclusion could develop or some other systemic compensation. Because of the cranio-caudal gradient of development and the kinetic chain, various conditions can be precipitated. Put simply, descending (craniofacial) developmental compensation proceeds from the top down, while ascending postural compensation proceeds from the bottom up. For example, when a child learns to control head movements through initial use of its neck muscles, various changes are elicited. The mastoid processes develop in association with sternocleidomastoid muscle function, while pneumatization of the mastoid air cells occurs around the same time. Moreover, lordosis of the cervical spine becomes apparent for the child to maintain horizontal gaze. When the child first learns to stand on its feet, postural compensation produces lordosis of the lumbar spine so the child can maintain balance while looking straight ahead. In fact, in adults, Chapman and Singh (2013) tested the effect of biomimetic oral appliance therapy combined with chiropractic cervical adjustment. Prior to treatment, leg lengths were measured for all subjects when lying supine on a chiropractic table: without the appliance in the mouth; with the appliance in situ, and again after chiropractic adjustment. The results showed that while the leg length discrepancy was approx. 12mm before treatment; the asymmetry was reduced to about 6mm with the device in situ and was further reduced to 2mm after the chiropractic adjustment. This preliminary study concluded that combination of a biomimetic oral appliance and cervical chiropractic adjustment appears to reduce postural compensation (leg length discrepancy) when occlusal decompensation is performed in adults. In a follow-up study, Singh *et al.* (2014) investigated changes in craniofacial alignment, using radiographic assessment. When deploying cervical chiropractic adjustment in combination with a biomimetic oral appliance, the craniofacial alignment improved, and the average decompensation was approx. 70%. It was therefore concluded that when a biomimetic appliance is used in conjunction with chiropractic adjustment, there appears to be a synergy resulting in improved craniofacial alignment in adults. Taken together, these two studies provide further support for the cranio-caudal kinetic chain. But, while structural equilibrium or homeostasis is achieved, functional balance needs to be addressed also. Many professionals seem to overlook the fact that the posterior boundary of the upper airway (posterior pharyngeal wall) is directly influenced by the cervical vertebrae. Therefore, the healthcare professional ought to be cognizant of upper airway changes and their impact on breathing and sleep. For these reasons, a home sleep apnea test (HSAT) or a polysomnographic sleep study by a sleep physician, pulmonologist, ENT specialist, etc., is suggested if clinically indicated in the PACE protocol. If sleep disordered breathing is diagnosed, pneumopedic therapy may be provided, even though orthodontists are undecided on the merits of early treatment in children. In fact, the position paper of the American Association of Orthodontists (2019) suggests that there is nothing an orthodontist can do to help in a diagnosis of pediatric OSA, which contrasts with the views of the American Dental Association (2017).

On the other hand, consider that there are three aspects to biomimetic correction. First, there needs to be a clinical correction of the size and shape of the midface. Following the cranio-caudal gradient of human development, the midface is located inferior to the cranial base. Thus, if the midface is underdeveloped, it will have a knock-on effect on the mandible, which develops after the midface. Some reports suggest that the midface reaches adult proportions by the age of 8–10yrs or so, while the mandible starts its growth spurt some 2–3yrs later. Thus, the second aspect of biomimetic correction is to correct the size, shape, and position of the mandible. Unlike the maxilla, the mandible is relatively easily to move. For this reason, numerous clinical protocols based on 'jumping the bite' evolved over centuries. One of the first of these procedures was called 'functional activation', which led to a whole host of 'functional appliances'. In fact, according to Singh (2010) the term 'functional appliances' may be an historical misnomer since these appliances rely upon craniofacial epigenetics to produce phenotypic variation, which is associated with clinical correction of various functional issues. It is now known that genes encode physiologic processes that involve bone development during tooth movement. The molecular and morphologic basis of craniofacial epigenetics can be explained by the spatial matrix hypothesis. Therefore, 'functional appliances' may be more preferably referred to as 'formational appliances' since bone deposition is a key component of biomimetic correction. In fact, it's important to note that a retruded mandible might be the result of midfacial hypoplasia, especially if a retrognathic maxilla is occupying the functional space of the mandible, resulting in a perturbed spatial matrix (Fig. 4). Therefore, the first two parts of biomimetic correction, which are integral to the PACE protocol, provide foundational correction of the skeleto-dental components, predominantly. For example, the bone of the maxilla is relatively easy to remodel with respect to the mandible. Thus, using a combination of remodeling and repositioning, a foundational correction can be achieved. The third part of biomimetic correction is to maintain the new maxillo-mandibular spatial relations. This aspect means paying attention to tongue, lip-posture, mode of breathing, swallowing, occlusion, etc. In other words, a functional correction must accompany the foundational correction, in order to maintain stability. Thus, a myo-spatial correction needs to be put into place with the muscles (mostly the tongue) acting as a physiologic 'retainer' for life. Consider a foundational correction whereby the hard palate is wide enough to accommodate the tongue, and the mandible is in a forward position to permit the tongue to occupy the hard palate. In this posture, the upper airway will most likely be optimized and functional. Therefore, a myo-spatial correction includes the functional spaces, such as the nasal airway, the maxillary sinuses and the upper airway. It is contended that these corrections can be achieved using biomimetic oral appliance therapy.

In previous studies, Singh and Clark (2001) showed how mandibular development can be enhanced in pediatric cases. Specifically, for teenage females, a 15% increase in size was localized at the condylar neck. It was concluded that, in growing patients, mandibular growth, remodeling, and osteogenesis may help in the correction of the underlying skeletal dysmorphology. In a similar study, Singh and Clark (2003) reported that in pubertal females, the orolabial fissure showed a 15% increase in size allied with a less prominent labiomental groove, which may help in nasal breathing, by providing a more effective lip seal. Based on these types of findings, Singh and Lipka (2009) presented optimization of a wire-based device for biomimetic correction. Using a single, upper Wireframe DNA appliance, which has six degrees of freedom, enhancement of craniofacial homeostasis was achieved in a 15yr-old girl (Fig. 4). In over 6 months of treatment, improvements were noticeable in facial symmetry, lip morphology, maxillo-mandibular relationship, as well as the occlusion, as predicted by the spatial matrix hypothesis. Further evidence for functional correction comes from a case of chronic rhinitis (Singh *et al.*, 2016). A 12yr-old girl reported to a dental office and medical history-taking revealed a previous diagnosis of chronic rhinitis. Other signs and symptoms included mouth breathing and mild fever, and a pediatric sleep disorder was suspected. After approx. 2yrs of biomimetic oral appliance therapy, the patient showed enhanced nasal breathing and regression of adenoidal hypertrophy. The patient's head posture, facial appearance and dental occlusion also improved. It was concluded that biomimetic oral appliance therapy was beneficial in this particular pediatric patient with chronic rhinitis, and further studies on this preliminary finding are noted below.

Adult cases can also present to the dental office with a variety of concerns. For example, some patients may be experiencing sleep or airway issues; some may have orthodontic problems, while others complain of craniofacial pain. The treatment of one such case was described by Singh and Utama (2013). A young female adult with a history of migraines attended for dental treatment. Following history taking and thorough investigation, a working diagnosis of Class I malocclusion (with a Class III tendency) was reached with differential diagnoses of TMD, UARS, and OSA. She was treated with upper and lower biomimetic appliances for about 12 months (Fig. 106). During this time, the transpalatal bone width increased from about 29mm to 35mm; and the lower posterior teeth were gradually vertically supra-erupted, by grinding sections of the upper appliance, starting with the premolars, and utilizing orthodontic elastics. Once the biomimetic oral appliance therapy was finished, the occlusion

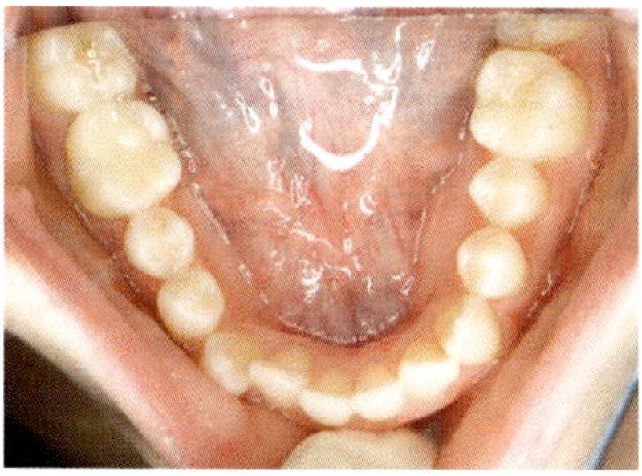

Figure 106a: Pre-treatment intra-oral photograph of lower arch showing crowding. Courtesy: Dr John Utama.

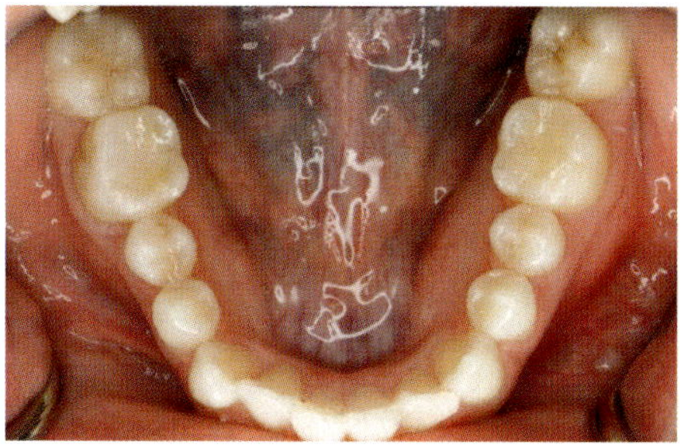

Figure 106b: Mid-treatment appearance of same patient. Note developmental decompensation after biomimetic oral appliance therapy and prior to final finishing with limited fixed orthodontics.

was fine-tuned for final occlusal interdigitation using standard orthodontic brackets (Fig. 97). Moreover, the patient reported that her headaches were gone, and generally she felt comfortable. She was followed for a further six months and it was noted that symptoms associated with migraine appeared to be resolved. Thus, in some cases, non-pharmaceutical and non-surgical treatments may yield health benefits. In fact, Singh and Ataii (2013) used a biomimetic oral appliance prior to the use of clear aligners to reduce the necessity for interproximal reduction in orthodontic correction. The results showed improved mandibular positioning and occlusion, and increased upper and lower arch widths, which resulted in functional and cosmetic improvements without any interproximal reduction or standard orthodontic brackets.

Some patients are primarily concerned about dentofacial esthetics when they attend a dental office. Harris and Singh (2013) presented a case of severe ‘gummy smile’ with an anterior open bite in an adult female who wanted to avoid the surgical options that she had been presented with previously (Fig. 1). The case was resolved in about 18 months, using biomimetic oral appliance therapy for the foundational correction, followed by limited orthodontic finishing. This case clearly illustrated the correlations of form, function, and behavior, supporting the notion of craniofacial homeostasis. The important question to ask in this case was: 'Why does this patient have a gummy smile and an anterior open bite?' rather than, 'How can this case be treated?'. On craniofacial examination, the answer became clear as it was apparent that the left naris was occluded (Fig. 1a), so that nasal breathing was obstructed. Due to the nasal cycle, when it was time to breathe through the left side, the patient would unconsciously become a mouth-breather. In this spatial position with the mouth open, the tongue left the roof of the mouth and resided in the floor of the mouth instead. This lack of support for the palate lead to palatal constriction, worsening the condition and, as the bone remodeled inferiorly into the available space, a 'gummy smile' or vertical maxillary excess was precipitated. This condition was, in turn, perpetuated/exacerbated by the tongue thrusting forward into the path of least resistance, instead of staying in contact with the hard palate. Therefore, oral myofunctional therapy was first instituted for habit correction. Next, during biomimetic oral appliance therapy, the transpalatal bone width was increased through bony remodeling to accommodate the tongue, which necessitated periodic device adjustments. After about 3 months of biomimetic oral appliance therapy, an improvement in the vertical maxillary excess was noted (Fig. 1b), likely due to improved nasal breathing. After a total of 9 months of biomimetic appliance therapy and a further 8 months of standard orthodontics, the 'gummy smile' was resolved (Fig. 1c), and improved anterior coupling of the teeth produced a result that was both esthetically pleasing and functionally acceptable.

In a similar study, Singh and Cress (2013) demonstrated how a biomimetic oral appliance might produce cosmetic facial enhancement. Post-treatment, this particular case showed a wider smile, as well as improved dental alignment without any interproximal reduction or orthodontic brackets; but increased bone volume (Fig. 12), and upper airway development (Fig. 13) was also achieved. Furthermore, 3D analysis of the CBCT scans before and after treatment localized the regions in which changes were produced by the biomimetic oral appliance (Fig. 12). It was, therefore, proposed that the biomimetic protocol may be used in cosmetic cases as an alternative to surgery or other invasive procedures to enhance facial esthetics, form, and function. To assess this proposal, another study was carried out by Singh and Kim (2016) who tested the hypothesis that facial enhancement can be achieved using biomimetic oral appliance therapy. In this study, 12 adults underwent treatment and various craniofacial parameters were measured on standardized lateral photographs before and after treatment. It was found that the labiomental angle improved statistically from 126° to 134° and the thyromandibular angle improved significantly from 126.5° to 118.5°. As noted earlier, the labiomental angle is an indicator of the degree of overbite. An increased overbite (associated with a relatively acute labiomental angle) often indicates a retruded mandible, which increases the risk of OSA. Conversely, a larger thyromandibular angle indicates an increased risk of OSA (Lam *et al.*, 2005). In our study, using finite-element analysis, the submandibular region showed a 30% decrease in size and the labiomental region showed a 20% size-decrease; in other words, both angles improved as anticipated. Thus, this study supports the notion that biomimetic oral appliance may not only enhance facial appearance non-surgically in adults but may also improve the upper airway. Therefore, as well as upper airway changes, TMJ, orthodontic, and craniofacial improvements can be obtained in adult and pediatric cases, using pneumopedics and craniofacial epigenetics. Taken as a whole, these findings suggest that genetically encoded developmental mechanisms may be epigenetically modulated by biomimetic oral appliances to help doctors and dentists in the management of certain craniofacial issues, including obstructive sleep apnea.

The biologic basis for biomimetic correction that has been introduced in this book uses two physiologic processes; pneumopedics and craniofacial epigenetics. Pneumopedics or non-surgical upper airway remodeling is an entirely new field of endeavor based on the well-recognized but under-utilized physiologic mechanism of pneumatization. In the first study of its kind, Singh *et al.* (2011) investigated the correlation between midfacial development and upper airway changes in a 38yr-old male diagnosed with

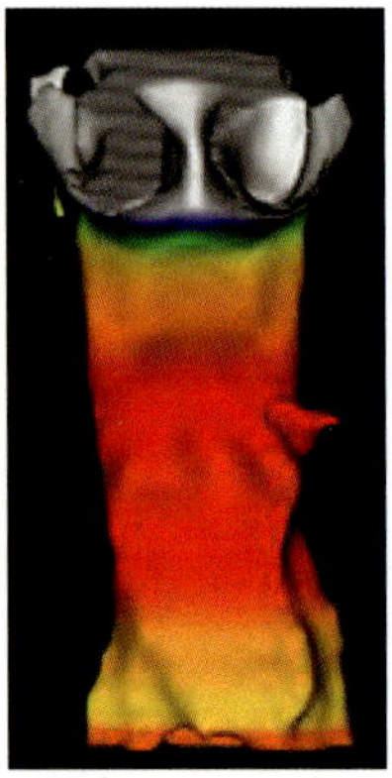

Figure 107a: Pseudo-colored 3D upper airway of an adult patient prior to treatment, showing a volume of 13.9cm^3.

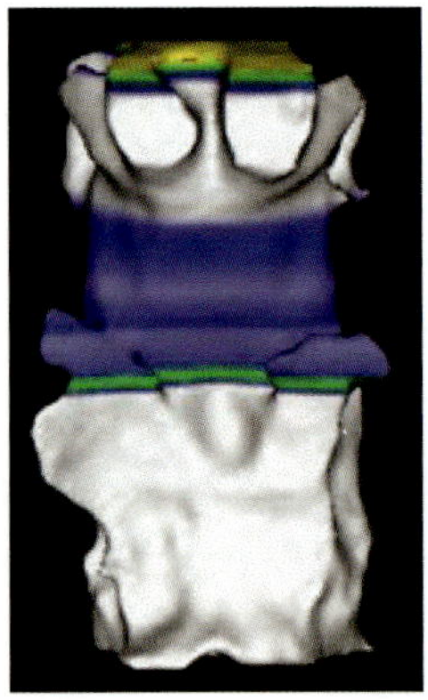

Figure 107b: Post-treatment appearance of same patient after biomimetic oral appliance therapy. Note the change in width and a volume of 29.1cm^3.

moderate OSA. After biomimetic oral appliance therapy, we found that the transpalatal bone width increased from approx. 34mm pre-treatment to 39mm (Fig. 8). More importantly perhaps, the upper airway volume increased by approx. 70% from 13cm^3 pre-treatment to 22cm^3 post-treatment even with no device in the mouth when the post-treatment CBCT scan was taken. Accompanying this size-change was a change in the shape of the mediolateral walls of the upper airway (Fig. 107), which has been reported on several occasions since (Morgan, 2016; Singh, 2018). Moreover, post-treatment, the initial AHI of 24 events/hr and an oxyhemoglobin saturation of 90% were improved to approx. 3 events/hr and 95%, respectively, with no device in the patient's mouth.

But some researchers have cast doubt on the efficacy of a maxillary appliance for the amelioration of OSA in adults. For example, in a pilot study, Gagnon *et al.* (2004) tested the use of a maxillary appliance for the treatment of OSA. They found no difference in AHI with or without the appliance in situ but some patients experienced increases in respiratory disturbances, and for those reasons maxillary appliances were not recommended for treating OSA. It can be ventured that, in their study, insufficient regard was paid to craniofacial phenotype. To test that conjecture, Singh and Callister (2013) deployed a maxillary biomimetic oral appliance in a 64yr-old male with moderate OSA. The initial AHI was approx. 25 events/hr with about 30 oxygen desaturation events/hr. After 6 months of treatment, the transpalatal bone width increased from approx. 35mm to 37mm, the oxygen desaturation events decreased to approx. 5 events/hr and the AHI normalized (to <5 events/hr). In addition, this patient was followed for a further 14 months, and it was found that the AHI remained within normal limits (<5 events/hour), the snoring decreased further, and the oxygen desaturation events remained at 5 events/hr. Thus, the AHI decreased by approx. 80% in this case, with less snoring and improvements in oxygen saturation using a maxillary device. But, the mechanism(s) by which biomimetic oral appliance therapy reached resolution of OSA in this case remained unknown at that time.

Maxillary bone changes during 'rapid maxillary expansion' (RME) in adults are controversial. In a systematic review, Verstraaten *et al.* (2010) investigated bone-borne maxillary expansion with corticotomies. Compared to tooth-borne surgically assisted RME (SARME), there was less tipping of the teeth, but details of the bony changes were lacking. Later, Nada *et al.* (2012) assessed the effects of tooth- and bone-borne SARME using CBCT scans. Post-treatment superimposition of the 3D models showed lateral expansion of the posterior alveolar segments, as expected. However, the anterior segment showed posterior displacement/remodeling of that region. Thus, both tooth- and bone-borne SARME produced tranverse bony expansion posteriorly but maxillary retrusion anteriorly. It remained unclear as to what types of bony changes, if any, could be achieved using a non-surgical technique. Therefore, Singh *et al.* (2014) investigated midfacial bony changes in adults undergoing biomimetic oral appliance therapy. Using 3D CBCT scans after approx. 18 months of treatment, it was found that the transpalatal bone width increased from about 33.5mm to 36mm. Similarly, Handelman *et al.* (2000) found that the arch width increase in adults undergoing non-surgical RME was similar to children, although the children achieved >50% of their expansion by an increase at the vault of the palate. In any case, their results indicated that non-surgical RME in adults to be both effective and safe. Moreover, in our study (Singh *et al.*, 2014), the pre-treatment midfacial bone volume of the sample was approx. 17cm^3 pre-treatment and increased significantly to about 19cm^3 post-treatment, an approx. 10% improvement. We concluded that biomimetic oral appliance therapy may be able to increase both maxillary bone width and midfacial volume in adults, and this prompted us to further investigate how this technique might help adults diagnosed with OSA.

In children, palatal expansion is more widely used, and its effects are still being understood. For example, Darsey *et al.* (2012) investigated the effects of the Hyrax appliance on maxillary expansion. Using CBCT scans they found dento-skeletal increases in the transverse axis, but the hard palate showed no changes in the vertical and antero-posterior axes. On the other hand, the nasal cavity width increased by approx. 1mm. For adults, Nada *et al.* (2013) studied the effects of tooth- and bone-borne SARME on the nasal airway volumes. In that study, 3D CBCT scans were taken prior to treatment and about 22 months later. They found that the nasal airway volume increased by 9.5% in the tooth-borne group and by 13% in the bone-borne group. Singh *et al.* (2016) also investigated nasal airway volume changes, using 3D CBCT scans in adult patients after 18 months of biomimetic oral appliance treatment. To acquire the nasal cavity, volumetric, 3-D reconstruction of the nasal cavity was undertaken between the anterior and posterior nasal spines, extending superiorly from the palatine process of the maxilla and the palatine bone to the cribriform plate of the ethmoid bone. Laterally, the maxillary sinuses were trimmed out at their junctions with the nasal cavity on the 3D CBCT data, and the nasal cavity volume was calculated in all cases. It was found that the mean nasal cavity volume was approx. 42cm^3 before treatment and increased significantly to 44cm^3 post-treatment. Although this increase represents only a 5% increase in nasal airway volume, it was achieved non-surgically and without any diastema formation, unlike the surgical alternatives. This study was repeated in Asian patients (Singh and Kim, 2020). We found that in Korean adults, the nasal airway volume increased significantly by 12.5% from approx. 22.4cm^3 before treatment to 25.6cm^3 post-treatment. Therefore, we concluded that the biomimetic oral appliance technique might help adults with OSA, by increasing the nasal cavity volume and decreasing nasal airflow resistance.

Sleep disordered breathing represents a spectrum of conditions, ranging from upper airway resistance syndrome (UARS) through to severe OSA, the pathogenesis of which is diverse. Singh (2010) suggested that torus palatinus, torus mandibularis, and other oral tori might be pathognomonic of OSA. In fact, Singh *et al.* (2012) were the first to describe the effects of surgical removal of mandibular tori in patients diagnosed with OSA. In a case of moderate OSA, we noted a 15% improvement in the AHI (from approx. 21 events/hr pre-operatively to 18 events/hr post-operatively), while the oxygen desaturation index improved by about 30%. Since this particular case also exhibited extreme dental wear patterns associated with sleep bruxism, Singh and Cress (2013) followed up with this case, reporting that after full mouth rehabilitation, an additional decrease in the AHI of some 30% was noted. After further biomimetic oral appliance therapy, an overall 60% decrease in the AHI and an 85% improvement in the oxygen desaturation index was found compared with the original baseline values in this particular case. In fact, further studies on the relationship between sleep bruxism and biomimetic oral appliance therapy are becoming available. For example, Liao and Singh (2015) described a case where sleep bruxism was resolved in a young female adult who had previously been using a dental night-guard. It can be suggested that if the bruxing habit had not been addressed in this case, the development of oral tori associated with OSA might have been expected at an older age. Indeed, Ruangsri *et al.* (2016) concluded that dentists may play an important role in screening patients at risk of OSA, since torus mandibularis is an important anatomical risk factors for OSA, as predicted by Singh (2010). Furthermore, Ahn *et al.* (2019) in a study of patients diagnosed with OSA, found that those with torus mandibularis showed an increase in the parameters associated with OSA, such as AHI. Taken together, these studies support the notion of evaluating and addressing oral tori in patients diagnosed with OSA, and further studies are required to investigate the consequences of the surgical outcome. In this respect, Singh *et al.* (2019) described a case of a 56yr-old male with moderate OSA. Following surgical reduction of bilateral torus mandibularis, and in combination with biomimetic oral appliance therapy, the AHI was reduced to within normal limits with no device in the patient's mouth, but the amount of REM sleep was also normalized, indicating that perhaps the underlying etiology of the condition had been addressed.

In fact, in a series of studies, the effect of biomimetic oral appliance therapy in adults with mild, moderate and even severe OSA was investigated. Singh *et al.* (2014) tested the hypothesis that the upper airway can be enhanced in adults diagnosed with OSA so that long-term CPAP therapy might potentially become avoidable. The pilot study consisted of 11 consecutive adults aged >21yrs who had been diagnosed with mild to moderate OSA, following an HSAT interpreted by a board-certified sleep physician. Each subject was treated using biomimetic oral appliance therapy by a dentist with advanced training in craniofacial sleep medicine. The mean AHI of the study sample was calculated prior to and after treatment with no appliance in the mouth when both sleep studies were done. It was found that approx. 9mths of biomimetic appliance treatment reduced the AHI by 65% with no device in the mouth when the overnight sleep study was performed. This was the first study to suggest that biomimetic oral appliance therapy may be able to reduce the AHI to within normal limits, and that life-long CPAP therapy might perhaps become avoidable. However, long-term follow up studies are still needed to determine the veracity of these initial upper airway improvements. In a similar study, Singh and Cress (2017) also reported that after approx. 9mths of biomimetic appliance treatment, the AHI decreased to 6 events/hr in a sample of adults with mild to moderate OSA, representing a fall in the AHI by 51.5% on average. Since the medical criteria for successful treatment is generally accepted as an AHI of <10 events/hr allied with a 50% reduction in AHI compared to the pre-treatment values, these findings corroborated the findings of our previous study, and laid the ground work for helping those patients who have been diagnosed with OSA but are unable to comply with CPAP use.

In a combined study, Singh *et al.* (2016) investigated the effect of biomimetic oral appliance treatment in adults with severe OSA. In that study, the approx. treatment time was 9.5mths and the initial AHI of 45 events/hr was decreased by almost 65% with no appliance in the patient's mouth, according to the post-treatment sleep studies. These results also suggest that biomimetic oral appliance therapy may be a useful alternative in managing severe OSA in adults who are unable to comply with CPAP, which is currently the preferred method or first line of treatment. Again, long-term follow-up is needed to reach more definitive conclusions on these initial findings, but in a case of very severe OSA (Heit *et al.*, 2016), a 27yr-old female reported to a dental office with TMD symptoms. Following screening for OSA, she was diagnosed with severe OSA with an AHI of 105 events/hr. Referral was, therefore, made to the sleep specialists who repeated the sleep study and confirmed an AHI of 118 events/hr. The physicians then referred the patient to the ENT specialists for tonsillectomy. Post-operatively, the AHI was reduced 70 events/hr and further controlled using CPAP, but the patient was unable to tolerate the CPAP pressure. Therefore, biomimetic oral appliance therapy was initiated. After approx. 9 mths of combined CPAP and biomimetic oral appliance use, the pulmonologist reported that the AHI fell to 1 event/hr without CPAP or the biomimetic oral appliance in situ when the final sleep study was performed. In fact, Abdullatif *et al.* (2016) undertook a systematic review and meta-analysis of maxillo-mandibular expansion as a potential solution for adults with OSA. On average, they found that while the AHI decreased significantly, the oxygen saturation nadir improved correspondingly; however, given the dearth of studies available, additional research on this approach is warranted. These preliminary studies support the novel pneumopedic approach advocated here but the molecular details of the corrective mechanism(s) still need to be elucidated.

Biomimetic oral devices rely on the natural human model (32 teeth, bilateral symmetry, etc.) to address sleep disordered breathing through non-surgical upper airway remodeling. The biologic basis for this correction uses two physiologic processes: pneumopedics and craniofacial epigenetics. Pneumopedics is an entirely new field of endeavor based on the well-recognized but under-utilized physiologic mechanism of pneumatization. This natural phenomenon has been known and studied for centuries (Withalm, 1950; Nowak and Mehlis, 1975) but has rarely been deployed therapeutically. Wehrbein and Diedrich (1992) quantified progressive pneumatization of the maxillary sinus after tooth extraction and orthodontic space closure, noting that the pneumatization tendency was significantly higher after molar extraction compared with the premolar region. In fact, Re *et al.* (2001) were able to orthodontically move a premolar tooth through the maxillary sinus, using an implant placed in the retromolar region as anchorage. After 6mths of treatment, an implant was inserted into the vacated premolar region, followed by an appropriate restoration of the crown. Moreover, the premolar that was relocated through the sinus maintained its supporting bone and periodontal tissues, while the implant used for anchorage also remained osseo-integrated. This result is not surprising since it has been shown, at least in vitro, that osteogenic mesenchymal stem cells within the human maxillary sinus membrane can produce bone (Berbéri *et al.*, 2017) and that maxillary sinus membrane tissues contain stem cells that show the potential of bone regeneration (Guo *et al.*, 2015). Therefore, pneumatization of the maxillary sinus may be amenable to novel clinical protocols, but the paranasal sinuses remain enigmatic in terms of both function and development.

Smith *et al.* (2005) studied the development of maxillary sinuses in primates. Using histologic and immunohistochemical techniques, they described the distribution of osteoclasts, osteoblasts, and osteopontin. Their findings indicated patterns of bone resorption/deposition that were consistent with expansion of the roof and floor of the sinus, correlating to vertical midfacial growth. However, the lateral and medial walls were more variable, likely related to development of adjacent structures, such as the orbits and alveolar processes. The results of their study supported those of Witmer (1997), who suggested that sinus expansion occurred by default into regions unopposed by developing adjacent structures, by simply replacing bone tissue with air spaces. In a later study, Smith *et al.* (2010) further investigated the notion that the paranasal sinuses are simply opportunistic spatial cavities within the craniofacial complex. They compared new world monkeys that form maxillary sinuses to squirrel monkeys, which do not. Using micro-CT scans and histo-morphometric techniques, the size and location of the paranasal spaces were assessed. They found that in the new world monkeys, pneumatization extended the maxillary sinus alongside the developing deciduous premolars, but in squirrel monkeys, the homologous cavities did not extend posteriorly. This morphologic difference was likely due to increased tooth size and orbital volumes, which encroached on the spatial matrix, limiting the space available for posterior expansion of the maxillary sinus. The authors concluded that pneumatization is a secondary growth mechanism that resorbs bony tissue, resulting in sinus formation. Therefore, this pneumatization occurs in association with skeletal elements that border on functional matrices, the spatial dynamics of which act as developmental constraints on pneumatic expansion of the paranasal sinuses. But, the origins of pneumaticity remain both elusive and intriguing.

Márquez (2008) reviewed the diversity of paranasal sinus pneumatization in a wide range of vertebrates and presented not only the ontogenetic complexity of paranasal sinus growth and development, but also a deeper understanding and greater appreciation of these craniofacial functional spaces. Starting with sauropodomorph and theropod dinosaurs, Wedel (2006) described postcranial (cervical) skeletal pneumaticity, somewhat homologous to the pneumatization of cervical air sacs in birds. On the other hand, Rauhut and Fechner (2005) discovered an isolated maxilla of the non-avian theropod dinosaur, Allosaurus. The specimen exhibited a well-developed paranasal pneumatic system. This finding suggested that craniofacial pneumatization might simply be opportunistic, playing a non-significant role in the evolution of craniofacial architecture. However, in a sample of birds, crocodilians, and lizards, O'Connor (2006) inferred that postcranial pneumaticity in extinct taxa indicated heterogeneous evolution of pulmonary systems with distinct exchange and non-exchange (air sacs) regions. These findings, in combination with other skeletal features, might be indicative of evolution of a flow-through pulmonary system even in non-avian dinosaurs. In fact, regional pneumaticity in extant birds shows consistent patterns of bone invasion, and thus provides grounds for identifying components of the pulmonary air sac system in their non-avian ancestors. Modern birds have a heterogeneous pulmonary system, consisting of a rigid, dorsally attached lung and several air sacs that act as bellows, directing inspired air through it. Sereno *et al.* (2008) described a predatory dinosaur that demonstrated significant skeletal pneumatization producing air sacs, which are also used for pulmonary ventilation in birds. Empirically, this model might represent the evolution of avian air sacs and lung ventilation in extant birds. Indeed, Butler *et al.* (2009) reported that pterosaurs also possess a bird-like respiratory system, including ventilatory air sacs. These patterns of postcranial skeletal pneumatization suggest that air sacs were probably present in the common ancestor of pterosaurs, and thus have wider implications for the evolution of respiratory systems in bird-like dinosaurs. In addition, Reidenberg and Laitman (2008) reviewed the cetacean (whale, dolphin, porpoise) air sac system, which may be related to the paranasal sinuses in mammals. The cetaceans lack paranasal sinuses, likely as an evolutionary adaptation for diving. While bony-walled chambers might fracture during diving due to changes in air pressure/volumes, flexible-walled extracranial diverticula are better adapted for diving. Nevertheless, cetacean air sacs do not appear to be homologous to paranasal sinuses, but may serve some other respiratory functions, such as gaseous exchange, increasing inspiratory volume and facilitating subaquatic sound production. I surmise, the mammalian paranasal air sinuses might represent vestigial organs of respiration to some extent, and if so, appropriate clinical protocols might be able to enhance this functional potential in a variety of ways.

Clinically, using CT imaging, Lawson *et al.* (2008) reported that maxillary sinus hypoplasia can occur unilaterally or bilaterally. They noted that that even when hypoplastic, the sinus retains its typical pyramidal configuration. In addition, although the sinus was rarely excessively pneumatized, surgical intervention frequently altered the size and shape of the sinus by osteogenesis, which might have a subsequent effect on midfacial bone volume. Nevertheless, the authors suggested that, clinically-speaking, the maxillary sinus appears to have a limited range of biologic responses. In a study on chronic rhinosinusitis, Deeb *et al.* (2011) assessed the maxillary sinus on CT scans of 50 control subjects. It was found that the volume of the right sinus was approx. 24cm^3, and 24.5cm^3 on the left side in healthy individuals. In contrast, in a study on Korean subjects, Park *et al.* (2010) reported normal adult values using CT scans of the maxillary sinuses. They determined that the mean sinus volume after growth was completed was approx. 15cm^3. The differences in these two studies might be explained by climatic variation since Butaric (2015) suggested that in diverse populations the relationship of the maxillary sinus and nasal cavity are variable, and epigenetic factors, such as climate, are needed to explain variations of these structures. On the other hand, Selcuk *et al.* (2015) demonstrated that the maxillary sinus varies in volume from approx. 15.5 cm^3 to 18cm^3, and although the sinus volumes are greater in males compared to females, no differences can be attributed to changes in climate.

In another clinical study, Tikku *et al.* (2013) measured volumetric changes of the maxillary sinuses as a compensatory mechanism to altered functional matrices in mouth breathers. They reported that the maxillary sinus volume was smaller in mouth breathers with a history of nasal obstruction, implying a developmental and/or functional relationship between the maxillary sinus and the nasal cavity. Later, Almuzian *et al.* (2018) studied the effects of rapid maxillary expansion (RME) on the upper airway in children. Using CBCT scans, they found approx. 3.5mm of palatal expansion in males and approx. 3mm in females with a correlation between dentoalveolar expansion and changes in the maxillary sinus volume. On the other hand, Darsey *et al.* (2012) used a Hyrax appliance for maxillary expansion in teenagers aged approx. 14yrs. Post-treatment, although increases in dentoskeletal structures and nasal cavity width were found, the volume of the maxillary sinus remained unchanged, and it was concluded that palatal expansion using a Hyrax appliance does not affect maxillary sinus volume. More recently, Singh and Kim (2020) investigated changes in maxillary sinus pneumatization in young Korean adults with a mean age of approx. 25yrs. Following biomimetic oral appliance therapy, the transpalatal bone width increased from approx. 35mm to 38.5mm while the maxillary air sinus volume on the left side increased significantly from approx. 19cm^3 to 20cm^3, and from 18.5cm^3 to 19.5cm^3 on the right side. Thus, biomimetic oral appliance therapy may be able to increase the maxillary air sinus volume in adults, and this finding might represent the pneumopedic phenomenon.

Singh (2018) reviewed the medical literature and surmised that upper airway remodeling can occur in both pathologic conditions such as asthma, chronic obstructive pulmonary disease, emphysema, as well as physiologically in healthy individuals. These naturally occurring and treatment-induced changes can be described as physiologic remodeling of the upper airway or pneumopedics, but the developmental dynamics of upper airway remodeling are not fully understood and require further investigation. For example, Forno *et al.* (2019) suggest that epigenetic processes can alter nasal airway epithelium. Thus, in a recent study, Hwang *et al.* (2019) investigated craniofacial changes associated with biomimetic oral appliance therapy to test the hypothesis of non-surgical remodeling of the maxillary air sinuses in pediatric rhinosinusitis. In a pediatric case series, we noted that 3D cone-beam CT scans before treatment of the maxillary sinuses showed: circumferential mucosal thickening and inflammatory disease; obstruction of the ostiomeatal complex; and enlarged inferior turbinates. Ten months after treatment, the transpalatal bone width increased slightly; the paranasal sinuses were aerated without mucosal thickening; the sinus walls were intact; and the ostiomeatal units were patent. In addition, the inferior nasal concha distance increased on both sides. We suspect that enhancement of maxillary air sinuses in cases of pediatric rhinosinusitis occurred through epigenetic, non-surgical remodeling (pneumopedics), although some might argue that these changes were due to normal growth and development. Further studies on the effect of this novel finding on endothelial dysfunction and sleep parameters are now needed.

References

Abdullatif J, Certal V, Zaghi S, Song SA, Chang ET, Gillespie MB, Camacho M. Maxillary expansion and maxillomandibular expansion for adult OSA: A systematic review and meta-analysis. *J Craniomaxillofac Surg*. 2016;44(5):574–578.

Ahn SH, Ha JG, Kim JW, Lee YW, Yoon JH, Kim CH, Cho HJ. Torus mandibularis affects the severity and position-dependent sleep apnoea in non-obese patients. *Clin Otolaryngol*. 2019;44(3):279–285.

Almuzian M, Ju X, Almukhtar A, Ayoub A, Al-Muzian L, McDonald JP. Does rapid maxillary expansion affect nasopharyngeal airway? A prospective Cone Beam Computerised Tomography (CBCT) based study. *Surgeon*. 2018;16:1–11.

American Association of Orthodontists. https://www1.aaoinfo.org/wp-content/uploads/2019/03/sleep-apnea-white-paper-amended-March-2019.pdf.

American Dental Association, 2017. https://www.ada.org/en/member-center/leadership-governance/councils-commissions-and-committees/dentistry-role-in-sleep-related-breathing-disorders.

Berbéri A, Al-Nemer F, Hamade E, Noujeim Z, Badran B, Zibara K. Mesenchymal stem cells with osteogenic potential in human maxillary sinus membrane: an in vitro study. *Clin Oral Investig*. 2017;21(5):1599–1609.

Butaric LN. Differential scaling patterns in maxillary sinus volume and nasal cavity breadth among modern humans. *Anat Rec* (*Hoboken*). 2015;298(10):1710–1721.

Butler RJ, Barrett PM, Gower DJ. Postcranial skeletal pneumaticity and air-sacs in the earliest pterosaurs. *Biol Lett*. 2009;5(4):557–560.

Chapman C, Singh GD. Combined effect of a biomimetic oral appliance and atlas orthogonist cervical adjustment on leg lengths in adults. *Annals Vert Sub Res*. 2013;46–50.

Coura GS, Garcez RC, de Aguiar CB, Alvarez-Silva M, Magini RS, Trentin AG. Human periodontal ligament: a niche of neural crest stem cells. *J Periodontal Res*. 2008;43(5):531–536.

Darsey DM, English JD, Kau CH, Ellis RK, Akyalcin S. Does hyrax expansion therapy affect maxillary sinus volume? A cone-beam computed tomography report. *Imaging Sci Dent*. 2012;42(2):83–8.

Deeb R, Malani PN, Gill B, Jafari-Khouzani K, Soltanian-Zadeh H, Patel S, Zacharek MA. Three-dimensional volumetric measurements and analysis of the maxillary sinus. *Am J Rhinol Allergy*. 2011;25(3):152–156.

Forno E, Wang T, Qi C, Yan Q, Xu CJ, Boutaoui N, Han YY, Weeks DE, Jiang Y, Rosser F, Vonk JM, Brouwer S, Acosta-Perez E, Colón-Semidey A, Alvarez M, Canino G, Koppelman GH, Chen W, Celedón JC. DNA methylation in nasal epithelium, atopy, and atopic asthma in children: a genome-wide study. *Lancet Respir Med*. 2019;7(4):336–346.

Fuentes MA, Opperman LA, Buschang P, Bellinger LL, Carlson DS, Hinton RJ. Lateral functional shift of the mandible: Part II. Effects on gene expression in condylar cartilage. *Am J Orthod Dentofacial Orthop*. 2003;123(2):160–166.

Gagnon Y, Mayer P, Morisson F, Rompré PH, Lavigne GJ. Aggravation of respiratory disturbances by the use of an occlusal splint in apneic patients: a pilot study. *Int J Prosthodont*. 2004;17(4):447–453.

Guo J, Weng J, Rong Q, Zhang X, Zhu S, Huang D, Li X, Chen S. Investigation of multipotent postnatal stem cells from human maxillary sinus membrane. *Sci Rep*. 2015;5:11660.

Handelman CS, Wang L, BeGole EA, Haas AJ. Nonsurgical rapid maxillary expansion in adults: report on 47 cases using the Haas expander. *Angle Orthod*. 2000;70(2):129–144.

Harris WG, Singh GD. Resolution of 'gummy smile' and anterior open bite using the DNA appliance™: Case Report. *J Amer Orthod Soc*. 2013;13(4):30–34.

Heit T, Sebastian J, Singh GD. A novel combined protocol for the resolution of severe obstructive sleep apnea. *J Sleep Disord Ther*. 2016;5(5):251–254.

Hwang H, Hwang C, West J, Singh GD. Changes in pediatric paranasal sinuses following biomimetic oral appliance therapy: 3 case reports. *Cranio*. 2019;2:1–6.

Lam B, Ip MS, Tench E, Ryan CF. Craniofacial profile in Asian and white subjects with obstructive sleep apnoea. *Thorax*. 2005;60(6):504–510.

Lawson W, Patel ZM, Lin FY. The development and pathologic processes that influence maxillary sinus pneumatization. *Anat Rec* (*Hoboken*). 2008;291(11):1554–1563.

Liao F, Singh GD. Resolution of sleep bruxism using biomimetic oral appliance therapy: A case report. *J Sleep Disord Ther*. 2015;4(4):1–5.

Magne P, Douglas WH. Porcelain veneers: dentin bonding optimization and biomimetic recovery of the crown. *Int J Prosthodont*. 1999;12(2):111–121.

Márquez S. The paranasal sinuses: the last frontier in craniofacial biology. *Anat Rec* (*Hoboken*). 2008;291(11):1350–1361.

Morgan TD. Novel approaches to the management of sleep-disordered breathing. *Sleep Medicine Clinics*. 2016;11:173–187.

Nada RM, Fudalej PS, Maal TJ, Bergé SJ, Mostafa YA, Kuijpers-Jagtman AM. Three-dimensional prospective evaluation of tooth-borne and bone-borne surgically assisted rapid maxillary expansion. *J Craniomaxillofac Surg*. 2012;40(8):757–762.

Nada RM, van Loon B, Schols JG, Maal TJ, de Koning MJ, Mostafa YA, Kuijpers-Jagtman AM. Volumetric changes of the nose and nasal airway 2 years after tooth-borne and bone-borne surgically assisted rapid maxillary expansion. *Eur J Oral Sci*. 2013;121(5):450–456.

Nowak R, Mehlis G. Studies on the state of pneumatization of the sinus maxillaris. *Anat Anz*. 1975;138(3):143–151.

O'Connor PM. Postcranial pneumaticity: an evaluation of soft-tissue influences on the postcranial skeleton and the reconstruction of pulmonary anatomy in archosaurs. *J Morphol*. 2006;267(10):1199–1226.

Park IH, Song JS, Choi H, Kim TH, Hoon S, Lee SH, Lee HM. Volumetric study in the development of paranasal sinuses by CT imaging in Asian: a pilot study. *Int J Pediatr Otorhinolaryngol*. 2010;74(12):1347–1350.

Rauhut OW, Fechner R. Early development of the facial region in a non-avian theropod dinosaur. *Proc Biol Sci*. 2005;272(1568):1179–1183.

Re S, Cardaropoli D, Corrente G, Abundo R. Bodily tooth movement through the maxillary sinus with implant anchorage for single tooth replacement. *Clin Orthod Res*. 2001;4(3):177–181.

Reidenberg JS, Laitman JT. Sisters of the sinuses: cetacean air sacs. *Anat Rec* (*Hoboken*). 2008;291(11):1389–1396.

Ruangsri S, Jorns TP, Puasiri S, Luecha T, Chaithap C, Sawanyawisuth K. Which oropharyngeal factors are significant risk factors for obstructive sleep apnea? An age-matched study and dentist perspectives. *Nat Sci Sleep*. 2016;8:215–219.

Salminen S, Gibson GR, McCartney AL, Isolauri E. Influence of mode of delivery on gut microbiota composition in seven year old children. *Gut*. 2004; 53(9): 1388–1389.

Schmidt JB, Chen K, Tranquillo RT. Effects of intermittent and incremental cyclic stretch on ERK signaling and collagen production in engineered tissue. *Cell Mol Bioeng*. 2016;9(1):55–64.

Selcuk OT, Erol B, Renda L, Osma U, Eyigor H, Gunsoy B, Yagci B, Yılmaz D. Do altitude and climate affect paranasal sinus volume? *J Craniomaxillofac Surg*. 2015;43(7):1059–1064.

Sereno PC, Martinez RN, Wilson JA, Varricchio DJ, Alcober OA, Larsson HC. Evidence for avian intrathoracic air sacs in a new predatory dinosaur from Argentina. *PLoS One*. 2008;3(9):e3303.

Singh GD, Ataii P. Combined DNA appliance™ and Invisalign™ therapy without interproximal reduction: A preliminary case series. *J Clin Case Rep*. 2013;3(5):2–3.

Singh GD, Callister JD. Use of a maxillary oral appliance for the resolution of obstructive sleep apnea. *Cranio*. 2013;31(3):171–179.

Singh GD, Chapman C, Preble M. Craniofacial changes after combined atlas-orthogonal and biomimetic oral appliance therapy. *Annals Vert Sub Res*. 2014;4:112–118.

Singh GD, Clark WJ. Localization of mandibular changes in patients with class II division 1 malocclusions treated with twin-block appliances: finite element scaling analysis. *Am J Orthod Dentofacial Orthop*. 2001;119(4):419–425.

Singh GD, Clark WJ. Soft tissue changes in patients with Class II Division 1 malocclusions treated using Twin Block appliances: Finite-element scaling analysis. *Eur J Orthod*. 2003;25(3):225–230.

Singh GD, Cress SE, McGuire MK, Chandrashekhar R. Case report: Effect of mandibular tori removal on obstructive sleep apnea parameters. *Dialogue*. 2012;1:22–24.

Singh GD, Cress SE. Biomimetic oral appliance therapy in adults with mild to moderate obstructive sleep apnea using combined maxillo-mandibular correction. *J Sleep Disord Mang*. 2017;3(1):1–7.

Singh GD, Cress SE. Case presentation: Effect of full mouth rehabilitation and oral appliance therapy on obstructive sleep apnea. *Dialogue*. 2013;2:18–20.

Singh GD, Cress SE. Craniofacial enhancement using a biomimetic oral appliance: Case report. *Dent Today*. 2013;329(12):92–94.

Singh GD, Griffin TM, Chandrashekhar R. Biomimetic oral appliance therapy in adults with mild to moderate obstructive sleep apnea. *Aust J Sleep Dis*. 2014;1(1);1–5.

Singh GD, Griffin TM, Cress SE. Biomimetic oral appliance therapy in adults with severe obstructive sleep apnea. *J Sleep Disord Ther*. 2016;5(1):1–5.

Singh GD, Heit T, Preble D, Chandrashekhar R. Changes in 3D nasal cavity volume after biomimetic oral appliance therapy in adults. *Cranio*. 2016;34(1):6–12.

Singh GD, Heit T, Preble D. Changes in 3D midfacial parameters after biomimetic oral appliance therapy in adults. *J Ind Orthod Soc*. 2014;48(2):104–108.

Singh GD, Jung SC, Chandrashekhar R. Resolution of pediatric chronic rhinitis using biomimetic oral appliance therapy: a case report. *Open J Clin Med Case Rep*. 2016;2(4):1082.

Singh GD, Kim HN. Changes in pneumatization of the maxillary air sinuses in Korean adults following biomimetic oral appliance therapy. *World J Otorhinolaryngol Head Neck Surg*. 2020. doi.org/10.1016/j.wjorl.2020.07.007.

Singh GD, Kim HN. Upper oropharyngeal airway changes in Korean adults following biomimetic oral appliance therapy. *Sleep Med.* 2019;64(1):s353–s354.

Singh GD, Kim KY. Facial enhancement using biomimetic oral appliance therapy in adults. *Dent Oral Craniofac Res*. 2016;2(4):313–317.

Singh GD, Kraver M, Chernyshev O. Restoration of sleep using a novel biomimetic protocol for adult OSA: Clinical case report. *Cranio*. 2019;37(2):136–139.

Singh GD, Lipka G. Case Report: Introducing the Wireframe DNA appliance™. *J Am Acad Gnathol Orthop*. 2009;26(4):8–1.

Singh GD, Utama J. Effect of the DNA appliance™ on migraine headache: Case report. *Int J. Orthod*. 2013;24(1):45–49.

Singh GD, Wendling S, Chandrashekhar R. Midfacial development in adult obstructive sleep apnea. *Dent. Today*. 2011;30(7):124–127.

Singh GD. Epigenetic orthodontics: Developmental mechanisms of functional (formational) orthodontic appliances. *J Amer Orthod Soc*. 2010;10(6):16–26.

Singh GD. On the etiology and significance of palatal and mandibular tori: Guest Editorial. *Cranio*. 2010;28(4):213–215.

Singh GD. Physiologic remodeling of the upper airway: Pneumopedics. *J Sleep Disord Treat Care*. 2018;7(2):1–6.

Smith TD, Rossie JB, Cooper GM, Carmody KA, Schmieg RM, Bonar CJ, Mooney MP, Siegel MI. The maxillary sinus in three genera of new world monkeys: factors that constrain secondary pneumatization. *Anat Rec* (*Hoboken*). 2010;293(1): 91–107.

Smith TD, Rossie JB, Cooper GM, Mooney MP, Siegel MI. Secondary pneumatization of the maxillary sinus in callitrichid primates: insights from immunohistochemistry and bone cell distribution. *Anat Rec A Discov Mol Cell Evol Biol*. 2005;285(2): 677–689.

Tikku T, Khanna R, Sachan K, Srivastava K, Munjal N. Dimensional changes in maxillary sinus of mouth breathers. *J Oral Biol Craniofac Res*. 2013;3(1):9–14.

Verstraaten J, Kuijpers-Jagtman AM, Mommaerts MY, Bergé SJ, Nada RM, Schols JG. A systematic review of the effects of bone-borne surgical assisted rapid maxillary expansion. *J Craniomaxillofac Surg*. 2010;38(3):166–174.

Vizzotto MB, de Araújo FB, da Silveira HE, Boza AA, Closs LQ. The quad-helix appliance in the primary dentition — orthodontic and orthopedic measurements. *J Clin Pediatr Dent*. 2008;32(2):165–170.

Wedel MJ. Origin of postcranial skeletal pneumaticity in dinosaurs. *Integr Zool*. 2006;1(2):80–85.

Wehrbein H, Diedrich P. Progressive pneumatization of the basal maxillary sinus after extraction and space closure. *Fortschr Kieferorthop*. 1992;53(2):77–83.

Withalm A. Influence of nasal respiration in the development of the paranasal sinuses; a contribution to the problem of the inhibition of pneumatization in the sinuses. *Monatsschr Ohrenheilkd Laryngorhinol*. 1950;84(7–9):201–207.

Witmer LM. The evolution of the antorbital cavity of Archosaurs: A study in soft-tissue reconstruction in the fossil record with an analysis of the function of pneumaticity. *J Vert Paleont Suppl*. 1997;17:1–73.

Wu Y, Zhuang J, Zhao D, Zhang F, Ma J, Xu C. Cyclic stretch-induced the cytoskeleton rearrangement and gene expression of cytoskeletal regulators in human periodontal ligament cells. *Acta Odontol Scand*. 2017;75(7):507–516.

Zhao H, Feng J, Ho TV, Grimes W, Urata M, Chai Y. The suture provides a niche for mesenchymal stem cells of craniofacial bones. *Nat Cell Biol*. 2015;17(4):386–396.

Epilogue

Synopsis: Two recent events have gripped the world's attention. The first is the novel corona virus (COVID-19) pandemic and the second is the "I can't breathe" movement. Both events have a significant bearing on airway, breathing, and sleep issues. The pandemic has initiated intense research into the prevention and treatment of COVID-19, which is essentially a viral pneumonia of unknown origin caused by the SARS-CoV-2 virus mutation. Generic epidemiologic approaches have been implemented, such as social distancing, hygiene awareness, and the use of personal protective equipment, including facemasks to prevent droplet transmission, etc. In addition, generic therapeutic approaches have been tried, including the use of dexamethasone and nitric oxide. On the other hand, the 'black lives matter' movement directly implicates biomimetic oral appliance therapy since the critical airway collapsing pressure (Pcrit) is dependent, at least in part, on the physical dynamics of the upper airway, including its caliber and muscle tone to prevent induced airway collapse. This Epilogue provides an overview of both of these current issues.

SARS-CoV-2

As noted in the previous chapters, nasal breathing has many beneficial effects, which include warming and humidifying inhaled air. Nocera *et al.* (2019) described an exosome-mediated, intrinsic immune defense mechanism in the anterior, middle, and posterior regions of the nasal airway, which provides some initial protection of the lower airway. In addition, the paranasal sinuses are a major source of nitric oxide (NO) biosynthesis and large amounts are released into the nasal airway. After inhalation, nasal NO has important effects in the distal airway, such as regulation of pulmonary function, and may therefore be clinically useful in the treatment of respiratory disorders (Lundberg and Weitzberg, 1999). In fact, some studies indicate that NO may help to reduce respiratory infections, while mouth breathing may attenuate antiviral responses, bypassing the filtering effect of the nasal airway and decreasing NO levels (Martel *et al.*, 2020). Kimberly *et al.* (1996) had concluded that most NO originates in the nasopharynx since exhaled NO is quantitatively greater during nasal breathing compared with mouth breathing, and they suggested that nasal NO is taken up by the lower respiratory tract. In an early study on severe acute respiratory syndrome (SARS), associated with a corona virus infection, Chen *et al.* (2004) reported that inhaled NO had a pulmonary vasodilator effect that improved arterial oxygenation, which consequently reduced the need for inspired oxygen and airway pressure therapy in adults diagnosed with SARS. Thus, patients with SARS who were hospitalized with hypoxia had their pulmonary hypertension corrected with NO therapy and were less reliant on ventilators. Later, in vitro tissue culture (Akerstrom *et al.*, 2005) showed that not only did NO indirectly inhibit the replication of the SARS corona virus in a dose-dependent fashion but NO also inhibited viral protein and RNA synthesis, while NO synthase inhibited the replication of the corona virus in Vero E6 cells.

Similarly, in the COVID-19 pandemic due to infection with the novel corona virus (SARS-CoV-2), clinical trials are underway to test the notion that inhaled NO improves oxygenation in patients with refractory hypoxemia (Lei *et al.*, 2020). In fact, recently, Zamanian *et al.* (2020) described a case of severe respiratory illness associated with COVID-19. The pulmonary arterial hypertension was successfully controlled using inhaled NO (20ppm) with supplemental oxygen delivered via a nasal canula. Over 17 days, the patient was gradually weaned off therapy and showed symptomatic recovery. Similarly, Patel *et al.* (2020) presented a pediatric case report of a young girl with severe thrombocytopenia and respiratory failure associated with COVID-19. She was treated with a combination of intravenous immunoglobulin and steroids for the platelet disorder, while the SARS was managed with both airway ventilation and inhaled NO since Thomassen *et al.* (1997) had earlier shown that alveolar macrophages are inhibited from producing inflammatory cytokines by NO. Later, Wishah *et al.* (2002) confirmed the inhibitory effect of upregulated NO in asthma as an anti-inflammatory agent modulating cytokine production. Earlier still, Swift *et al.* (1988) had found that obligate nasal breathing (achieved through interdental fixation) resulted in increased total lung capacity, functional residual capacity, and residual volume; but these parameters were decreased with total nasal obstruction. It was therefore concluded that nasal resistance to expiration maintains lung volumes and may determine arterial oxygenation. Since biomimetic oral appliance therapy has been shown to enhance the nasal airway (Singh *et al.*, 2016; Singh and Kim, 2020), sinus health (Hwang *et al.*, 2019), and sinus pneumatization (Singh and Kim, 2020), biomimetic oral appliance therapy, which targets the nasal airway and paranasal sinuses to increase NO biosynthesis, might be preferable in the management of SDB (Singh, 2020).

Induced upper airway collapse

The second recent issue involving the upper airway, breathing and sleep is the "I can't breathe" and 'black lives matter' movement. This issue indirectly implicates biomimetic oral appliance therapy since the critical airway collapsing pressure (Pcrit) is dependent, at least in part, on the physical dynamics of the upper airway, including its caliber and muscle tone to prevent induced airway collapse. If breathing is completely prevented, within < 5mins neuronal function starts failing from a lack of oxygenation.

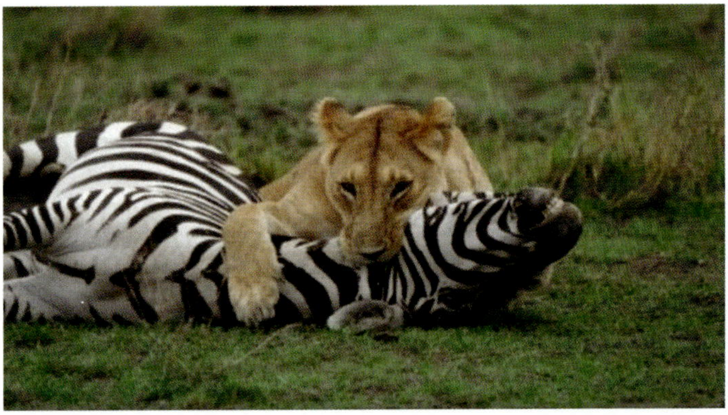

Figure 108: After the hunt, the lioness (predator) is shown inducing upper airway collapse in the zebra (prey).

Breathing can be forcefully arrested in cases of strangulation. The interruption of cerebral blood flow, coupled with hypoxia from respiratory arrest, leads to a loss of consciousness and later, death (Fig. 108). Other physical signs that indicate the use of excessive force to the neck include superficial abrasions of the skin, hemorrhage in the underlying soft tissues, and fracture of the hyoid bone/thyroid cartilage. However, at autopsy, the medical examiner may find no fatal injuries to the bronchial tree, brain, or heart (Lerner and Burns, 1986). Other causes of death from induced airway collapse include suffocation, which can be caused by physical entrapment or environmental suffocation, such as smothering, choking, suffocating gases, or mechanical asphyxia. In asphyxiation, the medical examiner may also report the finding of bloodshot eyes, high levels of carbon dioxide in the blood of the victim, or displacement of oxygen by poisoning gases (CO, CO_2, etc). Note that mechanical stimulation of the carotid sinus, which is found in the neck, results in bradycardia and a subsequent decrease in blood pressure. However, carotid sinus stimulation, coupled with drugs known to alter the carotid sinus reflex, might result in a catastrophic fall in blood pressure that could ultimately lead to death. Intoxicated individuals, therefore, may be at a higher risk of lethal complications through neck holds that cause carotid compression.

Airflow through the oropharyngeal airway simulates fluid flow through a narrow tube, which varies obeying Poiseuille's law. In this case, flow is directly proportional to the pressure differential and inversely proportional to the fourth power of the radius. Put simply, a small change in the radius of the tube or airway will have a dramatic effect on airflow. Bernoulli's principle also applies since, in fluid dynamics, a change in a fluid's speed must be matched by a change in pressure (force). Clinically, findings support the notion of a correlation between craniofacial morphology and upper airway structure. In fact, Guilleminault and Stoohs (1990) suggested that there is a noticeable relationship between craniofacial morphology and upper airway sufficiency. Furthermore, Carberry *et al.* (2016) surmise that a narrow upper airway or one that is highly collapsible is an important cause of OSA. If so, one might pose the question: Why don't smaller diameter pediatric airways collapse in the same way as those of adults with OSA? Although the answer is complex, the pediatric airway has a higher tonicity, lower arousal threshold, and growth potential. However, the ability to remodel the airway, even in adults, may reside in local stem cell populations that have been identified throughout the upper airway (Bravo *et al.*, 2013; Wang *et al.*, 2015; Wang *et al.*, 2019). Singh *et al.* (2020) investigated 3D changes in craniofacial architecture, to test the hypothesis that the upper airway can be non-surgically improved in adults using biomimetic oral appliance therapy. They found that the nasal cavity volume increased by 14%; the retropalatal airway distance increased by 25%; the retropalatal airway area increased by 24%; the retroglossal airway distance increased by 20%; the medio-lateral retroglossal airway width increased by 11%; while retroglossal airway area increased by 25% with no device in the patient's mouth. Multivariate tests showed a significant treatment effect on the upper airway parameters. It can be concluded that craniofacial architecture and upper airway morphology can potentially be non-surgically enhanced in non-growing adults, and this may represent a technique of preventing upper airway collapse in adults.

References

Akerström S, Mousavi-Jazi M, Klingström J, Leijon M, Lundkvist A, Mirazimi A. Nitric oxide inhibits the replication cycle of severe acute respiratory syndrome coronavirus. *J Virol*. 2005;79(3):1966–1969.

Bravo DT, Soudry E, Edward JA, Le W, Nguyen AL, Hwang PH, Sanyal M, Nayak JV. Characterization of human upper airway epithelial progenitors. *Int Forum Allergy Rhinol*. 2013;3(10):841-847.

Carberry JC, Jordan AS, White DP, Wellman A, Eckert DJ. Upper airway collapsibility (Pcrit) and pharyngeal dilator muscle activity are sleep stage dependent. *Sleep*. 2016;39(3):511–521.

Chen L, Liu P, Gao H, *et al.* Inhalation of nitric oxide in the treatment of severe acute respiratory syndrome: A rescue trial in Beijing. *Clin Infect Dis*. 2004;39(10):1531–1535.

Guilleminault C, Stoohs R. Chronic snoring and obstructive sleep apnea syndrome in children. *Lung*. 1990;168:912–919.

Hwang H, Hwang C, West J, Singh GD. Changes in pediatric paranasal sinuses following biomimetic oral appliance therapy: 3 case reports. *Cranio*. 2019;2:1–6.

Kimberly B, Nejadnik B, Giraud GD, Holden WE. Nasal contribution to exhaled nitric oxide at rest and during breathholding in humans. *Am J Respir Crit Care Med*. 1996;153(2):829–836.

Lei C, Su B, Dong H, Bellavia A, DiFenza R, Fakhr BS, Gianni S, Grassi LG, Kacmarek R, Morais CCA, *et al.* Protocol of a randomized controlled trial testing inhaled nitric oxide in mechanically ventilated patients with severe acute respiratory syndrome in COVID-19 (SARS-CoV-2). https://doi.org/10.1101/2020.03.09.20033530

Lerner SE, Burns RS. Legal issues associated with PCP abuse--the role of the forensic expert. *NIDA Res Monogr*. 1986;64:229–236.

Lundberg JO, Weitzberg E. Nasal nitric oxide in man. *Thorax*. 1999;54(10):947–952.

Martel J, Ko YF, Young JD, Ojcius DM. Could nasal nitric oxide help to mitigate the severity of COVID-19? *Microbes Infect*. 2020;22(4–5):168–171.

Nocera AL, Mueller SK, Stephan JR, *et al.* Exosome swarms eliminate airway pathogens and provide passive epithelial immunoprotection through nitric oxide. *J Allergy Clin Immunol*. 2019;143(4):1525–1535.e1.

Patel PA, Chandrakasan S, Mickells GE, Yildirim I, Kao CM, Bennett CM. Severe pediatric COVID-19 presenting with respiratory failure and severe thrombocytopenia. *Pediatrics*. 2020;146(1):e20201437.

Singh GD, Heit T, Preble D, Chandrashekhar R. Changes in 3D nasal cavity volume after biomimetic oral appliance therapy in adults. *Cranio*. 2016;34(1):6–12.

Singh GD, Kim HN, Kim SH, Wang L. 3D craniofacial and upper airway changes after biomimetic oral appliance therapy in Korean adults. *J Otorhinolaryngol Head Neck Surg*. 2020 (submitted).

Singh GD, Kim HN. Changes in nasal airway volume after biomimetic oral appliance therapy in Korean adults. *Am J Respir Crit Care Med*. 2020;201:A2442.

Singh GD, Kim HN. Changes in pneumatization of the maxillary air sinuses in Korean adults following biomimetic oral appliance therapy. *World J Otorhinolaryngol Head Neck Surg*. 2020. doi.org/10.1016/j.wjorl.2020.07.007.

Singh GD. Response to "Oral appliance therapy should be prescribed as a first-line therapy for OSA during the COVID-19 Pandemic". *J Dent Sleep Med*. 2020;7(3).

Swift AC, Campbell IT, McKown TM. Oronasal obstruction, lung volumes, and arterial oxygenation. *Lancet*. 1988;1(8577):73–75.

Thomassen MJ, Buhrow LT, Connors MJ, Kaneko FT, Erzurum SC, Kavuru MS. Nitric oxide inhibits inflammatory cytokine production by human alveolar macrophages. *Am J Respir Cell Mol Biol*. 1997;17(3):279–283.

Wang DY, Li Y, Yan Y, Li C, Shi L. Upper airway stem cells: Understanding the nose and role for future cell therapy. *Curr Allergy Asthma Rep*. 2015;15(1):490.

Wang G, Lou HH, Salit J, Leopold PL, Driscoll S, Schymeinsky J, Quast K, Visvanathan S, Fine JS, *et al.* Characterization of an immortalized human small airway basal stem/ progenitor cell line with airway region-specific differentiation capacity. *Respir Res*. 2019;20(1):196.

Wishah K, Malur A, Raychaudhuri B, Melton AL, Kavuru MS, Thomassen MJ. Nitric oxide blocks inflammatory cytokine secretion triggered by CD23 in monocytes from allergic, asthmatic patients and healthy controls. *Ann Allergy Asthma Immunol*. 2002;89(1):78–82.

Zamanian RT, Pollack CV Jr, Gentile MA, *et al.* Outpatient inhaled Nitric Oxide in a patient with vasoreactive idiopathic pulmonary arterial hypertension and COVID-19 infection. *Am J Respir Crit Care Med*. 2020;202(1):130–132.

Appendix

Clinical algorithm

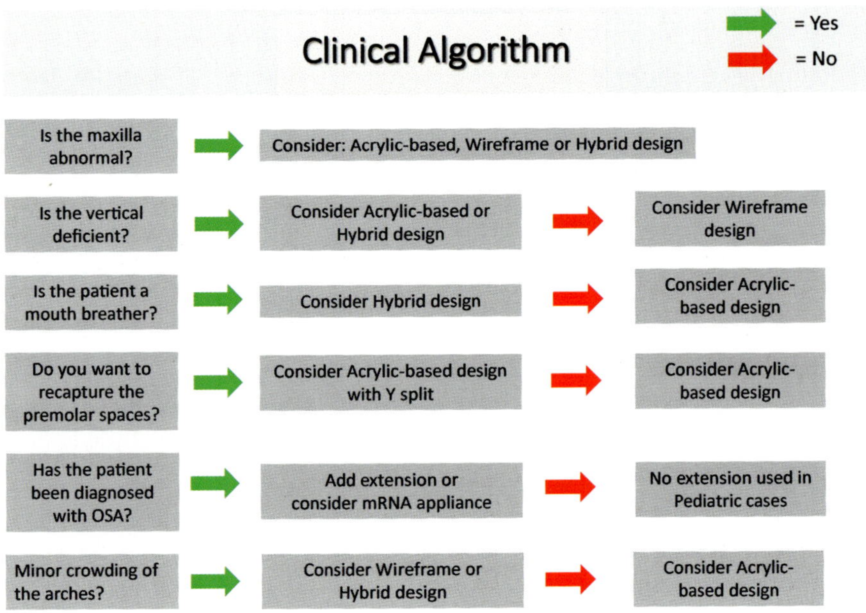

Device adjustments

Six device adjustments are required at each appointment.

1. Check retention and activation	Adjust Adams clasps, ball clasps, screw, Omega loops, etc.
2. Check the occlusion	Equilibrate, using articulating paper, flat plane, etc.
3. Check the Posterior Omega loop	Use 3-prong pliers to move it away from palate by 0.25mm
4. Check OSA extension	Adjust beaded extension for length, bend, turn its screw etc.
5. Check the labial bow	Needs to be approx. 0.25mm off the labial surfaces
6. Check 3D axial springs	Need to be in intimate contact with palatal surfaces

Epworth sleepiness scale

Can be used to assess daytime sleepiness.

0 = **No chance of dozing off**	2 = **Moderate chance of dozing off**
1 = **Slight chance of dozing off**	3 = **High chance of dozing off**

Rate the chance that you will doze off in the following situations:

Sitting and reading	
Watching television	
Sitting inactive in a public place (e.g. in a theater, during a meeting)	
As a passenger in a car driving for one hour without a break	
Lying down to rest in the afternoon when circumstances permit	
Sitting and talking to someone	
Sitting quietly after lunch without alcohol	
In a car while stopped for a few minutes in traffic	
Add above total score	

STOP-Bang questionnaire

Can be used to screen for obstructive sleep apnea (OSA) and will assess low, moderate, or high risk for OSA.

STOP

S	Do you **snore** loudly (loud enough to be heard through closed doors or louder than talking)?	YES	NO
T	Do you often feel **tired**, fatigued or sleepy during the daytime?	YES	NO
O	Has anyone **observed** you stop breathing or choking or gasping during your sleep?	YES	NO
P	Do you have or are you being treated for high blood **pressure**?	YES	NO

BANG

B	Is your **BMI** more than 35?	YES	NO
A	**Age** - over 50 years old?	YES	NO
N	**Neck** circumference - is it greater than 17" if you are a male or 16" if you are a female?	YES	NO
G	**Gender** - are you a male?	YES	NO

Pediatric sleep questionnaire

Contains questions about features of pediatric OSA.

Name	Age	Gender
		M F

While Sleeping, Does Your Child:

- ☐ Snore more than half the time?
- ☐ Always snore?
- ☐ Have heavy or loud breathing?
- ☐ Snore loudly?
- ☐ Have trouble breathing or struggles to breathe?
- ☐ Ever stop breathing at night?

Does Your Child?

- ☐ Tend to breath through the mouth during the day?
- ☐ Have a dry mouth upon waking up in the morning?
- ☐ Occasionally wet the bed?
- ☐ Grind his/her teeth while sleeping?
- ☐ Have any bite problems or crowded teeth?
- ☐ Wake up unrefreshed in the morning?
- ☐ Have a problem with daytime sleepiness?
- ☐ Have a teacher or anyone else who has commented about sleepiness during the day?
- ☐ Have difficulty waking up in the morning?
- ☐ Wake up with headaches?
- ☐ Have a history of growth problems?
- ☐ Have an overweight issue?

  Height ☐ Weight ☐
- ☐ Complain of restless or achy legs?
- ☐ Have arms and/or legs that twitch during sleep?
- ☐ Have nightmares? (more than one per week)

Epigenetic-Pneumopedic® protocol

Accords with the cranio-caudal gradient of human development.

- Oral sweep of a young baby soon after birth to inoculate oral flora; encourage breast feeding.
- An oral examination by a pediatrician or pediatric dentist of a young baby soon after birth. If ankylosis or tongue-tie is diagnosed, lingual frenectomy may be provided by a dentist/oral surgeon; encourage breast feeding.
- A cranial examination of a young baby soon after birth. If deformational plagiocephaly/cranial asymmetry is diagnosed, cranial therapy may be provided as indicated; review sleep hygiene.
- An oral examination by an oral myofunctional therapist, by the age of three years. If habits, such as digit-sucking, lip-sucking, etc. are diagnosed, OMT may be provided;
- A HSAT or PSG by a sleep specialist, pulmonologist, ENT, etc., by age three to six years. If sleep disordered breathing is diagnosed, epigenetic-pneumopedic therapy may be provided as indicated.
- A TMJ examination by a dentist, by the age of five years. If bruxism/ear infection is diagnosed or developing, a sleep study may be provided as indicated;
- An orthodontic examination by an orthodontist or general dentist, by the age of five years. If a malocclusion is diagnosed or developing, epigenetic-orthodontic therapy may be provided;
- A nutritional evaluation, by the age of five years. If food allergies/obesity are diagnosed, nutritional counseling may be provided.
- A cervical examination by a chiropractor, osteopath, etc., by the age of nine years. If cervical subluxation is diagnosed, physical therapy may be provided as indicated.

Index

D

E

M

N

O

P